NEONATAL UNIT, WOMEN'S PAVILLON

Drugs in Pregnancy and Lactation

A REFERENCE GUIDE TO FETAL AND NEONATAL RISK

Drugs in Pregnancy and Lactation

A REFERENCE GUIDE TO FETAL AND NEONATAL RISK

Gerald G. Briggs, B. Pharm.

Clinical Pharmacist, Women's Hospital
Memorial Hospital of Long Beach, California
Assistant Clinical Professor of Pharmacy
University of California, San Francisco
Clinical Instructor in Pharmacy
University of Southern California, Los Angeles

Thomas W. Bodendorfer, Pharm. D.

Detroit, Michigan
Formerly Clinical Pharmacist
Memorial Hospital of Long Beach, California
Assistant Clinical Professor of Pharmacy
University of California, San Francisco
Clinical Instructor in Pharmacy
University of Southern California, Los Angeles

Roger K. Freeman, M. D.

Medical Director, Women's Hospital
Memorial Hospital of Long Beach, California
Professor of Obstetrics and Gynecology
University of California, Irvine

Sumner J. Yaffe, M. D.

Director, Center for Research for Mothers and Children
National Institute of Child Health and Human Development
National Institutes of Health
Bethesda, Maryland

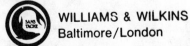

WILLIAMS & WILKINS
Baltimore/London

Copyright ©, 1983
Williams & Wilkins
428 East Preston Street
Baltimore, MD 21202, U.S.A.

Made in the United States of America

Library of Congress Cataloging in Publication Data

Main entry under title:

Drugs in pregnancy and lactation.

Includes index.
1. Fetus, Effect of drugs on the. 2. Milk, Human—Contamination. I. Briggs, Gerald G. [DNLM: 1. Catalogs, Drug—United States. 2. Lactation—Drug effects—Catalogs. 3. Pregnancy—Drug effects—Catalogs. 4. Fetus—Drug effects—Catalogs. 5. Infant Newborn—Drug effects. 6. Drug therapy—In pregnancy. QV 772 D795]
RG627.6.D79D79 1983   618.3′2071   82-13392
ISBN 0-683-01057-3

Composed and printed at the
Waverly Press, Inc.
Mt. Royal and Guilford Aves.
Baltimore, MD 21202, U.S.A.

Foreword

This book was written to be used by the clinician who deals with pregnant patients. Everyday in an obstetrical, pediatric or other medical practice, one encounters frequent questions about the use of drugs in pregnancy and lactation. These questions may involve the use of a drug for therapy of an associated condition, an inquiry about some drug a patient has already taken and then decides to ask about or the determination if an untoward pregnancy outcome or an adverse effect observed in the infant was caused by the consumption of some therapeutic agent by the patient. Other health professionals, such as nurses and pharmacists, also are often confronted with questions concerning drug usage in the pregnant or breast feeding woman.

Of course, this book is of necessity lacking in giving absolute answers on most drugs in question because experience in humans is not easy to gather. One seldom knows, even when the drug history is thought to be realistic, whether there is an actual cause-effect relationship between a specific drug and an adverse pregnancy outcome. Because the answers are generally inconclusive, physicians caring for pregnant patients should counsel their patients accordingly either when answering a question about some drug already ingested or when explaining the cost/benefit ratio to a patient who is being considered for some specific drug therapy.

For the breast feeding patient, the risks from a particular drug are usually much clearer although there are frequent examples where the risk must be inferred from related drugs. Unfortunately, many drugs have not been studied during nursing so the effects on the infant, if any, are completely unknown. A good rule to follow is *if the drug can safely be given directly to the infant, it is generally safe to give to the mother during lactation*.

This book allows the clinician to have at his or her fingertips an up-to-date summary of available data bearing on specific drugs. It is easy to read and organized in a logical manner to save the busy clinician time.

Roger K. Freeman, M.D.
Medical Director
Women's Hospital
Memorial Hospital Medical Center
Long Beach, California
Professor of Obstetrics and Gynecology
University of California, Irvine

Preface

We have always been amazed by the number of drugs and chemicals the fetus is exposed to during its nine month sojourn in the womb. Perhaps just as surprising is the realization that in spite of this chemical bath, the vast majority of newborns enter the world with the correct number of parts, all functioning properly. Teratology and, to a lesser extent, drugs in breast milk are and have been a major topic of interest and worry to the pregnant woman, to her relatives, and to the health professionals who care for her and her child. Over the past decade, we have been frequently confronted with questions concerning this area from physicians, nurses, pharmacists, patients, and the lay public. Almost all of the health professionals wanted more information on a specific drug than they could find in available reviews. Spurred on by this continued interest, we gradually accumulated a large number of primary references on drugs and the fetus. As we accumulated, we summarized the experiences contained in these reports into brief monographs to facilitate answering future questions. From this background, the idea to publish our monographs emerged in 1979. The breast milk sections were added due to the number of inquiries on this subject and its close relationship to drug effects on the developing fetus. Unfortunately, the passage of many drugs into breast milk has not been studied, and the cryptic "No data available" appears often. Individuals wishing to contribute to this area of knowledge have many opportunities to do so.

We have attempted to include all of the pertinent articles on a specific drug. On a few occasions, due to a large number of references, we have resorted to the use of a recent review (e.g., Coumadin). The use of reviews has been kept to a minimum since we believe one of the values of our work lies in the citation of the available literature so that readers can arrive at their own conclusions as to the risk a particular drug poses to the fetus or newborn. Although we frequently used case reports as our only source of information, knowledgeable readers will be painfully aware that most reports of this type are biased in several aspects. For example, their lack of reporting the total drug exposure history and its timing; the fact that they are retrospective and must rely on the memory of the patient at a very depressing moment; their lack of reporting nonteratogenic exposures so that results are weighted toward the negative side; their omission of important factors such as the reason for taking the drug, the relevant family history, and the general state of the mother's health. Inclusion of this data would certainly make evaluation of the literature easier.

Frequent use of one reference source (Heinonen OP, Slone D, Shapiro S. Birth defects and drugs in pregnancy. Littleton: Publishing Sciences Group, 1977) has been employed in our work. This prospective study often provided the only available information on some drugs. We extend our apologies in advance to authors whose work we inadvertently omitted. In any work of this magnitude, some important citations will be overlooked. Also, many drugs have not been included due to time and space limitations. We have attempted, however, to include those agents and classes of agents that have generated the most inquiries in our experience. With your assistance and the blessings of time, future editions will hopefully eliminate these shortcomings. We wish to express our sincere thank you to the many people who assisted us in putting this book together, including: Dr William E. Smith, Administrator of the Pharmacy Department at Memorial Hospital, for making available to us what time that he could so we could work on this project; Mrs Frances Lyon, Librarian at Memorial and her staff, Emi Kosaka, Lisa Ginsbarg, Mori Higa, Ellen Phillips, and David Downing; Dr Byron Schweigert, Director of the Drug Information Service at Memorial and his staff, Dr Philip Towne and Barbara Matthias; all of the manufacturers who responded to our pleas for information on their products and especially to Dr John J. Whalen, Director of Professional Information at Merck Sharpe & Dohme, who probably answered more of our letters than he cares to remember; the personnel at Auto-Type Word Processing Center, in particular Ms Irene Mendoza, Office Manager, for their typing of the manuscript; Susan and Leslee Briggs for the many hours they spent assembling the Index. Finally, and most important, our special thanks to our families, Susan and Leslee, and Kathleen and Derek, who have suffered through our long hours away from home, late dinners, cancelled vacations, and irritable husbands/fathers over the past three years.

                                                                    GGB
                                                                    TWB

Introduction

Sumner J. Yaffe, M.D. and Albert Bedell, M.A.

Parturition of the perfectly formed and mentally sound infant is a most wonderful, natural function. Postnatally, the natural ability of the mother to nurture her infant is manifested through breast feeding. Every requisite for successful childbearing and the ability to breast-feed exists within most women. When a woman lives under circumstances favorable to her full physical and behavioral development and health, she is usually able to experience pregnancy and lactation with few or no difficulties for herself or her child.

With changes in the organization and requirements of society, in response to new social, cultural, and ecological conditions, the experiences of today's pregnant woman have become very different from what they would have been in the past. In many respects her lot is much improved, but new problems have risen to supplant some of the old ones.

Women are constitutionally more sensitive throughout gestation to various debilitating influences. The advances of civilization are, on one hand, responsible for some of these conditions in women, yet these same advances have, on the other hand, done much to make childbearing safer and more agreeable. Many disorders associated with pregnancy can now be treated or cured, and many of the difficulties attendant to childbirth have been overcome through the high degree of obstetrical skill that has been attained.

Notwithstanding these advances, the problems are still great. The level of technical and scientific skill which medicine has attained will do little toward effectively relieving human suffering and eradicating disease as long as the practice of medicine is limited to curative and palliative measures. Physicians must acknowledge their responsibility to communicate to other physicians, pharmacologists, mothers and mothers-to-be, and the general public the risks attendant to these new techniques and treatment modalities. Effective communication is the only way to avoid the problems brought forth by ignorance or lack of knowledge.

Every day physicians and midwives usher newborns into the world with the full expectation that the care they administer, through advice and medicines, will be adhered to by the new mothers and will result in infants of sound mind and body. In addition the mother is presumed ready, if she so chooses, for nursing the newborn.

Special responsibilities are vested in the partnership between the pregnant woman and her physician. The physician has the responsibility to provide all the medical knowledge and skills available to him, including the latest emanations from the laboratories and pharmaceutical houses. The pregnant woman is expected to follow the physician's advice and prescriptions.

This has been the established arrangement since physicians began attending childbirth. The primary difference between those early times and today is what is expected of the physician. Hippocrates, Soranus, Aetios, and Avicenna, whose time ranged from the fourth century before the common era through the first millenium AD, maintained highly authoritative positions within their communities and provided their ministrations in a categorical fashion. That is to say, the practice of medicine was extremely pedagogical and it was the responsibility of the patient to follow the physician's advice or suffer the consequences.

Soranus of Ephesus (2), representing the consumate thinking of the time (second century AD), wrote in a threatening autocratic manner, "Even if a woman transgresses some or all of the rules mentioned (re: administration of drugs, sternutatives, pungent substances, and drunkenness, especially during the first trimester) and yet miscarriage of the fetus does not take place, let no one assume that the fetus has not been injured at all. For it has been harmed: it is weakened, becomes retarded in growth, less well nourished, and in general, more easily injured and susceptible to harmful agents; it becomes misshapen and of ignoble soul."

DRUGS IN PREGNANCY

Today's physician does not have the authoritative luxury of yesterday's practitioner. In particular, the present-day obstetrician has suffered a diminution of confidence because of the thalidomide catastrophe.

In 1941 Gregg (1) demonstrated that rubella infection in the mother could result in anatomic malformation in the fetus. This raised the concept that environment could affect fetal outcome. In spite of this, physicians continued to practice their profession with little concern to the empirical observations.

Because of its sedative and hypnotic effects, physicians administered thalidomide to the pregnant woman for her discomfort. Thalidomide had been evaluated for safety in several animal species, had been given a clean bill of health and had come to be regarded as a good pharmacologic agent. Yet the catastrophic and distinct embryopathic effects resulting from thalidomide administration to the human mother during early pregnancy are well-known.

It is important to note that even though thalidomide induces a distinct cluster of anatomic defects that are virtually pathognomonic for this agent, it required several years of thalidomide use and the birth of many thousands of grossly malformed infants before the cause and effect relationship between thalidomide administration in early pregnancy and its harmful effects was recognized. This serves to emphasize the difficulties that exist in incriminating drugs and chemicals that are harmful when administered during pregnancy. Hopefully, we will never have another drug prescribed for use during pregnancy whose teratogenicity is as potent as thalidomide (about one-third of women taking this agent during the first trimester gave birth to infants with birth defects).

Concern about the safety of foreign compounds administered to pregnant women has been increasingly evident since thalidomide. It was the direct response to this misadventure which led to the promulgation of the drug regulations of 1962 in the United States. According to these regulations, a drug must be demonstrated to be safe and effective for the conditions of use prescribed in its labeling. The regulations concerning this requirement state that a drug should be investigated for the conditions of use specified in the labeling, including dosage levels and patient populations for whom the drug is intended. In addition, appropriate information must be provided in the labeling in cases in which the drug is prescribed. The intent of the regulations is not only to ensure adequate labeling information for the safe and effective administration of the drug by the physician but also to ensure that marketed drugs have an acceptable benefit-to-risk ratio for their intended uses.

It is clear that any drug or chemical substance administered to the mother is able to cross the placenta to some extent unless it is destroyed or altered during passage. Placental transport of maternal substrates to the fetus and of substances from the fetus to the mother is established at about the fifth week of fetal life. Substances of low molecular weight diffuse freely across the placenta, driven primarily by the concentration gradient. It is important to note, therefore, that almost every substance used for therapeutic purposes can and does pass from the mother to the fetus. Of greater importance is whether the rate and extent of transfer are sufficient to result in significant concentrations within the fetus. We must discard the concept that there is a placental barrier.

Experiments with animals have provided considerable information concerning the teratogenic effects of drugs. Unfortunately, these experimental findings cannot be extrapolated from species to species, or even from strain to strain within the same species, much less from animals to humans. Research in this area and the prediction of toxicity in the human are further hampered by a lack of specificity between cause and effect.

Traditionally, teratogenic effects of drugs have been noted as anatomic malformations. It is clear that these are dose and time related and that the fetus is at great risk during the first three months of gestation. However, it is possible for drugs and chemicals to exert their effects upon the fetus at other times during pregnancy.

This was also understood by Hippocrates who, in the Corpus (3), maintained the second trimester as a safe stage of fetal development for the administration of drugs. In the Aphorisms, that collection of short medical truths, he prescribed, "Drugs may be administered to pregnant women from the fourth to the seventh month of gestation. After that period, the dose should be less."

The mechanisms of teratogenic agents are poorly understood, particularly in the human. Drugs may affect maternal tissues with indirect effects upon the fetus or they may have a direct effect on the embryonic cells and result in specific abnormalities. Drugs may affect the nutrition of the fetus by interfering with the passage of nutrients across the placenta. Alterations in placental metabolism influence the development of the fetus since placental integrity is a determinant of fetal growth.

Administration of a drug to a pregnant woman presents a unique problem for the physician. Not only must maternal pharmacologic mechanisms be taken into consideration when prescribing a drug but also the fetus must always be kept in mind as a potential recipient of the drug.

Recognition of the fact that drugs administered during pregnancy can affect the fetus should lead to decreased drug consumption. Nonetheless, studies conducted in the past few years indicate drug consumption during pregnancy is increasing. This may be due to several reasons. Most people in the Western world are unaware of their drug and chemical exposure. Many are uninformed as to the potentially harmful effects of drugs on the fetus. Also, there are some who feel that many individuals in modern society are overly concerned with their own comfort.

Whatever the reasons, exposure to drugs, both prescribed and over the counter, among mothers-to-be continues unabated throughout pregnancy. It is possible that this exposure to drugs and chemicals may be responsible for the large numbers of birth defects which are seen in the newborn infant and in later development.

It is crucial that concern also be given to events beyond the narrow limits of congenital anatomic malformations; evidence exists that intellectual, social and functional development also can be adversely affected. There are examples that toxic manifestations of intrauterine exposure to environmental agents may be subtle, unexpected and delayed.

Concern for the delayed effects of drugs, following intrauterine exposure, was first raised following the tragic discovery that female fetuses exposed to diethylstilbestrol (DES) are at an increased risk for adenocarcinoma of the vagina. This type of malignancy is not discovered until after puberty. Additional clinical findings indicate that male offspring were not spared from the effects of the drug. Some have abnormalities of the reproductive system such as epididymal cysts, hypotrophic testes, capsular induration, and pathologic semen.

The concept of long-term latency has been confirmed by investigations conducted in the research laboratories. Researchers found that when the widely used hypnotic-sedative agent phenobarbital was administered to pregnant rats it resulted in the birth of offspring who were significantly smaller than normal and who experienced delays in vaginal opening. Sixty percent of the females of these animals were infertile (4).

Recently, investigators in a laboratory at Children's Hospital of Philadelphia reported their research results with male animals (5). They found lower-than-normal testosterone levels in the brain and bloodstream of male rats whose mothers were given low doses of phenobarbital late in pregnancy. Even at 120 days of age, these male rats showed abnormal testosterone synthesis. It is felt by the investigators that phenobarbital, encountered in fetal life, may alter brain programming which results in permanent changes in sexual function. Phenobarbital is an old drug that is widely prescribed. It is also a component of many multiingredient pharmaceuticals whose use does not abate during pregnancy. The clinical significance of these experiments in animals is admittedly unknown, but the striking effects upon reproductive function warrant careful scrutiny of the safety of these agents during human pregnancy before prescribing them.

The physician is confronted with two imperatives in treating the pregnant woman: alleviate maternal suffering and do not harm the fetus. Until now the emphasis has been on the amelioration of suffering, but the time has come to concentrate on not harming the fetus. The simple equation to be applied here is weighing the therapeutic benefits of the drug to the mother against its risk potential to the developing fetus.

When one considers that more than 1.2 billion drug prescriptions are written each year, that there is unlimited self-administration of over-the-counter drugs, and that approximately 500 new pharmaceutical products are introduced annually, the need for prudency in the administration of pharmaceuticals has reached a critical point. Pregnancy is a symptom-producing event. Pregnancy has the potential of causing women to increase their intake of drugs and chemicals, with the potential being that the fetus will be nurtured in a sea of drugs.

In today's society the physician cannot stand alone in the therapeutic decision-making process. It now has become the responsibility of each woman of childbearing age to carefully consider her use of drugs. In a pregnant woman, the decision to administer a drug should be made only after a collaborative appraisal between the woman and her physician of the benefits-to-risk ratio.

BREAST FEEDING AND DRUGS

Between 1930 and the late 1960's there was a dramatic decline in the percentage of American mothers who breast-fed their babies. This was accompanied by a reduction in the length of breast feeding for those who did nurse. The incidence of breast feeding declined from approximately 80% of the children born between 1926 and 1930 to 49% of children born some 25 years later. For children born between 1966 and 1970, 28% were breast-fed. As data have become available for the decade of the seventies, it is clear the decline has been reversed (6). By 1975, the percentage of first born who were breast-fed rose to 37. At the present time in the United States, it appears (from a number of surveys) that about 50% of babies discharged from the hospital are breast-fed.

Any number of hypotheses can be made regarding the decline and recent increase in breast feeding in this country. A fair amount of credit can be given to the biomedical research of the past 15 years which has demonstrated the benefits of breast feeding.

Breast feeding is known to possess nutritional and immunologic properties superior to those found in infant formulas (6–9). The American Academy of Pediatrics has published a position paper emphasizing a return to breast feeding as the best nutritional mode for infants for the first six months of age (6). In addition to those qualities, some studies also suggest significant psychological benefits for both the mother and the infant in breast feeding.

The upswing in breast feeding, together with a markedly increased concern about health needs on the part of parents, has led to increased questioning of the physician, pharmacist, and other health professionals about the safety and potential toxicity of drugs and chemicals that may be excreted in breast milk.

Answers to these questions are not very apparent. Our knowledge concerning the long- and short-term effects and safety of maternally ingested drugs on the suckling infant is meager. We know little more now than Soranus did in 150 AD when he admonished wet nurses to refrain from the use of drugs and alcohol lest it have an adverse effect on the nursing infant.

It would be easy to recommend that the medicated mother not nurse, but it is likely that this recommendation would be ignored by the mother in discomfort and may well offend many health providers as well as their patients on both psychosocial and physiologic grounds.

It must be emphasized that virtually all investigations concerned with milk secretion and synthesis have been carried out in animals. The difficulty in studying human lactation employing histological techniques and the adminis-tration of radioactive isotopes is obvious. There are considerable differences in the composition of milk in different species. Some of these differences in composition would obviously bring about changes in drug elimination. Of great importance in this regard are the differences in the pH of human milk (pH usually >7.0) as contrasted to the pH of cows milk (pH usually <6.8) where drug excretion has been extensively studied.

Human milk is a suspension of fat and protein in a carbohydrate-mineral solution. A nursing mother easily makes 600 cc of milk per day containing sufficient protein, fat, and carbohydrate to meet the nutritional demands of the developing infant. Milk proteins are fully synthesized from substrates delivered from the maternal circulation. The major proteins are casein and lactalbumin. The role of these proteins in the delivery of drugs into milk has not yet been completely elucidated. Drug excretion into milk may be accomplished by binding to the proteins or onto the surface of the milk fat globule.

There also exists the possibility for drug binding to the lipid as well as to the protein components of the milk fat globule. It is also possible that lipid soluble drugs may be sequestered within the milk fat globule. In addition to lipids and protein, carbohydrate is entirely synthesized within the breast. All of these nutrients achieve a concentration in human milk that is sufficient for the needs of the human infant for the first six months of life.

The transport of drugs into breast milk from maternal tissues and plasma may proceed by a number of different routes. In general, however, the mechanisms that determine the concentration of a drug in breast milk are similar to those existing elsewhere within the organism. Drugs traverse mem-branes primarily by passive diffusion and the concentration achieved will be dependent not only on the concentration gradient but also on the intrinsic lipid solubility of the drug and its degree of ionization as well as binding to protein and other cellular constituents.

A number of reviews (10–12) give tables of the concentration of drugs in breast milk. Many times these tables also give the milk to plasma ratio. Most of the values from which the tables are derived consist of a single measurement of the drug concentration. Important information such as the maternal dose, the frequency of dose, the time from drug administration to sampling, the frequency of nursing, and the length of lactation is not given.

What these concentrations mean to the physician concerned about the infant is that the drug is present in the milk. This fact is apparent since, with few exceptions, all drugs that are present in the maternal circulation will be transferred into milk. Because the drug in the nursing infant's blood or urine is not measured, we have no information about the amount that is actually absorbed by the infant from the milk and, therefore, have no way of determining the possible pharmacologic effect on the infant. In fact, a critical examination of the tables that have been published reveals that much of the information was gathered decades ago when analytical methodology was not as sensitive as it is today. Since the discipline of pharmacokinetics was not developed until recently, many of the studies quoted in the tables in the review articles do not look precisely at the time relationship between drug administration and disposition.

Certain things are clear with regard to drugs administered during lactation. It is clear that physicians will have to become aware of the results of animal studies in this area and of the potential risk of maternal drug ingestion to the suckling infant. It is clear that a great many other drugs employed at this time need to be thoroughly studied in order to assess their safety during lactation. It is clear that if the mother needs the drugs for therapeutic purposes, then she should consider not nursing. The ultimate decision must be individualized according to the specific illness and the therapeutic modality. It is clear that nursing should be avoided following the administration of radioactive pharmaceuticals that are usually given to the mother for diagnostic purposes.

The situation with the excretion of drugs into human breast milk might well be considered analogous to the prethalidomide era when the effects on the fetus from maternally ingested drugs were recognized only as a result of a catastrophe. Objective evaluation of the efficacy and safety of drugs in breast milk must be undertaken. Until such data are available, the physician should always weigh the risk/benefit ratio when prescribing any maternal medication. It is also obligatory upon the nursing mother to become aware of the same factors and apply a measure of self-control before ingesting over-the-counter drugs. As stated before, it is quite evident that nearly all drugs will be present in breast milk following maternal ingestion. It is prudent to minimize maternal exposure, although very few drugs are currently known to be hazardous to the suckling child. If, after examining the benefit/risk factor, the physician decides that maternal medication is necessary, drug exposure to the infant may be minimized by scheduling the maternal dose just after a nursing period. More often than not, drugs are prescribed to the nursing mother for the relief of symptoms that do not require drug therapy. It is probable if the mothers were apprised by the physician of the potential risk to the infant, most would endure the symptoms rather than take the drug and discontinue breast feeding.

CONCLUSIONS

We have two basic situations being dealt with throughout this book: 1) risk potential to the fetus of maternal drugs ingested during the course of pregnancy and 2) risk potential to the infant of drugs taken by the mother while nursing.

The obvious solution to fetal and nursing infant risk avoidance is maternal abstinence. However, from a pragmatic standpoint, that would be impossible to implement. Another solution is to disseminate knowledge, in an authoritative manner, to all those involved in the pregnancy and breast feeding processes: physician, mother, midwife, nurse, father, and pharmacist.

This book helps fill a communication/information gap. We have carefully evaluated the research literature, animal and human, applied and clinical. We have established a risk factor for each of the more than 500 drugs, in keeping with the Food and Drug Administration guidelines, which may be administered during pregnancy and lactation. We feel that this book will be helpful to all concerned parties in developing the benefit/risk decision.

This is but a beginning. It is our fervent hope that the information gained from the use of this book will cause the concerned parties to be more trenchant in their future decision-making, either before prescribing or before ingesting drugs during pregnancy and lactation.

References

1. Gregg NM. Congenital cataract following German measles in the mother. Trans Ophthalmol Soc Aust 3:35–41, 1941.
2. Soranus. *Gynecology* (translation). Baltimore, Johns Hopkins Press, 1956.
3. Chadwick J, Mann WN. *The Medical Works of Hippocrates.* Springfield, Ill., Charles C Thomas, 1935.
4. Gupta C, Sondwane BR, Yaffe SJ, Shapiro BH. Phenobarbital exposure in utero: Alterations in female reproductive functions in rats. Science 208:508–510, 1980.
5. Gupta C, Yaffe SJ, Shapiro BH. Prenatal exposure to phenobarbital permanently decreases testosterone and causes reproductive dysfunction. Science 216:640–642, 1982.
6. Nutrition Committee of the Canadian Pediatric Society and the Committee on Nutrition of the American Academy of Pediatrics. Breast feeding. Pediatrics 62:591–601, 1978.
7. Fomon SJ. *Infant Nutrition*, 2nd ed. Philadelphia, W. B. Saunders, 1974, pp 360–370.
8. Jelliffe DB, Jelliffe EFP. Breast is best: Modern meanings. N Engl J Med 297:912–915, 1977.
9. Applebaum RM. The obstetricians approach to the breasts and breast feeding. J Reprod Med 14:98–116, 1975.
10. Knowles JA. Excretion of drugs in milk: A review. J Pediatr 66:1068–1082, 1965.
11. Hervada AR, Feit E, Sagrames R. Drugs in breast milk. Perinatal Care 2:19–25, 1978.
12. O'Brien TE. Excretion of drugs in human milk. Am J Hosp Pharm 31:844–854, 1974.

Instructions for Use of the Reference Guide

The Reference Guide is arranged so that the user can quickly locate a monograph. If the American generic name is known, go directly to the monograph, which is listed in alphabetical order. If only the trade or foreign name is known, refer to the Index for the appropriate American generic name. Foreign trade names have been included in the Index. To the best of our knowledge, all trade and foreign generic names are correct as shown, but since these may change, the reader should check other reference sources if there is any question as to the identity of an individual drug. Combination products are generally not listed in the Index. The user should refer to the manufacturer's product information for the specific ingredients and then use the Reference Guide as for single entities.

Each monograph contains six parts:
- —Generic name (United States)
- —Pharmacologic class
- —Risk Factor
- —Fetal Risk Summary
- —Breast Feeding Summary
- —References (omitted from some monographs)

Fetal Risk Summary

The Fetal Risk Summary is a brief review of the literature concerning the drug. The intent of the Summary is to provide clinicians and other individuals with sufficient data to counsel patients and to arrive at conclusions on the risk/benefit ratio a particular drug poses for the fetus. Since few absolutes are possible in the area of human teratology, the reader must carefully weigh the evidence, or lack thereof, before utilizing any drug in a pregnant woman. Animal datum has been excluded from most monographs unless it contributes, in our opinion, significantly to the total information. Readers who require more details than are presented should refer to the specific references listed at the end of the monograph.

Breast Feeding Summary

The Breast Feeding Summary is a brief review of the literature concerning the passage of the drug into human breast milk and the effects, if any, on the nursing infant. In many studies of drugs in breast milk, infants were not allowed to breast-feed. Readers should pay close attention to this distinction (i.e., excretion into milk vs effects on the nursing infant) when using a Summary. Those who require more details than are presented should refer to the specific references listed at the end of the monograph.

Risk Factors

Risk Factors (A, B, C, D, X) have been assigned to all drugs, based on the level of risk the drug poses to the fetus. They are designed to help the reader quickly classify a drug for use during pregnancy. They do not refer to breast feeding risk. Because they tend to oversimplify a complex topic, they should always be used in conjunction with the Fetal Risk Summary. The definitions used for the Factors are the same as those put forth by the Food and Drug Administration (Federal Register 1980;44:37434-67). Since most drugs have not yet been given a letter rating by their manufacturers, the Risk Factor assignments were usually made by the authors. If the manufacturer rated its product in its professional literature, the Risk Factor on the monograph will be shown with a subscript M (e.g., C_M). There were no instances in which the manufacturer and the authors differed in their assignment of a risk factor but the possibility for this exists. Some Risk Factors have an asterisk (e.g., sulfonamides, morphine, etc). These are drugs that present different risks to the fetus depending on when or for how long they are used. In these cases, a second Risk Factor will be found with a short explanation at the end of the Fetal Risk Summary. We hope this will increase the usefulness of these ratings. The definitions used for the Risk Factors are presented below.

Category A: Controlled studies in women fail to demonstrate a risk to the fetus in the first trimester (and there is no evidence of a risk in later trimesters), and the possibility of fetal harm appears remote.

Category B: Either animal-reproduction studies have not demonstrated a fetal risk but there are no controlled studies in pregnant women or animal-reproduction studies have shown an adverse effect (other than a decrease in fertility) that was not confirmed in controlled studies in women in the first trimester (and there is no evidence of a risk in later trimesters).

Category C: Either studies in animals have revealed adverse effects on the fetus (teratogenic or embryocidal or other) and there are no controlled studies in woman or studies in women and animals are not available. Drugs should be given only if the potential benefit justifies the potential risk to the fetus.

Category D: There is positive evidence of human fetal risk, but the benefits from use in pregnant women may be acceptable despite the risk (e.g., if the drug is needed in a life-threatening situation or for a serious disease for which safer drugs cannot be used or are ineffective).

Category X: Studies in animals or human beings have demonstrated fetal abnormalities or there is evidence of fetal risk based on human experience or both, and the risk of the use of the drug in pregnant women clearly outweighs any possible benefit. The drug is contraindicated in women who are or may become pregnant.

Contents

Name: **ACETAMINOPHEN**

Class: **Analgesic/Antipyretic**   Risk Factor: **B**

Fetal Risk Summary

Acetaminophen is routinely used during all stages of pregnancy for pain relief
and to lower elevated body temperature. In therapeutic doses, it is apparently
safe for short term use. Continuous, high daily dosage in one mother probably
caused severe anemia (hemolytic?) in her and fatal kidney disease in her
newborn (1). The drug crosses the placenta (2). Theoretically, acetaminophen
may cause fetal liver damage if the mother consumed a very large dose,
especially early in pregnancy (3). A woman at 36 weeks gestation consumed
a single dose of 22.5 g of acetaminophen producing toxic blood levels of 200
μg/ml (4). She was treated with acetylcysteine,and approximately 6 weeks
later delivered a normal female infant. The Collaborative Perinatal Project
monitored 50,282 mother-child pairs, 226 of which had 1st trimester exposure
to acetaminophen (5). Although no evidence was found to suggest a relationship to large categories of major or minor malformations, a possible association, based on 3 cases, was found with congenital dislocation of the hip (6).
The statistical significance of this association is unknown, and independent
confirmation is required. For use anytime during pregnancy, 781 exposures
were recorded (7). With the same qualifications, possible associations with
congenital dislocation of the hip (8 cases) and clubfoot (6 cases) were found
(8). Unlike aspirin, acetaminophen does not affect platelet function and there
is no increased risk of hemorrhage if the drug is given to the mother at term
(9, 10). In a study examining intracranial hemorrhage in premature infants, the
incidence of bleeding after acetaminophen close to term was no different than
non-exposed controls (see also Aspirin) (11).

Breast Feeding Summary

Acetaminophen is excreted into breast milk in low concentrations (12, 13).
Elimination is slower from the milk than from the plasma (13). No adverse
effects in nursing infants have been reported.

Author (ref)	No. Pts.	Dose	Concentrations (μg/ml) Serum	Concentrations (μg/ml) Milk	M:P Ratio	Effect on Infant
Madison (12)	Not stated	650 mg	—	11	—	—
Findlay (13)	1	324 mg (as Phenacetin)	— —	0.89 —	0.81 0.91–1.42	—

References

1. Char VC, Chandra R, Fletcher AB, Avery GB. Polyhydramnios and neonatal renal failure—a possible association with maternal acetaminophen ingestion. J Pediatr 1975;86:638–9.
2. Levy G, Garrettson LK, Soda DM. Evidence of placental transfer of acetaminophen. Pediatrics 1975;55:895.
3. Rollins DE, Von Bahr C, Glaumann H, Moldens P, Rane H. Acetaminophen: potentially toxic metabolite formed by human fetal and adult liver microsomes and isolated fetal liver cells. Science 1979;205:1414–6.
4. Byer AJ, Traylor TR, Semmer JR. Acetaminophen overdose in the third trimester of pregnancy. JAMA 1982;247:3114–5.
5. Heinonen OP, Slone D, Shapiro S. *Birth Defects and Drugs in Pregnancy*, Littleton: Publishing Sciences Group, 1977:286–95.
6. *Ibid*, 471.
7. *Ibid*, 434.
8. *Ibid*, 484.
9. Pearson H. Comparative effects of aspirin and acetaminophen on hemostasis. Pediatrics 1978;62(Suppl):926–9.
10. Rudolph AM. Effects of aspirin and acetaminophen in pregnancy and in the newborn. Arch Intern Med 1981;141:358–63.
11. Rumack CM, Guggenheim MA, Rumack BH, Peterson RG, Johnson ML, Braithwaite WR. Neonatal intracranial hemorrhage and maternal use of aspirin. Obstet Gynecol 1981;58(Suppl):52S–6S.
12. Personal communication. Madison WL, McNeil Laboratories, 1979.
13. Findlay JWA, DeAngelis RL, Kearney MF, Welch RM, Findlay JM. Analgesic drugs in breast milk and plasma. Clin Pharmacol Ther 1981;29:625–33.

Name: **ACETAZOLAMIDE**

Class: **Carbonic Anhydrase Inhibitor**   Risk Factor: **C**

Fetal Risk Summary

Despite widespread usage, no reports linking the use of acetazolamide with congenital defects have been located. A single case of a neonatal sacrococcygeal teratoma has been described (1). The mother received 750 mg daily for glaucoma during the 1st and 2nd trimesters. A relationship between the drug and carcinogenic effects in the fetus has not been supported by other reports. Retrospective surveys of the use of acetazolamide during gestation have not demonstrated an increased fetal risk (2, 3). The Collaborative Perinatal Project monitored 50,282 mother-child pairs, 12 of which had 1st trimester exposure to acetazolamide (4). For use anytime during pregnancy, 1,024 exposures were recorded (5). In neither case was evidence found to suggest a relationship to large categories of major or minor malformations or to individual defects.

Author (ref.)	No. Pts.	Indication	Gestational Age	Dose	Other Drugs	Fetal Effects	Comment
Worsham (1)	1	Glaucoma	1st and 2nd trimester	750 mg/day p.o.	FeSO$_4$ Dicyclomine Folic acid	Sacrococcygeal teratoma	—

Breast Feeding Summary

No data available.

References

1. Worsham GF, Beckman EN, Mitchell EH. Sacrococcygeal teratoma in a neonate association with maternal use of acetazolamide. JAMA 1978;240:251–2.
2. Favre-Tissot. An original clinical study of the pharmacologic-teratogenic relationship. Ann Med Psychol 1967:389.
3. McBride WG. The teratogenic action of drugs. Med J Aust 1963;2:689–93.
4. Heinonen OP, Slone D, Shapiro S. *Birth Defects and Drugs in Pregnancy.* Littleton: Publishing Sciences Group, 1977:372.
5. *Ibid*, 441.

Name: **ACETOHEXAMIDE**

Class: **Oral Hypoglycemic** Risk Factor: **D**

Fetal Risk Summary

Acetohexamide is a sulfonylurea used for the treatment of adult-onset diabetes mellitus. It is not indicated for the pregnant diabetic. When administered near term, acetohexamide crosses the placenta and may persist in the neonatal serum for several days (1). One mother, who took 1 g per day throughout pregnancy, delivered an infant whose serum level was 4.4 mg/100 ml at 10 hours of life (1). Prolonged symptomatic hypoglycemia due to hyperinsulinism lasted for five days. If used in pregnancy, acetohexamide should be stopped at least 48 hours before delivery to avoid this complication (2).

Although teratogenic in animals, an increased incidence of congenital defects, other than that expected in diabetes mellitus, has not been found with acetohexamide (see also Chlorpropamide, Tolbutamide) (3–5). Maternal diabetes is known to increase the rate of malformations by two to four fold, but the mechanism(s) are not understood (see also Insulin). In spite of the lack of evidence for acetohexamide teratogenicity, the drug should not be used in pregnancy since it will not provide good control in patients who cannot be controlled by diet alone (2). The manufacturer recommends it not be used in pregnancy.

Breast Feeding Summary

No data available (see Tolbutamide).

References

1. Kemball ML, McIver C, Milnar RDG, Nourse CH, Schiff D, Tiernan JR. Neonatal hypoglycaemia in infants of diabetic mothers given sulphonylurea drugs in pregnancy. Arch Dis Child 1970;45:696–701.
2. Friend JR. Diabetes. Clin Obstet Gynaecol 1981;8:353–82.
3. Malins JM, Cooke AM, Pyke DA, Fitzgerald MG. Sulphonylurea drugs in pregnancy. Br Med J 1964;2:187.

4. Adam PAJ, Schwartz R. Diagnosis and treatment: should oral hypoglycemic agents be used in pediatric and pregnant patients? Pediatrics 1968;42:819–23.
5. Dignan PSJ. Teratogenic risk and counseling in diabetes. Clin Obstet Gynecol 1981; 24:149–59.
6. Product information. Dymelor. Eli Lilly and Company, 1981.

Name: **ACETOPHENAZINE**

Class: **Tranquilizer**   Risk Factor: **C**

Fetal Risk Summary

Acetophenazine is a piperazine phenothiazine in the same group as prochlorperazine (see Prochlorperazine). Phenothiazines readily cross the placenta (1). No specific information on the use of acetophenazine in pregnancy has been located. Although occasional reports have attempted to link various phenothiazine compounds with congenital malformations, the bulk of the evidence indicates these drugs are safe for the mother and fetus (see also Chlorpromazine).

Breast Feeding Summary

No data available.

References

1. Moya F, Thorndike V. Passage of drugs across the placenta. Am J Obstet Gynecol 1962;84:1778–98.

Name: **ACETYLCHOLINE**

Class: **Parasympathomimetic (Cholinergic)**   Risk Factor **C**

Fetal Risk Summary

Acetylcholine is used primarily in the eye. No reports of its use in pregnancy have been located. As a quaternary ammonium compound, it is ionized at physiologic pH and transplacental passage in significant amounts would not be expected.

Breast Feeding Summary

No data available.

Name: **ACETYLDIGITOXIN**

Class: **Cardiac Glycoside**   Risk Factor: **B**

Fetal Risk Summary

See Digitalis.

Breast Feeding Summary

See Digitalis.

Name: **ALBUTEROL**

Class: **Sympathomimetic (Adrenergic)**   Risk Factor: **B**

Fetal Risk Summary

Albuterol is a β-sympathomimetic used to prevent premature labor (see also Ritodrine) (1–10). In one patient, albuterol was infused over 17 weeks via a catheter placed in the right subclavian vein (10–12). A normal male infant was delivered within a few hours of stopping the infusion. Although no congenital malformations have been observed, the use of albuterol prior to the 20th week of gestation has not been reported. Albuterol may cause fetal and maternal tachycardia (1–3). Fetal rates may exceed 160 beats per minute. Major decreases in maternal blood pressure have been reported with both systolic and diastolic dropping more than 30 mm Hg (2, 4, 6). Fetal distress following maternal hypotension was not mentioned. Other maternal adverse effects associated with albuterol have been acute congestive heart failure, pulmonary edema and death (13–21). Like all β-mimetics, albuterol may cause transient maternal hyperglycemia followed by an increase in serum insulin (4, 22, 23). Neonatal hypoglycemia, although not reported for albuterol, should be expected if the maternal hyperglycemia has not terminated prior to delivery (see also Ritodrine). Albuterol has been used in pregnant diabetic patients (24, 25). Significant increases in glycogenolysis and lipolysis were observed, especially in patients with juvenile diabetes. Monitoring of maternal blood glucose is recommended. Albuterol decreases the incidence of neonatal respiratory distress syndrome similar to other β-mimetics (26, 27). Long term evaluation of infants exposed to *in utero* β-mimetics has been reported but not specifically for albuterol (28, 29). No harmful effects in the infants were observed.

Breast Feeding Summary

No data available.

References

1. Liggins GC, Vaghan GS. Intravenous infusion of salbutamol in the management of premature labor. J Obstet Gynaecol Br Commonw 1973;80:29–33.

2. Korda AR, Lynerum RC, Jones WR. The treatment of premature labor with intravenous administered salbutamol. Med J Aust 1974;1:744–6.
3. Hastwell G. Salbutamol aerosol in premature labour. Lancet 1975;2:1212–3.
4. Hastwell GB, Halloway CP, Taylor TLO. A study of 208 patients in premature labor treated with orally administered salbutamol. Med J Aust 1978;1:465–9.
5. Hastwell G, Lambert BE. A comparison of salbutamol and ritodrine when used to inhibit premature labour complicated by ante-partum haemorrhage. Curr Med Res Opin 1979;5:785–9.
6. Ng KH, Sen DK. Hypotension with intravenous salbutamol in premature labour. Br Med J 1974;3:257.
7. Pincus R. Salbutamol infusion for premature labour—the Australian trials experience. Aust NZ Obstet Gynaecol 1981;21:1–4.
8. Gummerus M. The management of premature labor with salbutamol. Acta Obstet Gynecol Scand 1981;60:375–7.
9. Crowhurst JA. Salbutamol, obstetrics and anaesthesia: a review and case discussion. Anaesth Intensive Care 1980;8:39–43.
10. Lind T, Godfrey KA, Gerrard J, Bryson MR. Continuous salbutamol infusion over 17 weeks to pre-empt premature labour. Lancet 1980;2:1165–6.
11. Boylan P, O'Discoll K. Long-term salbutamol or successful Shirodkar suture? Lancet 1980;2:1374.
12. Addis GJ. Long-term salbutamol infusion to prevent premature labor. Lancet 1981;1:42–3.
13. Whitehead MI, Mander AM, Hertogs K, Williams RM, Pettingale KW. Acute congestive cardiac failure in a hypertensive woman receiving salbutamol for premature labour. Br Med J 1980;280:1221–2.
14. Poole-Wilson PA. Cardiac failure in a hypertensive woman receiving salbutamol for premature labour. Br Med. J 1980;281:226.
15. Fogarty AJ. *Ibid.*
16. Davies PDO. *Ibid*, 226–7.
17. Robertson M, Davies AE, *Ibid*, 227.
18. Crowley P. *Ibid.*
19. Whitehead MI, Mandere AM, Pettingale KW. *Ibid.*
20. Davies AE, Robertson MJS. Pulmonary oedema after the administration of intravenous salbutamol and ergometrine—case report. Br J Obstet Gynaecol 1980;87:539–41.
21. Milliez, Blot Ph, Sureau C. A case report of maternal death associated with betamimetics and betamethasone administration in premature labor. Eur J Obstet Gynaecol Reprod Biol 1980;11:95–100.
22. Thomas DJB, Dove AF, Alberti KGMM. Metabolic effects of salbutamol infusion during premature labour. Br J Obstet Gynaecol 1977;84:497–9.
23. Wager J, Lunell NO, Nadal M, Ostman J. Glucose tolerance following oral salbutamol treatment in late pregnancy. Acta Obstet Gynecol Scand 1981;60:291–4.
24. Barnett AH, Stubbs SM, Mander AM. Management of premature labour in diabetic pregnancy. Diabetologia 1980;188:365–8.
25. Wager J, Fredholm BB, Lunell NO, Persson B. Metabolic and circulatory effects of oral salbutamol in the third trimester of pregnancy in diabetic and non-diabetic women. Br J Obstet Gynaecol 1981;88:352–61.
26. Hastwell GB. Apgar scores, respiratory distress syndrome and salbutamol. Med J Aust 1980;1:174–5.
27. Hastwell G. Salbutamol and respiratory distress syndrome. Lancet 1977;2:354.
28. Wallace RL, Caldwell DL, Ansbacher R, Otterson WN. Inhibition of premature labor by terbutaline. Obstet Gynecol 1978;51:387–92.
29. Freysz H, Willard D, Lehr A, Messer J, Boog G. A long term evaluation of infants who received a beta-mimetic drug while in utero. J Perinat Med 1977;5:94–9.

Name: **ALPHAPRODINE**

Class: **Narcotic Analgesic** Risk Factor: **B***

Fetal Risk Summary

No reports linking the use of alphaprodine with congenital defects have been located. Characteristic of all narcotics used in labor, alphaprodine may produce respiratory depression in the newborn (1–8). Suppression of collagen-induced platelet aggregation has been demonstrated but specific data was not given (9). However, abnormal bleeding following the use of the drug has not been reported even though the magnitude of platelet dysfunction was comparable to that found in hemorrhagic states.

[* Risk Factor D if used for prolonged periods or in high doses at term.]

Breast Feeding Summary

No data available.

References

1. Smith EJ, Nagyfy SF. A report on comparative studies of new drugs used for obstetrical analgesia. Am J Obstet Gynecol 1949;58:695–702.
2. Hapke FB, Barnes AC. The obstetric use and effect on fetal respiration of Nisentil. Am J Obstet Gynecol 1949;58:799–801.
3. Kane WM. The results of Nisentil in 1,000 obstetrical casese. Am J Obstet Gynecol 1953;65:1020–6.
4. Backner DD, Foldes FF, Gordon EH. The combined use of alphaprodine (Nisentil) hydrochloride and levallorphan (Lorfan) tartrate for analgesia in obstetrics. Am J Obstet Gynecol 1957;74:271–82.
5. Gillan JS, Hunter GW, Darner CB, Thompson GR. Meperidine hydrochloride and alphaprodine hydrochloride as obstetric analgesic agents; a double-blind study. Am J Obstet Gynecol 1958;75:1105–10.
6. Roberts H, Kuck MAC. Use of alphaprodine and levallorphan during labour. Can Med Assoc J 1960;83:1088–93.
7. Burnett RG, White CA. Alphaprodine for continuous intravenous obstetric analgesia. Obstet Gynecol 1966;27:472–7.
8. Anthinarayanan PR, Mangurten HH. Unusually prolonged action of maternal alphaprodine causing fetal depression. Quarterly Pediatric Bulletin (Winter) 1977;3:14–6.
9. Corby DG, Schulman I. The effects of antenatal drug administration on aggregation of platelets of newborn infants. J Pediatr 1971;79:307–13.

Name: **AMANTADINE**

Class: **Antiviral/Antiparkinsonism** Risk Factor: **C**

Fetal Risk Summary

Cardiovascular malformation has been reported in an infant exposed to amantadine during the 1st trimester (1). Other reports have not been located. The drug is embryotoxic and teratogenic in animals in high doses (1, 2). Theoretically, amantadine may be a human teratogen but the absence of reports may have more to do with the probable infrequency of use in pregnant patients than to its teratogenic potency (3).

Author (ref.)	No. Pts.	Indication	Gestational Age	Dose	Other Drugs	Fetal Effects	Comment
Nora (1)	1	Parkinson-like movement disorder	1st trimester	100 mg/day	Not stated	Cardiovascular defect (single ventricle with pulmonary atresia)	Association with drug unknown

Breast Feeding Summary

Amantadine is excreted into breast milk in low concentrations. Although no reports of adverse effects in nursing infants have been located, the manufacturer recommends the drug not be used in nursing mothers (2).

References

1. Nora JJ, Nora AH, Way GL. Cardiovascular maldevelopment associated with maternal exposure to amantadine. Lancet 1975;2:607.
2. Product information. In Physicians' Desk Reference, ed. 35. Oradell, N.J.: Medical Economics Company, 1981.
3. Coulson AS. Amantadine and teratogenesis. Lancet 1975;2:1044.

Name: **AMBENONIUM**

Class: **Parasympathomimetic (Cholinergic)**   Risk Factor: **C**

Fetal Risk Summary

Ambenonium is a quaternary ammonium chloride with anticholinesterase activity used in the treatment of myasthenia gravis. It has been used in pregnancy but too little data is available to analyze (1, 2). Because it is ionized at physiologic pH, it would not be expected to cross the placenta in significant amounts. McNall has cautioned that intravenous anticholinesterases should not be used in pregnancy for fear of inducing premature labor (1). Although apparently safe for the fetus, cholinesterase inhibitors may affect the condition of the newborn (1). Transient muscular weakness has been observed in about 20% of newborns whose mothers were treated with these drugs during pregnancy.

Breast Feeding Summary

Because it is ionized at physiologic pH, ambenonium would not be expected to be excreted into breast milk (3).

References

1. McNall PG, Jafarnia MR. Management of myasthenia gravis in the obstetrical patient. Am J Obstet Gynecol 1965;92:518–25.

2. Heinonen OP, Slone D, Shapiro S. *Birth Defects and Drugs in Pregnancy*. Littleton: Publishing Sciences Group, 1977:345–56.
3. Wilson JT. Pharmacokinetics of drug excretion. In Wilson JT, ed. *Drugs in Breast Milk*. Australia: ADIS Press, 1981:17.

Name: **AMIKACIN**

Class: **Antibiotic**   Risk Factor: **C$_M$**

Fetal Risk Summary

Amikacin is an aminoglycoside antibiotic. The drug rapidly crosses the placenta into the fetal circulation and aminotic fluid (1–4). Studies in patients undergoing elective abortions in the 1st and 2nd trimesters indicate that amikacin distributes to most fetal tissues except the brain and cerebrospinal fluid (1, 3). The highest fetal concentrations were found in the kidneys and urine. At term, cord serum levels were ⅓ to ½ of maternal serum levels while measurable amniotic fluid levels did not appear until almost 5 hours post-injection (2).

No reports linking the use of amikacin to congenital defects have been located. Ototoxicity, which is known to occur after amikacin therapy, has not been reported as an effect of *in utero* exposure. However, eighth cranial nerve toxicity in the fetus is well known following exposure to other aminoglycosides (see Kanamycin and Streptomycin) and may potentially occur with amikacin.

Breast Feeding Summary

Amikacin is excreted into breast milk in low concentrations. Following 100- and 200-mg intramuscular doses, only traces of amikacin could be found over six hours in 2 of 4 patients (2, 5). Since oral absorption of this antibiotic is poor, ototoxicity in the infant would not be expected. However, three potential problems exist for the nursing infant: modification of bowel flora, direct effects on the infant and interference with the interpretation of culture results if a fever work-up is required.

References

1. Bernard B, Abate M, Ballard C, Wehrle P. Maternal-fetal pharmacology of BB-K8. Antimicrob Agents Chemother 14th Ann Conf: Abstr 71, 1974.
2. Matsuda C, Mori C, Maruno M, Shiwakura T. A. study of amikacin in the obstetrics field. Jap J Antibiot 1974; 27:633–6.
3. Bernard B, Abate M, Thielen P, Attar H, Ballard C, Wehrle P. Maternal-fetal pharmacological activity of amikacin. J Infect Dis 1977;135:925–31.
4. Flores-Mercado F, Garcia-Mercado J, Estopier-Jauregin C, Galindo-Hernandez E, Diaz-Gonzalez C. Clinical pharmacology of amikacin sulphate: blood, urinary and tissue concentrations in the terminal stage of pregnancy. J Int Med Res 1977;5;292–4.
5. Yuasa M. A study of amikacin in obstetrics and gynecology. Jap J Antibot 1974;27;377–81.

Name: **AMILORIDE**

Class: **Diuretic**   Risk Factor: B_M

Fetal Risk Summary

Amiloride is a potassium-conserving diuretic. Animal studies have not shown adverse effects in the fetus (1). Only one report of fetal exposure to amiloride has been located. In this case, a malformed fetus was discovered following voluntary abortion in a patient with renovascular hypertension (2). The patient had been treated during the 1st trimester with amiloride, propranold and captopril. The left leg of the fetus ended at mid-thigh without distal development and no obvious skull formation was noted above the brain tissue. The authors attributed the defects to captopril.

Breast Feeding Summary

No data available.

References

1. Product information. Midamor. Merck Sharpe & Dohme, 1982.
2. Duminy PC, Burger PT. Fetal abnormality associated with the use of captopril during pregnancy. S Afr Med J 1981;60:805.

Name: **AMINOCAPROIC ACID**

Class: **Hemostatic**   Risk Factor: **C**

Fetal Risk Summary

No data available.

Breast Feeding Summary

No data available.

References

1. Nilsson IM. Epsilon-aminocaproic acid (E-ACA) as a therapeutic agent based on 5 years clinical experience. Acta Medica Scand 1966;180:Suppl No. 448.

Name: **AMINOGLUTETHIMIDE**

Class: **Anticonvulsant/Anti-Steroidogenic**   Risk Factor: **D**

Fetal Risk Summary

Aminoglutethimide when given throughout pregnancy has been suspected of causing virilization in the fetus (1, 2). No adverse effect was seen when exposure was limited to the 1st and early 2nd trimesters (3, 4). Virilization may be due to inhibition of adrenocortical function.

Breast Feeding Summary

No data available.

References

1. Iffy L, Ansell JS, Bryant FS, Hermann WL. Nonadrenal female pseudohermaphroditism: an unusual case of fetal masculinization. Obstet Gynecol 1965;26;59–65.
2. Marek J, Horky K. Aminoglutethimide administration in pregnancy. Lancet 1970;2:1312–3.
3. Le Maire WJ, Cleveland WW, Bejar RL, Marsh JM, Fishman L. Aminoglutethimide: a possible cause of pseudohermaphroditism in females. Am J Dis Child 1972;124:421–3.
4. Hanson TJ, Ballonoff LB, Northcutt RC. Aminoglutethimide and pregnancy. JAMA 1974;230:963–4.

Name: **AMINOPHYLLINE**

Class: **Spasmolytic/Vasodilator**   Risk Factor: **C**

Fetal Risk Summary

See Theophylline.

Breast Feeding Summary

See Theophylline.

Name: **AMINOPTERIN**

Class: **Antineoplastic**   Risk Factors: **X**

Fetal Risk Summary

Aminopterin is an antimetabolite antineoplastic agent. It is structurally similar to and has been replaced by methotrexate (amethopterin). Several reports have described fetal anomalies when the drug was used as an unsuccessful abortifacient (1–8). The malformations included:

Meningocephalocele	Cleft lip/palate
Cranial anomalies	Low set ears
Abnormal positioning of extremities	Hypoplasia of thumb and
Short forearms	fibula
Hydrocephaly	Brachycephaly
Talipes	Anecephaply
Incomplete skull ossification	Clubfoot
Mental retardation	Syndactyly
	Hypognathia or retrognathia

Use of aminopterin in the 2nd and 3rd trimesters has not been associated with congenital defects (8). Long term studies of growth and mental development in offspring exposed to aminopterin during the 2nd trimester, the period of neuroblast multiplication, have not been conducted (9).

Breast Feeding Summary

No data available.

References

1. Meltzer HJ. Congenital anomalies due to attempted abortion with 4-aminopteroglutamic acid. JAMA 1956;161:1253.
2. Warkany J, Beaudry PH, Hornstein S. Attempted abortion with aminopterin (4-amino-pteroyl glutamic acid). Am J Dis Child 1959;97:274–81.
3. Shaw EB, Steinbach HL. Aminopterin-induced fetal malformation. Am J Dis Child 1968;115:477–82.
4. Brandner M, Nussle D. Foetopathic due a l'aminopterine avec stenose cogenitale de l'espace medullaire des os tubulaires ongs. Ann Radiol 1969;12:705–10.
5. Shaw EB. Fetal damage due to maternal aminopterin ingestion: follow-up at age 9 years. Am J Dis Child 1972;124:93–4.
6. Reich EW, Cox RP, Becker MH, et al. Recognition in adult patients of malformations induced by folic acid antagonists. Birth Defects 1978;14:139–60.
7. Shaw EB, Rees EL. Fetal damage due to aminopterin ingestion: follow-up at 17½ years of age. Am J Dis Child 1980;134:1172–3.
8. Nicholson HO. Cytotoxic drugs in pregnancy; review of reported cases. J Obstet Gynaecol Br Commonw 1968;75:307–12.
9. Dobbing J. Pregnancy and leukaemia. Lancet 1977;1:1155.

Name: *para*-AMINOSALICYLIC ACID
Class: **Antitubercular**   Risk Factor: **C**

Fetal Risk Summary

The Collaborative Perinatal Project monitored 50,282 mother-child pairs, 43 of which had 1st trimester exposure to aminosalicylic acid (1). Congenital defects were found in 5 infants. This incidence (11.6%) was nearly twice the expected frequency. No major category of malformations or individual defects were identified. An increased malformation rate for ear, limb and hypospadias has been reported for 123 patients taking 7 to 14 g of aminosalicylic acid per day with other antitubercular drugs (2). Confirmation of an increased risk of congenital defects has not been demonstrated by other studies (3–5).

Breast Feeding Summary

No data available.

References

1. Heinonen OP, Slone D, Shapiro S. *Birth Defects and Drugs in Pregnancy*. Littleton: Publishing Sciences Group, 1977:299.
2. Varpela E. On the effect exerted by first line tuberculosis medicines on the foetus. Acta Tuberc Scand 1964; 35:53–69.

3. Lowe CR. Congenital defects among children born to women under supervision or treatment for pulmonary tuberculosis. Br J Prev Soc Med 1964;18:14–6.
4. Wilson EA, Thelin TJ, Ditts PV. Tuberculosis complicated by pregnancy. Am J Obstet Gynecol 1973; 115;526–9.
5. Scheinhorn DJ, Angelillo VA. Antituberculosis therapy in pregnancy. Risk to the fetus. West J Med 1977;127;195–8.

Name: **AMITRIPTYLINE**

Class: **Antidepressant**   Risk Factor: **D**

Fetal Risk Summary

Limb reduction anomalies have been reported with amitriptyline (1). Analysis of 522,630 births, 86 with 1st trimester exposure to amitriptyline, did not confirm an association with this defect (2–9). Reported malformations other than limb reduction include (4, 8, 9):

Micrognathia, anomalous right mandible, left pes equinovarus (1 case)
Swelling of hands and feet (1 case)
Hypospadias (1 case)

These reports indicate that amitriptyline is not a major cause of congenital limb deformities. Urinary retention in the neonate has been associated with maternal use of nortriptyline (metabolite of amitriptyline) (10).

Breast Feeding Summary

Amitriptyline and its metabolite, nortriptyline, are excreted into breast milk in low concentrations (11–13). In one patient, estimates indicated the baby received about 1% of the mother's dose (13). No clinical signs of drug activity were observed in the infant. Although levels of amitriptyline and its metabolite have been undetectable in infant serum, the effects of exposure to small amounts in the milk are not known (11–13).

Author (ref.)	No. Pts.	Dose	Concentrations (μg/ml)		M:P Ratio	Effect on Infant
			Serum	Milk		
Bader (11)	1	—	0.14	0.15	1.0	No drug detected in infant's serum
Erickson (14)	1	—	0.09	—	—	No drug detected in infant's serum

References

1. McBride WG. Limb deformities associated with iminodibenzyl hydrochloride. Med J Aust 1972;1:492.
2. Australian Drug Evaluation Committee. Tricyclic antidepressants and limb reduction deformities. Med J Aust 1973;1:768–9.
3. Heinonen OP, Slone D, Shapiro S. *Birth Defects and Drugs in Pregnancy*. Littleton: Publishing Sciences Group, 1977:336–7.
4. Idanpaan-Heikkila J, Saxen L. Possible teratogenicity of Imipramine/chloropyramine. Lancet 1973;2:282–3.

5. Rachelefsky GS, Flynt JW, Ebbin AJ, Wilson MG. Possible teratogenicity of tricyclic antide-pressants. Lancet 1972;1:838.
6. Banister P, Dafoe C, Smith ESO, Miller J. Possible teratogenicity of tricyclic antidepressants. Lancet 1972;1:838–9.
7. Scanlon FJ. Use of antidepressant drugs during the first trimester. Med J Aust 1969;2:1077.
8. Crombie DL, Pinsent R, Fleming D. Imipramine in pregnancy. Br Med J 1972;1:745.
9. Kuenssberg EV, Knox JDE. Imipramine in pregnancy. Br Med J 1972;2:292.
10. Shearer WT, Schreiner RL, Marshall RE. Urinary retention in a neonate secondary to maternal ingestion of nortriptyline. J Pediatr 1972;81:570–2.
11. Bader TF, Newman K. Amitriptyline in human breast milk and the nursing infants serum. Am J Psychiatry 1980;137;855–6.
12. Wilson JT, Brown D, Cherek DR, et al. Drug excretion in human breast milk. Principles, pharmacokinetics and projected consequences. Clin Pharmacokinet 1980;5:1–66.
13. Brixen-Rasmussen L, Halgrener J, Jorgensen A. Amitriptyline and nortriptyline excretion in human breast milk. Psychopharmacology (Berlin) 1982;76:94–5.
14. Erickson SH, Smith GH, Heidrich F. Tricyclics and breast feeding. Am J Psychiatry 1979;136:1483.

Name: **AMMONIUM CHLORIDE**

Class: **Expectorant/Urinary Acidifier**   Risk Factor: **B**

Fetal Risk Summary

The Collaborative Prenatal Project monitored 50,282 mother-child pairs, 365 of which had 1st trimester exposure to ammonium chloride from its use as an expectorant in cough medications (1). For use anytime during pregnancy, 3,401 exposures were recorded (2). In neither case was evidence found to suggest a relationship to large categories of major or minor malformations. Three possible associations with individual malformations were found but the statistical significance of these is unknown (3, 4). Independent confirmation is required to determine the actual risk.

Inguinal hernia (1st trimester only) (11 cases)
Cataract (6 cases)
Any benign tumor (17 cases)

When consumed in large quantities near term, ammonium chloride may cause acidosis in the mother and the fetus (5, 6). In some cases, the decreased pH and pCO_2, increased lactic acid, and reduced oxygen saturation were as severe as those seen with fatal apnea neonatorum. However, the newborns did not appear in distress.

Breast Feeding Summary

No data available.

References

1. Heinonen OP, Slone D, Shapiro S. *Birth Defects and Drugs in Pregnancy*. Littleton: Publishing Sciences Group, 1977:378–81.
2. *Ibid*, 442.
3. *Ibid*, 478.
4. *Ibid*, 496.

5. Goodlin RC, Kaiser IH. The effect of ammonium chloride induced maternal acidosis on the human fetus at term. I. pH, hemoglobin, blood gases. Am J Med Sci 1957;233:666–74.
6. Kaiser IH, Goodlin RC. The effect of ammonium chloride induced maternal acidosis on the human fetus at term. II. Electrolytes. Am J Med Sci 1958;235:549–54.

Name: **AMOBARBITAL**

Class: **Sedative/Hypnotic**   Risk Factor: **D**

Fetal Risk Summary

Amobarbital is a member of the barbiturate class. The drug crosses the placenta achieving levels in the cord serum similar to the maternal serum (1, 2). Single or continuous dosing of the mother near term does not induce amobarbital hydroxylation in the fetus as demonstrated by the prolonged elimination of the drug in the newborn (half-life 2.5 times maternal). An increase in the incidence of congenital defects in infants exposed *in utero* to amobarbital has been reported (3, 4). One survey of 1,369 patients exposed to multiple drugs found 273 who received amobarbital during the 1st trimester (3). Ninety-five of the exposed infants delivered infants with major or minor abnormalities. Malformations associated with barbiturates, in general, were:

Anencephaly	Congenital dislocation of the hip
Congenital heart disease	Soft-tissue deformity of the neck
Severe limb deformities	Hypospadias
Cleft lip and palate	Accessory auricle
Intersex	Polydactyly
Papilloma of the forehead	Naevus
	Hydrocele

The Collaborative Perinatal Project monitored 50,282 mother-child pairs, 298 of which had 1st trimester exposure to amobarbital (4). For use anytime during pregnancy, 867 exposures were recorded (5). A possible association was found between the use of the drug in the 1st trimester and the following:

Cardiovascular (7 cases)
Polydactyly in Blacks (2 cases in 29 Blacks)
Genitourinary other than hypospadias (3 cases)
Inguinal hernia (9 cases)
Clubfoot (4 cases)

In contrast to the above reports, a 1964 survey of 187 pregnant patients who had received various neuroleptics, including amobarbital, found a 3.1% incidence of malformations in the offspring (6). This is approximately the expected incidence of abnormalities in a non-exposed population. Arthrogryposis and multiple defects were reported in an infant exposed to amobarbital during the 1st trimester (7). The defects were attributed to immobilization of the limbs at the time of joint formation, multiple drug use and active tetanus.

Breast Feeding Summary

No data available.

References

1. Kraver B, Draffan GH, Williams FM, Calre RA, Dollery CT, Hawkins DF. Elimination kinetics of amobarbital in mothers and newborn infants. Clin Pharmacol Ther 1973;14:442–7.
2. Draffan GH, Dollery CT, Davies DS, et al. Maternal and neonatal elimination of amobarbital after treatment of the mother with barbiturates during late pregnancy. Clin Pharmacol Ther 1976;19:271–5.
3. Nelson MM, Forfar JO. Associations between drugs administered during pregnancy and congenital abnormalities of the fetus. Br Med J 1971;1:523–7.
4. Heinonen OP, Slone D, Shapiro S. *Birth Defects and Drugs in Pregnancy*. Littleton: Publishing Sciences Group, 1977:336, 344.
5. *Ibid*, 438.
6. Favre-Tissot. An original clinical study of the pharmacologic-teratogenic relationship. Ann Med Psychol (Paris) 1967:389.
7. Jago RH. Arthrogryposis following treatment of maternal tetanus with muscle relaxants. Arch Dis Child 1970;45:277–9.

Name: **AMOXAPINE**

Class: **Antidepressant**   Risk Factor: **C$_M$**

Fetal Risk Summary

No reports linking the use of amoxapine with congenital defects have been located. Animal studies have not demonstrated a teratogenic effect (1).

Breast Feeding Summary
No data available.

Reference

1. Product information. Asendin. Lederle Laboratories: Pearl River, New York, 1981.

Name: **AMOXICILLIN**

Class: **Antibiotic**   Risk Factor: **B**

Fetal Risk Summary

Amoxicillin is a penicillin antibiotic similar to ampicillin (see also Ampicillin). No reports linking its use to congenital defects have been located. The Collaborative Perinatal Project monitored 50,282 mother-child pairs, 3,546 of which had 1st trimester exposure to penicillin derivatives (1). For use anytime during pregnancy, 7,171 exposures were recorded (2). In neither case was evidence found to suggest a relationship to large categories of major or minor malformations or to individual defects.

Amoxicillin depresses both plasma-bound and urinary excreted estriol (see also Ampicillin) (3). Urinary estriol was formerly used to assess the condition of the fetoplacental unit but this is now made by measuring plasma unconjugated estriol which is not usually affected by amoxicillin.

Breast Feeding Summary

Amoxicillin is excreted into breast milk in low concentrations. Following a 1-g oral dose given to 6 mothers, peak milk levels occurred at 4 to 5 hours, average 0.9 μg/ml (range 0.68 to 1.3 μg/ml) (4). Mean milk:plasma ratios at 1, 2 and 3 hours were 0.014, 0.013 and 0.043, respectively. Although no adverse effects have been recorded, three potential problems exist for the nursing infant: modification of bowel flora, direct effects on the infant (e.g., allergy/sensitization) and interference with the interpretation of culture results if a fever work-up is required.

References

1. Heinonen OP, Slone D, Shapiro S. *Birth Defects and Drugs in Pregnancy.* Littleton: Publishing Sciences Group, 1977:297–313.
2. *Ibid*, 435.
3. Van Look PFA, Top-Huisman M, Gnodde HP. Effect of ampicillin or amoxycillin administration on plasma and urinary estrogen levels during normal pregnancy. Eur J Obstet Gynaecol Reprod Biol 1981;12:225–33.
4. Kafetzis D, Siafas C, Georgakopoulos P, Papadatos C. Passage of cephalosporins and amoxicillin into the breast milk. Acta Paediatr Scand 1981; 70:285–8.

Name: # AMPHOTERICIN B

Class: **Antifungal Antibotic** Risk Factor: **B**

Fetal Risk Summary

No reports linking the use of amphotericin B with congenital defects have been located. The Collaboratorive Perinatal Project monitored 50,282 mother-child pairs, 9 of which had 1st trimester exposure to amphotericin B (1). Numerous other reports have also described the use of amphotericin B during various stages of pregnancy, including the 1st trimester (2–17). No evidence of adverse fetal effects was found by these studies. Amphotericin B can be used during pregnancy in those patients who will clearly benefit from the drug.

Breast Feeding Summary

No data available.

References

1. Heinonen OP, Slone D, Shapiro S. *Birth Defects and Drugs in Pregnancy.* Littleton: Publishing Sciences Group, 1977;297.
2. Neiberg AD, Maruomatis F, Dyke J, Fayyad A. Blastomyces dermatitidis treated during pregnancy. Am J Obstet Gynecol 1977;128:911–2.
3. Philpot CR, Lo D. Crytococcal meningitis in pregnancy. Med J Aust 1972;2:1005–7.
4. Aitken GWE, Symonds EM. Cryptococcal meningitis in pregnancy treated with amphotericin. Br J Obstet Gynaecol 1962;69:677–9.
5. Feldman R. Cryptococcosis of the CNS treated with amphotericin B during pregnancy. South Med J 1959;2:1415–7.
6. Kuo D. A case of torulosis of the central nervous system during pregnancy. Med J Aust 1962;1:558–60.

7. Crotty JM. Systemic mycotic infections in northern territory aborigines. Med J Aust 1965;1:184.
8. Littman ML. Cryptococcosis (torulosis) current concepts and therapy. Am J Med 1959;27:976–8.
9. Mick R, Muller-Tyle, Neufeld T. Comparison of the effectiveness of Nystatin and amphotericin B in the therapy of female genital mycoses. Wien Med Wochenschr 1975:125:131–5.
10. Silberfarb PM, Sarois GA, Tosh FE. Cryptococcosis and pregnancy. Am J Obstet Gynecol 1972;112:714–20.
11. McCoy MJ, Ellenberg JF, Killam AP. Coccidioidomycosis complicating pregnancy. Am J Obstet Gynecol 1980;137:739–40.
12. Curole DN. Cryptococcal meningitis in pregnancy. J Reprod Med 1981;26:317–9.
13. Sanford WG, Rasch JR, Stonehill RB. A therapeutic dilemma: The treatment of disseminated coccidioidomycosis with amphotericin B. Ann Intern Med 1962;56:553–63.
14. Harris RE. Coccidioidomycosis complicating pregnancy. Report of 3 cases and review of the literature. Obstet Gynecol 1966;28:401–5.
15. Smale LE, Waechter KG. Dissemination of coccidioidomycosis in pregnancy. Am J Obstet Gynecol 1970;107:356–9.
16. Hadsall FJ, Acquarelli MJ. Disseminated coccidioidomycosis presenting as facial granulomas in pregnancy: a report of two cases and a review of the literature. Laryngoscope 1973;83:51–8.
17. Ismail MA, Lerner SA. Disseminated blastomycosis in a pregnant woman. Review of amphotericin B usage during pregnancy. Am Rev Resp Dis 1982;126:350–3.

Name: **AMPICILLIN**

Class: **Antibiotic**   Risk Factor: **B**

Fetal Risk Summary

Ampicillin is a penicillin antibiotic (see also Penicillin G). The drug rapidly crosses the placenta into the fetal circulation and amniotic fluid (1–6). Fetal serum levels can be detected within 30 minutes and equilibrate with maternal serum in 1 hour. Amniotic fluid levels can be detected in 90 minutes, reaching 20% of the maternal serum peak in about 8 hours. The pharmacokinetics of ampicillin during pregnancy have been reported (7).

Ampicillin depresses both plasma-bound and urinary excreted estriol by inhibiting steroid conjugate hydrolysis in the gut (8–12). Urinary estriol was formerly used to assess the condition of the fetoplacental unit, depressed levels being associated with fetal distress. This assessment is now made by measuring plasma-unconjugated estriol, which is not usually affected by ampicillin. An interaction between ampicillin and oral contraceptives resulting in pregnancy has been suspected, but in a study assessing hormone levels, all cycles appeared to be anovulatory (13, 14).

No reports linking the use of ampicillin with congenital defects have been located. The drug apparently does not exert a toxic effect on the developing fetus (14). The Collaborative Perinatal Project monitored 50,282 mother-child pairs, 3,546 of which had 1st trimester exposure to penicillin derivatives (15). For use anytime during pregnancy, 7,171 exposures were recorded (16). In neither case was evidence found to suggest a relationship to large categories of major or minor malformations or to individual defects. Based on this data, it is unlikely that ampicillin is teratogenic.

Breast Feeding Summary

Ampicillin is excreted into breast milk in low concentrations. Milk:plasma ratios have been reported up to 0.2 (17, 18). Although adverse effects are apparently rare, three potential problems exist for the nursing infant: modification of bowel flora, direct effects on the infant (e.g., allergic response/sensitization) and interference with the interpretation of culture results if a fever work-up is required. Candidiasis and diarrhea have been reported in an infant whose mother was receiving ampicillin (19).

References

1. Bray R, Boc R, Johnson W. Transfer of ampicillin into fetus and amniotic fluid from maternal plasma in late pregnancy. Am J Obstet Gynecol 1966;96:938–42.
2. MacAulay M, Abou-Sabe M, Charles D. Placental transfer of ampicillin. Am J Obstet Gynecol 1966;96:943–50.
3. Biro L, Ivan E, Elek E, Arr M. Data on the tissue concentration of antibotics in man. Tissue concentrations of semi-synthetic penicillins in the fetus. Int Z Klin Pharmakol Ther Toxikol 1970;4:321–4.
4. Elek E, Ivan E, Arr M. Passage of penicillins from mother to foetus in humans. Int J Clin Pharmacol Ther Toxicol 1972;6:223–8.
5. Kraybill EN, Chaney NE, McCarthy LR. Transplacental ampicillin: inhibitory concentrations in neonatal serum. Am J Obstet Gynecol 1980;138:793–6.
6. Jordheim O, Hagen AG. Study of ampicillin levels in maternal serum, umbilical cord serum and amniotic fluid following administration of pivampicillin. Acta Obstet Gynecol Scand 1980;59:315–7.
7. Philipson A. Pharmacokinetics of ampicillin duing pregnancy. J Infect Dis 1977;136:370–6.
8. Willman K, Pulkkinen M. Reduced maternal plasma and urinary estriol during ampicillin treatment. Am J Obstet Gynecol 1971;109:893–6.
9. Boehn F, DiPietro D, Goss D. The effect of ampicillin administration on urinary estriol and serum estradiol in the normal pregnant patient. Am J Obstet Gynecol 1974;119:98–101.
10. Sybulski S, Maughan G. Effect of ampicillin administration on estradiol, estriol and cortisol levels in maternal plasma and on estriol levels in urine. Am J Obstet Gynecol 1976;124:379–81.
11. Aldercreutz H, Martin F, Lehtinen T, Tikkanen M, Pulkkinen M. Effect of ampicillin adminis-tration on plasma conjugated and unconjugated estrogen and progesterone levels in preg-nancy. Am J Obstet Gynecol 1977;128:266–71.
12. Van Look PFA, Top-Huisman M, Gnodde HP. Effect of ampicillin or amoxycillin administration on plasma and urinary estrogen levels during normal pregnancy. Eur J Obstet Gynecol Reprod Biol 1981;12:225–33.
13. Dossetor J. Drug interactions with oral contraceptives. Br Med J 1975;4:467–8.
14. Friedman CI, Huneke AL, Kim MH, Powell J. The effect of ampicillin on oral contraceptive effectiveness. Obstet Gynecol 1980;55:33–7.
15. Heinonen OP, Slone D, Shapiro S. Birth Defects and Drugs in Pregnancy. Littleton: Publishing Sciences Group, 1977:297–313.
16. Ibid, 435.
17. Wilson J, Brown R, Cherek D, et al. Drug excretion in human breast milk: principles, pharmacokinetics and projected consequences. Clin Pharmacol Ther 1980;5:1–66.
18. Knowles J. Excretion of drugs in milk—a review. J Pediatr 1965;66:1068–82.
19. Williams M. Excretion of drugs in milk. Pharm J 1976;217:219.

Name: **AMYL NITRITE**

Class: **Vasodilator**   Risk Factor: **C**

Fetal Risk Summary

Amyl nitrate is a rapid acting, short duration vasodilator used primarily for the treatment of angina pectoris. Due to the nature of its indication, experience in pregnancy is limited. The Collaborative Perinatal Project recorded 7 1st trimester exposures to amyl nitrite and nitroglycerin plus 8 other patients exposed to other vasodilators (1). From this small group of 15 patients, 4 malformed children were produced, a statistically significant incidence ($p <$ 0.02). It was not stated if amyl nitrite was taken by any of the mothers of the affected infants. Although the data serves as a warning, the number of patients is so small that conclusions as to the relative safety of amyl nitrite in pregnancy cannot be made.

Breast Feeding Summary

No data available.

References

1. Heinonen OP, Slone D, Shapiro S. *Birth Defects and Drugs in Pregnancy.* Littleton: Publishing Sciences Group, 1977:371–3.

Name: **ANGIOTENSIN**

Class: **Sympathomimetic (Adrenergic)**   Risk Factor: **C**

Fetal Risk Summary

Angiotensin is no longer available in the United States. No reports of its use in pregnancy have been located.

Breast Feeding Summary

No data available.

Name: **ANILERIDINE**

Class: **Narcotic Analgesic**   Risk Factor: **B***

Fetal Risk Summary

No reports linking the use of anileridine with congenital defects have been located. Withdrawal may occur in infants exposed *in utero* to prolonged maternal ingestion of anileridine. The drug's usage in pregnancy is primarily confined to labor. Respiratory depression in the neonate similar to that produced by meperidine or morphine should be expected (1).

[* Risk Factor D if used for prolonged periods or in high doses at term.]

Breast Feeding Summary

No data available.

Reference

1. **Bonica J.** *Principles and Practice of Obstetric Analgesia and Anesthesia.* Philadelphia: FA Davis Company. 1967:250.

Name: **ANISINDIONE**

Class: **Anticoagulant**   Risk Factor: **D**

Fetal Risk Summary

See Coumarin Derivatives.

Breast Feeding Summary

See Coumarin Derivatives.

Name: **ANISOTROPINE**

Class: **Parasympatholytic**   Risk Factor: **C**

Fetal Risk Summary

Anisotropine is an anticholinergic quaternary ammonium methylbromide. In a large prospective study, 2,323 patients were exposed to this class of drugs during the first trimester, 2 of whom took anisotropine (1). A possible association was found between the total group and minor malformations.

Breast Feeding Summary

No data available (see also Atropine).

References

1. Heinonen OP, Slone D, Shapiro S. *Birth Defects and Drugs in Pregnancy.* Littleton: Publishing Sciences Group, 1977:346–53.

Name: **APROBARBITAL**

Class: **Sedative/Hypnotic**   Risk Factor: **C**

Fetal Risk Summary

No data available.

Breast Feeding Summary

No data available.

Name: **APROTININ**

Class: **Hemostatic**   Risk Factor: **D**

Fetal Risk Summary

No reports linking the use of aprotinin and congenital defects have been located. The drug crosses the placenta and decreased fibrinolytic activity in the newborn (1). The drug has been used safely in severe accidental hemorrhage with coagulation where labor has not been established (2).

Breast Feeding Summary

No data available

References

1. Hoffhauer H, Dobbeck P. Untersuchungen uber die plactapassage des kallikrenin inhibitors. Klin Wochenschr 1970;48:183–4.
2. Sher G. Trasylol in cases of accidental hemorrhage with coagulation disorder and associated uterine inertia. S Afr Med J 1974;48:1452–5.

Name: **ASPIRIN**

Class: **Analgesic/Antipyretic**   Risk Factor: **C***

Fetal Risk Summary

Aspirin is the most frequently ingested drug in pregnancy either as a single agent or in combination with other drugs (1). The terms Aspirin and Salicylates are used interchangeably in this monograph unless specifically separated. In eight surveys totaling over 54,000 patients, aspirin was consumed sometime during gestation by slightly over 33,000 (61%) (2–9). The true incidence is probably much higher than this since many patients either do not remember taking aspirin or consume drug products without realizing they contain large amounts of salicylates (2, 4, 8). Evaluation of the effects of aspirin on the fetus is very difficult due to this common, and often hidden, exposure.

However, some toxic effects on the mother and fetus from large doses of salicylates have been known since 1893 (10).

Aspirin consumption during pregnancy may produce adverse effects in the mother: anemia, antepartum and/or postpartum hemorrhage, prolonged gestation, and prolonged labor (5, 11, 48). The increased length of labor and frequency of postmaturity result from the inhibition of prostaglandin synthetase by aspirin. Aspirin has been shown to significantly delay the induced abortion time in nulliparous patients, but not multiparous, by this same mechanism (12). In an Australian study, regular aspirin ingestion was also found to increase the number of complicated deliveries (cesarean sections, breech, and forceps) (5). Small doses of aspirin may decrease urinary estriol excretion (13).

Fetal and newborn effects, other than congenital defects, from aspirin exposure *in utero* may include increased perinatal mortality, intrauterine growth retardation, congenital salicylate intoxication, and depressed albumin-binding capacity (2, 5, 14–16, 48). For the latter effect, no increase in the incidence of jaundice was observed (2). Perinatal mortality in the Australian study was usually a result of stillbirths more than neonatal deaths (5, 14). Some of the stillborns were associated with antepartum hemorrhage while others may have been due to closure of the ductus arteriosus *in utero* (18). Closure of the ductus has been shown in animals due to aspirin inhibition of prostaglandin synthetase. However, a large prospective American study involving 41,337 patients, 64% of whom used aspirin sometime during gestation, failed to show that aspirin was a cause of stillbirths, neonatal deaths, or reduced birth weight (17). The difference between these findings probably relates to the chronic or intermittent use of higher doses by the patients in the Australian study (18). Excessive use of aspirin was blamed for the stillbirth of a fetus where salicylate levels in the fetal blood and liver were 25–30 mg/100 ml and 12 mg/100 ml, respectively (19). Congenital salicylate intoxication was found in two newborns exposed to high aspirin doses prior to delivery (15, 16). Although both infants survived, one infant exhibited withdrawal symptoms beginning on the second neonatal day consisting of hypertonia, agitation, a shrill piercing cry, and increased reflex irritability (16). Serum salicylate level was 31 mg/100 ml. Most of the symptoms gradually subsided over 6 weeks but some mild hypertonia may have persisted.

Aspirin given in low doses during the week prior to delivery may effect the clotting ability of the newborn (20–26). In the initial studies by Bleyer and Breckenridge, 3 of 14 newborns exposed to aspirin within 1 week of delivery had minor hemorrhagic phenomena *versus* only 1 of 17 non-exposed controls (20). Collagen-induced platelet aggregation was absent in the aspirin group and, although of less clinical significance, Factor XII activity was markedly depressed. A direct correlation was found between Factor XII activity and the interval between the last dose of aspirin and birth. Neonatal purpuric rash with depressed platelet function has also been observed after maternal use of aspirin close to term (26). Salicylates, other than aspirin, may not be a problem since the acetyl moiety is apparently required to depress platelet function (27–29).

An increased incidence of intracranial hemorrhage (ICH) in premature or low birth weight infants may occur after maternal aspirin use near birth (30).

Computed tomographic screening for ICH was conducted on 108 infants 3 to 7 days after delivery. All of the infants were either 34 weeks or less in gestation, or 1500 g or less in birth weight. A total of 53 (49%) developed ICH, including 12 (71%) of the 17 aspirin-exposed newborns. This incidence was statistically significant ($p < 0.05$) when compared to the 41 (45%) non-aspirin-exposed who developed ICH. The conclusions of this study have been challenged and defended (31, 32). In view of the potentially serious outcome, however, aspirin should be used with extreme caution by patients in danger of premature delivery.

Aspirin readily crosses the placenta (10). When given near term, higher concentrations are found in the neonate than in the mother (33). The kinetics of salicylate elimination in the newborn have been studied (33–35).

The relationship between aspirin and congenital defects is controversial. Several studies have examined this question with findings either supporting or denying a relationship. In two large retrospective studies, mothers of 1,291 malformed infants were found to have consumed aspirin during pregnancy more frequently than mothers of normal infants (36, 37). In a retrospective survey of 599 children with oral clefts, use of salicylates in the 1st trimester was almost three times more frequent in the mothers of children with this defect (38). Reviewing these studies, Collins noted several biases, including the fact they were retrospective, that could account for the results (18). Three other reports of aspirin teratogenicity involving a total of 10 infants have been located (39–41). In each of the cases, other drugs and factors were present. The Collaborative Perinatal Project monitored 50,282 mother-child pairs, 14,864 of which used aspirin during the 1st trimester (6). For use anytime during pregnancy, 32,164 (64%) aspirin exposures were recorded. This prospective study did not find evidence of a teratogenic effect with aspirin. However, the data did not exclude the possibility that grossly excessive doses of aspirin may be teratogenic. An Australian study of 144 infants of mothers who took aspirin regularly in pregnancy also failed to find an association between salicylates and malformations (14). Based on these studies, and the fact that aspirin usage in pregnancy is so common, it is not possible to determine the teratogenic risk of salicylates, if indeed it exists.

In summary, the use of aspirin during pregnancy, especially of chronic or intermittent high doses, should be avoided. The drug may effect maternal and newborn hemostasis mechanisms leading to an increased risk of hemorrhage. High doses may be related to increased perinatal mortality, intrauterine growth retardation, and teratogenic effects. Low doses do not seem to carry these risks. Near term, aspirin may prolong gestation and labor even in very low doses. If an analgesic or antipyretic is needed, acetaminophen should be considered.

[* Risk Factor D if used in the 3rd trimester.]

Breast Feeding Summary

Aspirin and other salicylates are excreted into breast milk in low concentrations. Sodium salicylate was first demonstrated in human milk in 1935 (42). One study of a mother taking 4 g daily found no detectable salicylate in her milk or in her infant's serum, but the test sensitivity was only 50 μg/ml (43).

Reported milk concentrations are much lower than this level. Following single or repeated oral doses, peak milk levels occur at around 3 hours ranging from 1.1 to 10 μg/ml (44, 45). This represented a milk:plasma ratio of 0.03 to 0.08 at 3 hours. Since salicylates are eliminated more slowly from milk than from plasma, the ratio increased to 0.34 at 12 hours (45). Peak levels have also been reported to occur at 9 hours (46). Only one report has attributed infant toxicity to salicylates obtained in mother's milk (47). A 16-day-old female developed severe salicylate intoxication, with a serum salicylate level of 24 mg/100 ml on the third hospital day. Milk and maternal serum levels were not obtained. Although the parents denied giving the baby aspirin or other salicylates, it is unlikely, based on the above reports, that she could have received the drug from the milk in the quantities found. Adverse effects on platelet function in the nursing infant exposed to aspirin via the milk have not been reported but are a potential risk.

References

1. Corby DG. Aspirin in pregnancy: maternal and fetal effects. Pediatrics 1978;62(Suppl): 930–7.
2. Palmisano PA, Cassady G. Salicylate exposure in the perinate. JAMA 1969;209:556–8.
3. Forfar JO, Nelson MM. Epidemiology of drugs taken by pregnant women: drugs that may affect the fetus adversely. Clin Pharmacol Ther 1973;14:632–42.
4. Finnigan D, Burry AF, Smith IDB. Analgesic consumption in an antenatal clinic survey. Med J Aust 1974;1:761–2.
5. Collins E, Turner G. Maternal effects of regular salicylate ingestion in pregnancy. Lancet 1975;2:335–7.
6. Slone D, Heinonen OP, Kaufman DW, Siskind V, Monson RR, Shapiro S. Aspirin and congenital malformations. Lancet 1976;1:1373–5.
7. Hill RM, Craig JP, Chaney MD, Tennyson LM, McCulley LB. Utilization of over-the-counter drugs during pregnancy. Clin Obstet Gynecol 1977;20:381–94.
8. Harrison K, Thomas I, Smith I. Analgesic use during pregnancy. Med J Aust 1978;2:161.
9. Bodendorfer TW, Briggs GG, Gunning JE. Obtaining drug exposure histories during pregnancy. Am J Obstet Gynecol 1979;135:490–4.
10. Jackson AV. Toxic effects of salicylate on the foetus and mother. J Path Bact 1948;60:587–93.
11. Lewis RN, Schulman JD. Influence of acetylsalicylic acid, an inhibitor of prostaglandin synthesis, on the duration of human gestation and labour. Lancet 1973;2:1159–61.
12. Niebyl JR, Blake DA, Burnett LS, King TM. The influence of aspirin on the course of induced midtrimester abortion. Am J Obstet Gynecol 1976;124:607–10.
13. Castellanos JM, Aranda M, Cararach J, Cararach V. Effect of aspirin on oestriol excretion in pregnancy. Lancet 1975;1:859.
14. Turner G, Collins E. Fetal effects of regular salicylate ingestion in pregnancy. Lancet 1975;2:338–9.
15. Earle R Jr. Congenital salicylate intoxication—report of a case. N Engl J Med 1961;265:1003–4.
16. Lynd PA, Andreasen AC, Wyatt RJ. Intrauterine salicylate intoxication in a newborn. A case report. Clin Pediatr (Phila) 1976;15:912–3.
17. Shapiro S, Monson RR, Kaufman DW, Siskind V, Heinonen OP, Slone D. Perinatal mortality and birth-weight in relation to aspirin taken during pregnancy. Lancet 1976;1:1375–6.
18. Collins E. Maternal and fetal effects of acetaminophen and salicylates in pregnancy. Obstet Gynecol 1981;58(Suppl):57S–62S.
19. Aterman K, Holzbecker M, Ellenberger HA. Salicylate levels in a stillborn infant born to a drug-addicted mother, with comments on pathology and analytical methodology. Clin Tox 1980;16:263–8.
20. Bleyer WA, Breckenridge RJ. Studies on the detection of adverse drug reactions in the

newborn. II. The effects of prenatal aspirin on newborn hemostasis. JAMA 1970;213:2049–53.

21. Corby DG, Schulman I. The effects of antenatal drug administration on aggregation of platelets of newborn infants. J Pediatr 1971;79:307–13.

22. Casteels-Van Daele M, Eggermont E, de Gaetano G, Vermijlen J. More on the effects of antenatally administered aspirin on aggregation of platelets of neonates. J Pediatr 1972;80:685–6.

23. Haslam RR, Ekert H, Gillam GL. Hemorrhage in a neonate possible due to maternal ingestion of salicylate. J Pediatr 1974;84:556–7.

24. Ekert H, Haslam RR. Maternal ingested salicylate as a cause of neonatal hemorrhage. Reply. J Pediatr 1974;85:738.

25. Pearson H. Comparative effects of aspirin and acetaminophen on hemostasis. Pediatrics 1978;62(Suppl):926–9.

26. Haslam RR. Neonatal Purpura secondary to maternal salicylism. J Pediatr 1975;86:653.

27. O'Brien JR. Effects of salicylates on human platelets. Lancet 1968;1:779–83.

28. Weiss HJ, Aledort ML, Shaul I. The effect of salicylates on the haemostatic properities of platelets in man. J Clin Invest 1968;47:2169–80.

29. Bleyer WA. Maternal ingested salicylates as a cause of neonatal hemorrhage. J Pediatr 1974;85:736–7.

30. Rumack CM, Guggenheim MA, Rumack BH, Peterson RG, Johnson ML, Braithwaite WR. Neonatal intracranial hemorrhage and maternal use of aspirin. Obstet Gynecol 1981;58(Suppl):52S–6S.

31. Soller RW, Stander H. Maternal drug exposure and perinatal intracranial hemorrhage. Obstet Gynecol 1981;58:735–7.

32. Corby DG. Editorial comment. Obstet Gynecol 1981;58:737–40.

33. Levy G, Procknal JA, Garrettson LK. Distribution of salicylate between neonatal and maternal serum at diffusion equilibrium. Clin Pharmacol Ther 1975;18:210–4.

34. Levy G, Garretson LK. Kinetics of salicylate elimination by newborn infants of mothers who ingested aspirin before delivery. Pediatrics 1974;53:201–10.

35. Garrettson LK, Procknal JA, Levy G. Fetal acquisition and neonatal elimination of a large amount of salicylate. Study of a neonate whose mother regularly took therapeutic doses of aspirin during pregnancy. Clin Pharmacol Ther 1975;17:98–103.

36. Richards ID. Congenital malformations and environmental influences in pregnancy. Br J Prev Soc Med 1969;23:218–25.

37. Nelson MM, Forfar JO. Associations between drugs administered during pregnancy and congenital abnormalities of the fetus. Br Med J 1971;1:523–7.

38. Saxen I. Associations between oral clefts and drugs during pregnancy. Int J Epidemiol 1975;4:37–44.

39. Benawra R, Mangurten HH, Duffell DR. Cyclopia and other anomalies following maternal ingestion of salicylates. J Pediatr 1980;96:1069–71.

40. McNiel JR. The possible effect of salicylates on the developing fetus. Brief summaries of eight suggestive cases. Clin Pediatr (Phila) 1973;12:347–50.

41. Sayli BS, Asmaz A, Yemisci B. Consanguinity, aspirin, and phocomelia. Lancet 1966;1:876.

42. Kwit NT, Hatcher RA. Excretion of drugs in milk. Am J Dis Child 1935;49:900–4.

43. Erickson SH, Oppenheim GL. Aspirin in breast milk. J Fam Pract 1979;8:189–90.

44. Weibert RT, Bailey DN. Salicylate excretion in human breast milk (Abstract No. 7). Presented at the 1979 Seminar of the California Society of Hospital Pharmacists, Los Angeles, October 13, 1979.

45. Findlay JWA, DeAngelis RL, Kearney MF, Welch RM, Findley JM. Analgesic drugs in breast milk and plasma. Clin Pharmacol Ther 1981;29:625–33.

46. Anderson PO. Drugs and breast feeding—a review. Drug Intell Clin Pharm 1977;11:208–23.

47. Clark JH, Wilson WG. A 16-day-old breast-fed infant with metabolic acidosis caused by salicylate. Clin Pediatr (Phila) 1981;20:53–4.

48. Rudolph AM. Effects of aspirin and acetaminophen in pregnancy and in the newborn. Arch Intern Med 1981;141:358–63.

Name: **ASPIRIN, BUFFERED**

Class: **Analgesic/Antipyretic** Risk Factor: **C***

Fetal Risk Summary

See Aspirin.

[* Risk Factor D if used in the 3rd trimester.]

Breast Feeding Summary

See Aspirin.

Name: **ATROPINE**

Class: **Parasympatholytic** Risk Factor: **C**

Fetal Risk Summary

Atropine, an anticholinergic, rapidly crosses the placenta (1–3). The drug has been used to test placental function in high risk obstetrical patients by producing fetal vagal blockade and subsequent tachycardia (4). The Collaborative Perinatal Project monitored 50,282 mother-child pairs, 401 of which used atropine in the 1st trimester (5). For use anytime during pregnancy, 1,198 exposures were recorded (6). In neither case was evidence found for an association with malformations. However, when the group of parasympatholytics were taken as a whole (2,323 exposures), a possible association with minor malformations was found (5). Atropine has been used to reduce gastric secretions prior to cesarean section without producing fetal or neonatal effects (7, 8).

Breast Feeding Summary

The passage of atropine into breast milk is controversial (9). It has not been adequately documented if measurable amounts are excreted or, if excretion does occur, if this may affect the nursing infant. However, since infants are particularly sensitive to anticholinergic agents, breast feeding should probably be suspended if atropine or atropine-like drugs must be given to the mother.

References

1. Nishimura H, Tanimura T. *Clinical Aspects of the Teratogenicity of Drugs.* New York: American Elsevier, 1976:63.
2. Kivalo I, Saarikoski S. Placental transmission of atropine at full-term pregnancy. Br J Anaesth 1977;49:1017–21.
3. Kanto J, Virtanen R, Iisalo E, Maenpaa K, Liukko P. Placental transfer and pharmacokinetics of atropine after a single maternal intravenous and intramuscular administration. Acta Anaesth Scand 1981;25:85–8.
4. Hellman LM, Fillisti LP. Analysis of the atropine test for placental transfer in gravidas with toxemia and diabetes. Am J Obstet Gynecol 1965;91:797–805.

5. Heinonen OP, Slone D, Shapiro S. *Birth Defects and Drugs in Pregnancy*. Littleton: Publishing Sciences Group, 1977:346–53.
6. *Ibid*, 439.
7. Diaz DM, Diaz SF, Marx GF. Cardiovascular effects of glycopyrrolate and belladonna derivatives in obstetric patients. Bull NY Acad Med 1980;56:245–8.
8. Roper RE, Salem MG. Effects of glycopyrrolate and atropine combined with antacid on gastric acidity. Br J Anaesth 1981;53:1277–80.
9. Stewart JJ. Gastrointestinal drugs. In Wilson JT, ed. *Drugs in Breast Milk*. Australia: ADIS Press, 1981:65–71.

Name: **AZATHIOPRINE**

Class: **Antineoplastic/Immunosuppressant**   Risk Factor: **D**

Fetal Risk Summary

Azathioprine is used primarily in renal and liver transplant patients. The drug crosses the placenta and trace amounts of its active metabolite, mercaptopurine, have been found in fetal blood (see also Mercaptopurine) (1). Experience in pregnancy is limited but most investigators have found azathioprine to be relatively safe (2–14). Congenital defects have been associated with its use in two patients: pulmonary valvular stenosis, and preaxial polydactyly (type 1) (15, 16). Transient chromosomal aberrations has been observed (17). Immunosuppression of the newborn was observed in one infant whose mother received azathioprine (150 mg) and prednisone (30 mg) daily throughout pregnancy (8). The suppression was characterized by lymphopenia, decreased survival of lymphocytes in culture, absence of IgM, and reduced levels of IgG. Recovery occurred at about 15 weeks of age. Azathioprine has been reported to interfere with the effectiveness of an intrauterine contraceptive device (IUD) (18). Two renal transplant patients, maintained on azathioprine and prednisone, each received a copper IUD (Cu7). Both became pregnant with the IUD in place. No defects were noted in either newborn although one was delivered prematurely. The authors recommend other means of contraception in sexually active women receiving azathioprine/prednisone.

Breast Feeding Summary

No data available.

References

1. Sarrikoski S, Seppala M. Immunosuppression during pregnancy. Transmission of azathioprine and its metabolites from the mother to the fetus. Am J Obstet Gynecol 1973;115:1100–6.
2. Gillibrand PN. Systemic lupus erythematosus in pregnancy treated with azathioprine. Proc Roy Soc Med 1966;59:834.
3. Board JA, Lee HM, Draper DA, Hume DM. Pregnancy following kidney homotransplantation from a non-twin: report of a case with concurrent administration of azathioprine and prednisone. Obstet Gynecol 1967;29:318–23.
4. Kaufmann JJ, Dignam W, Goodwin WE, Martin DC, Goldman R, Maxwell MH. Successful, normal childbirth after kidney homotransplantation. JAMA 1967;200:338–41.
5. Anonymous. Eleventh annual report of human renal transplant registry. JAMA 1973;216:1197.

6. Nolan GH, Sweet RL, Laros RK, Roure CA. Renal cadaver transplantation followed by successful pregnancies. Obstet Gynecol 1974;43:732–8.

7. Sharon E, Jones J, Diamond H, Kaplan D. Pregnancy and azathioprine in systemic lupus erythematosus. Am J Obstet Gynecol 1974;118:25–7.

8. Cote CJ, Meuwissen HJ, Pickering RJ. Effects on the neonate of prednisone and azathioprine administered to the mother during pregnancy. J Pediatr (Phila) 1974;85:324–8.

9. Erkman J, Blythe JG. Azathioprine therapy complicated by pregnancy. Obstet Gynecol 1972;40:708–9.

10. Price HV, Salaman JR, Laurence KM, Langmaid H. Immunosuppressive drugs and the foetus. Transplantation 1976;21:294–8.

11. The Registration Committee of the European Dialysis and Transplant Association. Successful pregnancies in women treated by dialysis and kidney transplantation. Br J Obstet Gynaecol 1980;87:839–45.

12. Golby M. Fertility after renal transplantation. Transplantation 1970;10:201–7.

13. Rabau-Friedman E, Mashiach S, Cantor E, Jacob ET. Association of hypoparathyroidism and successful pregnancy in kidney transplant recipient. Obstet Gynecol 1982;59:126–8.

14. Myers RL, Schmid R, Newton JJ. Childbirth after liver transplantation. Transplantation 1980;29:432.

15. Nishimura H, Tanimura T. Clinical Aspects of the Teratogenicity of Drugs. New York: American Elsevier, 1976:106–7.

16. Williamson RA, Karp LE. Azathioprine teratogenicity: review of the literature and case report. Obstet Gynecol 1981;58:247–50.

17. Leb DE, Weisskopf B, Kanovitz BS. Chromosome aberrations in the child of a kidney transplant recipient. Arch Intern Med 1971;128:441–4.

18. Zerner J, Doil KL, Drewry J, Leeber DA. Intrauterine contraceptive device failures in renal transplant patients. J Reprod Med 1981;26:99–102.

b

Name: **BACAMPICILLIN**

Class: **Antibiotic**   Risk Factor: **B**

Fetal Risk Summary

Bacampicillin, a penicillin antibiotic, is converted to ampicillin during absorption from the gastrointestinal tract (see Ampicillin).

Breast Feeding Summary

See Ampicillin.

Name: **BACITRACIN**

Class: **Antibiotic**   Risk Factor: **C**

Fetal Risk Summary

No reports linking the use of bacitracin with congenital defects have been located. The drug is primarily used topically, although the injectable form is available. One study listed 18 patients exposed to the drug in the 1st trimester (1). The route of administration was not specified. No association with malformations was found.

Breast Feeding Summary

No data available.

References

1. Heinonen OP, Slone D, Shapiro S. *Birth Defects and Drugs in Pregnancy.* Littleton: Publishing Sciences Group, 1977:297, 301.

Name: **BELLADONNA**

Class: **Parasympatholytic**   Risk Factor: **C**

Fetal Risk Summary

Belladonna is an anticholinergic agent. The Collaborative Perinatal Project monitored 50,282 mother-child pairs, 554 of which used belladonna in the 1st trimester (1). Belladonna was found to be associated with malformations in general and with minor malformations. For use anytime during pregnancy, 1,355 exposures were recorded (2). No association was found in this case.

Breast Feeding Summary

See Atropine.

References

1. Heinonen OP, Slone D, Shapiro S. *Birth Defects and Drugs in Pregnancy*. Littleton: Publishing Sciences Group, 1977:346–53.
2. *Ibid.* 439.

Name: **BENDROFLUMETHIAZIDE**

Class: **Diuretic**   Risk Factor: **D**

Fetal Risk Summary

See Chlorothiazide.

Breast Feeding Summary

Bendroflumethiazide has been used to suppress lactation (see Chlorothiazide).

Name: **BENZENE HEXACHLORIDE, GAMMA**

Class: **Scabicide/Pediculicide**   Risk Factor: **B**

Fetal Risk Summary

Gamma-benzene hexachloride is used topically for the treatment of lice and scabies. Small amounts are absorbed through the intact skin and mucous membranes (1). No reports linking the use of this drug with toxic or congenital defects have been located, but one reference suggested it should be used with caution due to its potential to produce neurotoxicity, convulsions and aplastic anemia (2). Limited animal studies have not shown a teratogenic effect (3, 4). In one animal study, the drug seemed to have a protective effect when given with known teratogens (5).

Breast Feeding Summary

No data available.

References

1. American Hospital Formulary Service. Benzene Hexachloride, Gamma. American Society of Hospital Pharmacists, 1978.
2. Sanmiguel GS, Ferrer AP, Alberich MT, Genaoui BM. Considerociones sobre el tratamiento de la infancia y en el embarazo. Actas Dermosifilogr 1980;71:105–8.
3. Palmer AK, Cozens DD, Spicer EJF, Worden AN. Effects of lindane upon reproduction function in a 3-generation study of rats. Toxicology 1978;10:45–54.
4. Palmer AK, Bottomley AM, Worden AN, Frohberg H, Bauer A. Effect of lindane on pregnancy in the rabbit and rat. Toxicology 1978;10:239–47.
5. Shtenberg AI, Torchinski I. Adaptation to the action of several teratogens as a consequence of preliminary administration of pesticides to females. Biull Eksp Biol Med 1977;83:227–8.

Name: **BENZTHIAZIDE**

Class: **Diuretic** Risk Factor: **D**

Fetal Risk Summary

See Chlorothiazide.

Breast Feeding Summary

See Chlorothiazide.

Name: **BENZTROPINE**

Class: **Parasympatholytic** Risk Factor: **C**

Fetal Risk Summary

Benztropine is an anticholinergic agent structurally related to atropine (see also Atropine). It also has antihistaminic activity. In a large prospective study, 2,323 patients were exposed to this class of drugs during the 1st trimester, 4 of whom took benztropine (1). A possible association was found between the total group and minor malformations. Paralytic ileus has been observed in two newborns exposed to chlorpromazine and benztropine at term (2). In one of these infants, other anticholinergic drugs may have contributed to the effect (see Doxepin). The small left colon syndrome was characterized by decreased intestinal motility, abdominal distention, vomiting, and failure to pass meconium. The condition cleared rapidly in both infants following a Gastrografin enema.

Breast Feeding Summary

No data available (see Atropine).

References

1. Heinonen OP, Slone D, Shapiro S. *Birth Defects and Drugs in Pregnancy*. Littleton: Publishing Sciences Group, 1977:346–53.
2. Falterman CG, Richardson CJ. Small left colon syndrome associated with maternal ingestion of psychotropic drugs. J Pediatr 1980;97:308–10.

Name: **BETAMETHASONE**

Class: **Corticosteroid** Risk Factor: **C**

Fetal Risk Summary

No reports linking the use of betamethasone with congenital defects have been located. Betamethasone is often used in patients with premature labor at about 26 to 34 weeks gestation to stimulate fetal lung maturation (1–14). The benefits of this therapy are:

Reduction in incidence of respiratory distress syndrome (RDS)

Decreased severity of RDS if it occurs

Decreased incidence of and mortality from intracranial hemorrhage

Increased survival of premature infants

In patients with prolonged rupture of the membranes, administration of betamethasone to the mother did not reduce the frequency of RDS or perinatal mortality (15, 16). Betamethasone therapy is less effective in decreasing the incidence of RDS in male infants than in female infants (17). The reasons for this difference have not been discovered.

An increased incidence of hypoglycemia in newborns exposed to *in utero* betamethasone has been reported (18). Other reports have not observed this effect. In the initial study examining the effect of betamethasone on RDS, Liggins and Howie reported an increased risk of fetal death in patients with severe preeclampsia (1). They proposed that the corticosteroid had an adverse effect on placentas already damaged by vascular disease. A second study did not confirm these findings (7). Leukocytosis was observed in a 880 g, 30-weeks-gestation female infant whose mother received 12 mg of betamethasone 4 hours prior to delivery (19). The WBC count returned to normal in about one week. Although human studies have usually shown a benefit, the use of corticosteroids in animals has been associated with several toxic effects (20, 21):

Reduced fetal head circumference

Reduced fetal adrenal weight

Increased fetal liver weight

Reduced fetal thymus weight

Reduced placental weight

Fortunately, none of these effects have been observed in human investigations. Finally, a study was conducted in 4-year-old children born of mothers treated with betamethasone for premature labor (22). The encouraging results indicated there was no difference in cognitive and psychosocial development between treated and non-treated groups.

Breast Feeding Summary

No data available.

References

1. Liggins GC, Howie RN. A controlled trial of antepartum glucocorticoid treatment for prevention of the respiratory distress syndrome in premature infants. Pediatrics 1972;50:515-25.
2. Gluck L. Administration of corticosteroids to induce maturation of fetal lung. Am J Dis Child 1976;130:976-8.
3. Ballard RA, Ballard PL. Use of prenatal glucocorticoid therapy to prevent respiratory distress syndrome: a supporting view. Am J Dis Child 1976;130:982-7.
4. Mead PB, Clapp JF III. The use of betamethasone and timed delivery in management of premature rupture of the membranes in the preterm pregnancy. J Reprod Med 1977;19:3-7.
5. Block MF, Kling OR, Crosby WM. Antenatal glucocorticoid therapy for the prevention of respiratory distress syndrome in the premature infant. Obstet Gynecol 1977;50:186-90.
6. Ballard RA, Ballard PL, Granberg JP, Sniderman S. Prenatal administration of betamethasone for prevention of respiratory distress syndrome. J Pediatr 1979;94:97-101.
7. Nochimson DJ, Petrie RH. Glucocorticoid therapy for the induction of pulmonary maturity in severely hypertensive gravid women. Am J Obstet Gynecol 1979;133:449-51.
8. Eggers TR, Doyle LW, Pepperell RJ. Premature labour. Med J Aust 1979;1:213-6.
9. Doran TA, Swyer P, MacMurray B, et al. Results of a double-blind controlled study on the use of betamethasone in the prevention of respiratory distress syndrome. Am J Obstet Gynecol 1980;136:313-20.
10. Schutte MF, Treffers PE, Koppe JG, Breur W. The influence of betamethasone and orciprenaline on the incidence of respiratory distress syndrome in the newborn after preterm labour. Br J Obstet Gynaecol 1980;87:127-31.
11. Dillon WP, Egan EA. Aggressive obstetric management in late second-trimester deliveries. Obstet Gynecol 1981;58:685-90.
12. Johnson DE, Munson DP, Thompson TR. Effect of antenatal administration of betamethasone on hospital costs and survival of premature infants. Pediatrics 1981;68:633-7.
13. Bishop EH. Acceleration of fetal pulmonary maturity. Obstet Gynecol 1981;58(Suppl):48S-51S.
14. Ballard PL, Ballard RA. Corticosteroids and respiratory distress syndrome: status 1979. Pediatrics 1979;63:163-5.
15. Eggers TR, Doyle LW, Pepperell RJ. Premature rupture of the membranes. Med J Aust 1979;1:209-13.
16. Garite TJ, Freeman RK, Linzey EM, Braly PS, Dorchester WL. Prospective randomized study of corticosteroids in the management of premature rupture of the membranes and the premature gestation. Am J Obstet Gynecol 1981;141:508-15.
17. Ballard PL, Ballard RA, Granberg JP, et al. Fetal sex and prenatal betamethasone therapy. J Pediatr 1980;97:451-4.
18. Papageorgiou AN, Desgranges MF, Masson M, Colle E, Shatz R, Gelfand MM. The antenatal use of betamethasone in the prevention of respiratory distress syndrome: a controlled double-blind study. Pediatrics 1979;63:73-9.
19. Bielawski D, Hiatt IM, Hegyi T. Betamethasone-induced leukaemoid reaction in pre-term infant. Lancet 1978;1:218-9.
20. Taeusch HW Jr. Glucocorticoid prophylaxis for respiratory distress syndrome: a review of potential toxicity. J Pediatr 1975;87:617-23.
21. Johnson JWC, Mitzner W, London WT, Palmer AE, Scott R. Betamethasone and the rhesus fetus: multisystemic effects. Am J Obstet Gynecol 1979;133:677-84.
22. MacArthur BA, Howie RN, Dezoete JA, Elkins J. Cognitive and psychosocial development of 4-year-old children whose mothers were treated antenatally with betamethasone. Pediatrics 1981;68:638-43.

Name: **BETHANECHOL**

Class: **Parasympathomimetic (Cholinergic)** Risk Factor: **C**

Fetal Risk Summary

The use of bethanechol in pregnancy has been reported, but too little data is available to analyze (1).

Breast Feeding Summary

Although specific data on the excretion of bethanechol into breast milk is lacking, one author cautioned that mothers receiving regular therapy with this drug should not breast feed (2).

References

1. Heinonen OP, Slone D, Shapiro S. *Birth Defects and Drugs in Pregnancy*. Littleton: Publishing Sciences Group, 1977:345–56.
2. Platzker ACD, Lew CD, Stewart D. Drug "administration" via breast milk. Hosp Pract 1980;15:111–122.

Name: **BIPERIDEN**

Class: **Parasympatholytic** Risk Factor: **C$_M$**

Fetal Risk Summary

Biperiden is an anticholinergic agent used in the treatment of parkinsonism. No reports of its use in pregnancy have been located (see also Atropine).

Breast Feeding Summary

No data available (see also Atropine).

Name: **BLEOMYCIN**

Class: **Antineoplastic** Risk Factor: **D**

Fetal Risk Summary

No reports linking the use of bleomycin with congenital defects have been located. Chromosomal aberrations in human marrow cells have been reported but the significance to the fetus is not known (1).

Breast Feeding Summary

No data available.

References

1. Bornstein RS, Hungerford DA, Haller G, Engstrom PF, Yarbro JW. Cytogenic effects of bleomycin therapy in man. Cancer Res 1971;31:2004–7.

Name: **BRETYLIUM**

Class: **Antiarrhythmic**   Risk Factor: **C**

Fetal Risk Summary

Bretylium, a quaternary ammonium compound, is an adrenergic blocker used as an antiarrhythmic agent. No information on its use in pregnancy has been located. Hypotension has been observed in 50% of patients after bretylium (1). Although reports are lacking, reduced uterine blood flow with fetal hypoxia (bradycardia) is a potential risk. The manufacturer states that bretylium may be used in life-threatening situations if the expected benefits outweigh the unknown potential risks to the fetus (1).

Breast Feeding Summary

No data available.

References

1. Product information. Bretylol. American Critical Care, 1981.

Name: **BROMIDES**

Class: **Anticonvulsant/Sedative**   Risk Factor: **D**

Fetal Risk Summary

The Collaborative Perinatal Project monitored 50,282 mother-child pairs, 986 of which had 1st trimester exposure to bromides (1). For use anytime during pregnancy, 2,610 exposures were recorded (2). In neither case was evidence found to suggest a relationship to large categories of major or minor malformations. Four possible associations with individual malformations were found but the statistical significance of these are unknown and independent confirmation is required:

Polydactyly (14 cases)
Gastrointestinal (10 cases)
Clubfoot (7 cases)
Congenital dislocation of hip (anytime use) (92 cases)

There have been two case reports of intrauterine growth retardation and subsequent failure to thrive (3, 4). One of these affected infants also had congenital heart disease. More study is needed to establish a relationship between the use of bromides and congenital defects. Neonatal bromide intoxication from transplacental accumulation has been described (5, 6). Symptoms of neonatal bromism are generally nonspecific, and include poor suck response, diminished Moro reflex, and hypotonia. Monitoring of serum bromide concentrations is recommended in neonates with *in utero* exposure.

Breast Feeding Summary

Bromide appears in breast milk. Kwit reported breast milk concentrations of 16–66 μg/ml in 2 patients given 5 g daily for one month (7). A single case of drowsiness and rash in a breast-fed infant appeared in 1921 (8). However, nothing since these original reports has been located. Breast feeding is not recommended in patients receiving bromide-containing medications.

References

1. Heinonen OP, Slone D, Shapiro S. *Birth Defects and Drugs in Pregnancy.* Littleton: Publishing Sciences Group, 1977;;402–6.
2. *Ibid*, 444.
3. Rossiter EJR, Rendel-Short TJ. Congenital effects of bromism? Lancet 1972;2:705.
4. Opitz JM, Grosse RF, Haneberg B. Congenital effects of bromism? Lancet 1972;1:91.
5. Pleasure JR, Blackburn MG. Neonatal bromide intoxication: prenatal ingestion of a large quantity of bromides with transplacental accumulation in the fetus. Pediatrics 1975;55:503–6.
6. Mangurten HH, Ban R. Neonatal hypotonia secondary to transplacental bromism. J Pediatr 1974;85:426–8.
7. Kwit NT, Hatcher RA. Excretion of drugs in milk. Am J Dis Child 1935;49:900–4.
8. Van der Bogert F. Bromin poisoning through mother's milk. Am J Dis Child 1921;21:167.

Name: # BROMPHENIRAMINE

Class: **Antihistamine** Risk Factor: **C**

Fetal Risk Summary

The Collaborative Perinatal Project monitored 50,282 mother-child pairs, 65 of which had 1st trimester exposure to brompheniramine (1). Based on 10 malformed infants, a statistically significant association ($p < 0.01$) was found between this drug and congenital defects. This relationship was not found with other antihistamines. For use anytime during pregnancy, 412 exposures were recorded (2). In this case, no evidence was found for an association with malformations.

Breast Feeding Summary

Data on the excretion of brompheniramine into breast milk has not been located. One manufacturer considers the drug contraindicated for nursing mothers (3).

References

1. Heinonen OP, Slone D, Shapiro S. *Birth Defects and Drugs in Pregnancy.* Littleton: Publishing Sciences Group, 1977:322–5.
2. *Ibid*, 437.
3. Product information. Dimetane. AH Robins Company, 1982.

Name: **BUCLIZINE**

Class: **Antihistamine/Antiemetic**   Risk Factor: **C**

Fetal Risk Summary

Buclizine is a piperazine antihistamine which is used as an antiemetic (see also Cyclizine and Meclizine for closely related drugs). The drug is teratogenic in animals but its effects on the human fetus has not been thoroughly studied.

The Collaborative Perinatal Project monitored 50,282 mother-child pairs, 44 of which had 1st trimester exposure to buclizine (1). No evidence was found to suggest a relationship to large categories of major or minor malformations. For use anytime during pregnancy, 62 exposures were recorded (2). A possible association with congenital defects was found from this exposure based on 3 malformed children.

The manufacturer considers the drug to be contraindicated in early pregnancy (3).

Breast Feeding Summary

No data available.

References

1. Heinonen OP, Slone D, Shapiro S. *Birth Defects and Drugs in Pregnancy*. Littleton: Publishing Sciences Group, 1977:323–4.
2. *Ibid*, 437.
3. Product information. In *Physicians' Desk Reference*, ed. 35. Oradell, N.J.: Medical Economics Company, 1981.

Name: **BUSULFAN**

Class: **Antineoplastic**   Risk Factor: **D**

Fetal Risk Summary

Busulfan is an alkylating antineoplalstic agent. The use of this drug has been reported in 32 pregnancies, 22 in the 1st trimester (1). Four malformed infants have been observed (see table below) (1, 2). Data from one review indicated that 40% of the infants exposed to anticancer drugs were of low birth weight (1). This finding was not related to the timing of the exposure. Long term studies of growth and mental development in offspring exposed to busulfan during the 2nd trimester, the period of neuroblast multiplication, have not been conducted (3). Chromosomal damage has been associated with busulfan therapy but the potential for future teratogenicity is unknown (4). Irregular menses and amenorrhea, the latter at times permanent, have been reported in women receiving busulfan (5, 6).

Author (ref)	No. Pts.	Indica- tion	Gestational Age	Dose	Other Drugs	Fetal Effects	Comments
Nicholson (1)	3	Various	1st trimes- ter (2) 2nd trimes- ter (1)	Not stated	Not stated	1 Unspecified malformations; aborted at 20 weeks 1 Anomalous deviation, left lobe liver 1 Pyloric stenosis	
Diamond (2)	1	Granu- locytic leukemia	Throughout	4–6 mg/ day	Mercapto- purine Radiation	Cleft palate Microphthalmia Cytomegaly Hypoplasia of ovaries and thy- roid gland Corneal opacity Intrauterine growth retardation	

Breast Feeding Summary

No data available.

References

1. Nicholson HO. Cytotoxic drugs in pregnancy: review of reported cases. J Obstet Gynaecol Br Commonw 1968;75:307–12.
2. Diamond I, Anderson MM, McCreadie SR. Transplacental transmission of busulfan (Myleran) in a mother with leukemia: production of fetal malformation and cytomegaly. Pediatrics 1960;25:85–90.
3. Dobbing J. Pregnancy and leukaemia. Lancet 1977;1:1155.
4. Gebhart E, Schwanitz G, Hartwich G. Chromosomal aberrations during busulphan therapy. Dtsch Med Wochenschr 1974;99:52–6.
5. Galton DAG, Till M, Wiltshaw E. Busulfan: summary of clinical results. Ann NY Acad Sci 1958;68:967–73.
6. Schilsky RL, Lewis BJ, Sherins RJ, Young RC. Gonadal dysfunction in patients receiving chemotherapy for cancer. Ann Intern Med 1980;93:109–14.

Name: **BUTALBITAL**

Class: **Sedative**   Risk Factor: **C***

Fetal Risk Summary

Butalbital is a short-acting barbiturate that is contained in a number of analgesic mixtures. In a large prospective study, 112 patients were exposed to this drug during the 1st trimester (1). No association with malformations was found. Severe neonatal withdrawal was described in a male infant whose mother took 150 mg of butalbital daily during the last 2 months of pregnancy in the form of a proprietary headache mixture (Esgic—butalbital 50 mg, caffeine 40 mg and acetaminophen 325 mg per dose) (2). The infant was also exposed to oxycodone, pentazocine and acetaminophen during the 1st trimes- ter but apparently these had been discontinued prior to the start of the butalbital product. Onset of withdrawal occurred within 2 days of birth.

[*Risk Factor D if used for prolonged periods or in high doses near term.]

Breast Feeding Summary

No data available (see also Pentobarbital).

References

1. Heinonen OP, Slone D, Shapiro S. *Birth Defects and Drugs in Pregnancy.* Littleton: Publishing Sciences Group, 1977:336–7.
2. Ostrea EM. Neonatal withdrawal from intrauterine exposure to butalbital. Am J Obstet Gynecol 1982;143:597–9.

Name: **BUTAPERAZINE**

Class: **Tranquilizer**   Risk Factor: **C**

Fetal Risk Summary

Butaperazine is a piperazine phenothiazine in the same group as prochlorperazine (see Prochlorperazine). The phenothiazines readily cross the placenta (1). No specific information on the use of butaperazine in pregnancy has been located. Although occasional reports have attempted to link various phenothiazine compounds with congenital malformations, the bulk of the evidence indicates these drugs are safe for the mother and fetus (see also Chlorpromazine).

Breast Feeding Summary

No data available.

References

1. Moya F, Thorndike V. Passage of drugs across the placenta. Am J Obstet Gynecol 1962;84:1778–98.

Name: **BUTORPHANOL**

Class: **Analgesic**   Risk Factor: **B***

Fetal Risk Summary

No reports linking the use of butorphanol with congenital defects have been located. Since it has both narcotic agonist and antagonist properties, prolonged use during gestation may result in fetal addiction with subsequent withdrawal in the newborn (see also Pentazocine).

At term, butophanol rapidly crosses the placenta producing cord serum levels averaging 84% of maternal concentrations (1, 2). Depressant effects on the newborn from *in utero* exposure during labor are similar to those seen with meperidine (1–3).

A study comparing neonatal neurobehavior was conducted in 135 patients during their first day of life (4). Maternal analgesia consisted of 1 mg of butorphanol (68 patients) or 40 mg of meperidine (67 patients). No difference between the drugs was observed.

[*Risk Factor D if used for prolonged periods or in high doses at term.]

Breast Feeding Summary

Butorphanol passes into breast milk in concentrations paralleling levels in maternal serum (2). Milk:plasma ratios after intramuscular (IM) (1–2 mg) or oral (8 mg) doses were 0.7 and 1.9, respectively. Using 2 mg IM or 8 mg orally four times a day would result in 4 μg excreted in the full daily milk output (1000 ml). Although it has not been studied, this amount is probably insignificant.

References

1. Maduska AL, Hajghassemali M. A double-blind comparison of butorphanol and merperidine in labour: maternal pain relief and effect on the newborn. Can Anaesth Soc J 1978;25:398–404.
2. Pittman KA, Smyth RD, Losada M, Zighelboim I, Maduska AL, Sunshine A. Human perinatal distribution of butorphanol. Am J Obstet Gynecol 1980;138:797–800.
3. Quilligan EJ, Keegan KA, Donahue JM. Double-blind analgesic comparison of intravenous butorphanol and meperidine in obstetrical patients. Int J Gynaecol Obstet (accepted for publication).
4. Hodgkinson R, Huff RW, Hayashi RH, Husain FJ. Double-blind comparison of maternal analgesia and neonatal neurobehaviour following intravenous butorphanol and meperidine. J Int Med Res 1979;7:224–30.

Name: **BUTRIPTYLINE**

Class: **Antidepressant**   Risk Factor: **D**

Fetal Risk Summary

No data available (see Imipramine).

Breast Feeding Summary

No data available (see Imipramine).

Name: **CAFFEINE**

Class: **Central Stimulant**   Risk Factor: **B**

Fetal Risk Summary

Caffeine is one of the most popular drugs in North America and many other parts of the world. It is frequently used in combination products containing aspirin, phenacetin and codeine. Caffeine is present in a number of commonly consumed beverages, such as coffee, teas and colas. The Food and Drug Administration has removed caffeine from the list of drugs "generally regarded as safe" and has issued a warning regarding the consumption of caffeine during pregnancy (1, 2). Caffeine crosses the placenta and achieves fetal blood and tissue levels similar to maternal concentrations (3–5). Cord blood levels of 1 to 1.6 μg/ml have been measured (3). Caffeine has also been found in newborns exposed to theophylline *in utero* (6). The mutagenicity and carcinogenicity of caffeine has been evaluated in over 50 studies involving laboratory animals, human and animal cell tissue cultures, and human lympho- cytes *in vivo* (3). The significance of mutagenic and carcinogenic effects found in non-mammalian systems has not been established in man. The Collaborative Perinatal Project (CPP) monitored 50,282 mother-child pairs, 5,378 of which had 1st trimester exposure to caffeine (7). No evidence of a relationship to congenital defects was found. For use anytime during pregnancy, 12,696 exposures were recorded (8). In this case, a statistically significant association was found between caffeine and specific malformations:

Musculoskeletal defects (10 cases)

Hydronephrosis (23 cases)

Hemangiomas/granulomas (19 cases)

A follow-up analysis by the CPP on 2,030 malformed infants and maternal use of caffeine-containing beverages has recently been reported (9). The results do not support caffeine as a major teratogen. Several authors have associated high caffeine consumption (6 to 8 cups coffee per day) with decreased fertility, increased incidence of spontaneous abortion, and low birth weights (3, 10–14). Unfortunately, few of these studies have isolated the effects of caffeine from cigarette or alcohol use, both of which are positively associated with caffeine consumption (3). One German study has observed that high coffee use alone is associated with low birth weights (15). The Delivery Interview Program at the Boston Hospital for Women assessed the effects of coffee consumption in more than 12,400 women. Low birth weights and short gestation occurred more often among offspring of women who drank 4 or more cups of coffee per day and who were also smokers (16). No relationship between low birth weights/short gestation and caffeine was found after controlling for smoking, alcohol intake, and demographic characteristics. The altering of catecholamine levels by the presence of caffeine is of concern (17). However, the significance of this pharmacological effect in normal human development is not understood. Based on the available evidence, indiscriminate use of caffeine during pregnancy is not recommended, especially in the management of the infertile couple.

Breast Feeding Summary

Caffeine is excreted into breast milk (18, 19). A milk:plasma ratio of 0.5 has been measured. An estimated 170 μg of caffeine could be ingested by a nursing infant whose mother had consumed one cup of coffee (about 150 mg of caffeine per cup) (18). While this amount may be low, accumulation can occur in mothers with moderate to heavy use of caffeine. No reports of adverse effects in the nursing infant have been located.

References

1. Morris MB, Weinstein L. Caffeine and the fetus: is trouble brewing? Am J Obstet Gynecol 1981;140:607–10.
2. Goyan JE. Statement by the commissioner of Food and Drugs, FDA press release. Washington, DC. September 4,1980(P80-36):3.
3. Soyka LF. Caffeine ingestion during pregnancy: in utero exposure and possible effects. Semin Perinatol 1981;5:305–9.
4. Goldstein A, Warren R. Passage of caffeine into human gonadal and fetal tissue. Biochem Pharmacol 1962;17:166–8.
5. Parsons WD, Aranda JV, Neims AH. Elimination of transplacentally acquired caffeine in fullterm neonates. Pediatr Res 1976;10:333.
6. Brazier JL, Salle B. Conversion of theophylline to caffeine by the human fetus. Semin Perinatol 1981;5:315–20.
7. Heinonen OP, Slone D, Shapiro S. Birth Defects and Drugs in Pregnancy. Littleton: Publishing Sciences Group, 1977:366–70.
8. Ibid, 493–4.
9. Rosenberg L, Mitchell AA, Shapiro S, Slone D. Selected birth defects in relation to caffeine-containing beverages. JAMA 1982;247:1429–32.
10. Weathersbee PS, Olsen LK, Lodge JR. Caffeine and pregnancy. Postgrad Med 1977;62:64–9.
11. Anonymous. Caffeine and birth defects—another negative study. Pediatr Alert 1982;7:23–4.
12. Hogue CJ. Coffee in pregnancy. Lancet 1981;2:554.
13. Weathersbee PS, Lodge JR, Caffeine: its direct and indirect influence on reproduction. J Reprod Med 1977;19:55–63.
14. Lechat MF, Borlee I, Bouckaert A, Misson C. Caffeine study. Science 1980;207:1296–7.
15. Mau G, Netter P. Kaffee- und alkoholkonsum-riskofaktoren in der schwangerschaft? Geburtshilfe Frauenheilkd 1974;34:1018–22.
16. Linn S, Schoenbaum SC, Monson RR, Rosner B, Stubblefield PG, Ryan KJ. No association between coffee consumption and adverse outcomes of pregnancy. N Engl J Med 1982;306:141–5.
17. Bellet S, Roman L, DeCastro O, et al. Effect of coffee ingestion on catecholamine release. Metabolism 1969;18:288–91.
18. Berlin CM. Excretion of the methylxanthines in human milk. Semin Perinatol 1981;5:389–94.
19. Jobe PC. Psychoactive substances and antiepileptic drugs. In Wilson JT, ed. Drugs in Breast Milk. Australia: ADIS Press, 1981:40.

Name: **CALCITONIN**

Class: **Calcium Regulation Hormone**   Risk Factor: **B**

Fetal Risk Summary

No reports linking the use of calcitonin with congenital defects have been located. Marked increases of calcitonin concentrations in fetal serum over maternal levels has been demonstrated at term (1). The significance of this finding is unknown.

Breast Feeding Summary

No data available. Calcitonin has been shown to inhibit lactation in animals. Mothers wishing to breast feed should be informed of this potential complication (2).

References

1. Kovarik J, Woloszczuk W, Linkesch W, Pavelka R. Calcitonin in pregnancy. Lancet 1980;1:199–200.
2. Product information. Calcimar. Armour Laboratories. 1979.

Name: **CAMPHOR**

Class: **Antipruritic/Local Anesthetic**   Risk Factor: **C**

Fetal Risk Summary

No reports linking the use of topically applied camphor with congenital defects have been located. Camphor is toxic and potentially a fatal poison if taken orally in sufficient quantities. Four cases of fetal exposure after accidental ingestion, including a case of fetal death and neonatal respiratory failure, have been reported (1–4). The drug crosses the placenta (2).

Breast Feeding Summary

No data available.

References

1. Figgs J, Hamilton R, Homel S, McCabe J. Camphorated oil intoxication in pregnancy. Report of a case. Obstet Gynecol 1965;25:255–8.
2. Weiss J, Catalano P. Camphorated oil intoxication during pregnancy. Pediatrics 1973;52:713–4.
3. Blackman WB, Curry HB. Camphor poisoning: report of case occurring during pregnancy. J Fla Med Assoc 1957;43:99.
4. Jacobziner H, Raybin HW. Camphor poisoning. Arch Pediatr 1962;79:28.

Name: **CAPTOPRIL**

Class: **Antihypertensive** Risk Factor: **C**

Fetal Risk Summary

A malformed fetus was discovered following voluntary abortion in a patient with renovascular hypertension (1). The patient had been treated during the 1st trimester with captopril, propranolol and amiloride. The left leg ended at mid-thigh without distal development and no obvious skull formation was noted above the brain tissue. Captopril is embryocidal in animals and has been shown to cause an increase in stillbirths in some species (2).

Breast Feeding Summary

Captopril is excreted into breast milk in low concentrations. Twelve mothers given 100 mg three times a day produced average peak milk levels of 4.7 ng/ml 3.8 hours after their last dose (3). This represented an average milk:plasma ratio of 0.012. No differences were found in captopril levels in pre- and post-drug milk. No effects on the nursing infants were observed.

References
1. Duminy PC, Burger PT. Fetal abnormality associated with the use of captopril during pregnancy. S Afr Med J 1981;60:805.
2. Pipkin FB, Turner SR, Symonds EM. Possible risk with captopril in pregnancy: some animal data. Lancet 1980;1:1256.
3. Devlin RG, Fleiss PM. Selective resistance to the passage of captopril into human milk. Clin Pharmacol Ther 1980;27:250.

Name: **CARBACHOL**

Class: **Parasympathomimetic (Cholinergic)** Risk Factor: **C**

Fetal Risk Summary

Carbachol is used in the eye. No reports of its use in pregnancy have been located. As a quaternary ammonium compound, it is ionized at physiologic pH and transplacental passage in significant amounts would not be expected.

Breast Feeding Summary

No data available.

Name: CARBAMAZEPINE

Class: **Anticonvulsant**   Risk Factor: **D**

Fetal Risk Summary

Carbamazepine, a tricyclic anticonvulsant, has been in clinical use since 1962. The drug crosses the placenta and concentrates in fetal tissues (1, 2). Use of carbamazepine during the 1st trimester has been reported in 531 pregnancies (3–12). Multiple anomalies were found in one stillborn infant where carbamazepine was the only anticonvulsant used by the mother (see below) (11). Individual defects observed in this and other cases include talipes, meningomyelocele, anal atresia, ambiguous genitalia, congenital heart disease, hyperterolism, hypoplasia of the nose, cleft lip, congenital hip dislocation, inguinal hernia, hypoplasia of the nails, and torticollis (3–12). Nakane found no statistical relationship between carbamazepine in 129 patients and 11 malformed children (7). Carbamazepine has been recommended as the drug of choice in women at risk of pregnancy who require anticonvulsant therapy for the first time (13). However, since multiple anticonvulsant therapy is typical and consistent information on the defects observed is not always available, any conclusion regarding the safety or teratogenicity of carbamazepine is not possible.

Author (ref)	No. Pts.	Indication	Gestational Age	Dose	Other Drugs	Fetal Effects	Comment
Hicks (11)	1	Temporal lobe epilepsy	1st trimester	400 mg day	Not stated	Fetal death at 25 weeks Closely set eyes Flat nose with single nasopharynx Polydactylia Atrial septal defect Patent ductus arteriosus Absent gallbladder Absent thyroid Collapsed fontanel	

Breast Feeding Summary

Carbamazepine is excreted into breast milk producing milk:plasma ratios of 0.24 to 0.69 (1, 5, 10). The amount of carbamazepine available to an infant via the breast milk is low, but infant serum levels have been measured as high as 0.5 to 1.8 μg/ml (1). Accumulation of the drug in the infant is suggested by these values. Although reports of adverse effects from carbamazepine in the nursing infant have not been found, breast feeding is not recommended.

Author (ref.)	No. Pts.	Dose	Concentration (μg/ml) Serum	Milk	M:P Ratio	Effect on Infant
Pynnonen (1)	1	6 mg/kg/day	3.2	1.8	0.56	Infant serum = 1.8 μg/ml
	1	5.8 mg/kg/day	2.6	1.8	0.69	Infant serum = 0.5 μg/ml
	1	7.3 mg/kg/day	2.4	1.5	0.62	—
Niebyl (10)	1	1 g/day	5.8	2.3 (skim fraction)	0.4	—
				1.4 (lipid fraction)	0.24	—

References

1. Pynnonen S, Knato J, Stilanpaa M, Erkkola R. Carbamazepine: Placental transport, tissue concentrations in the foetus and newborns, and level milk. Acta Pharmacol Toxicol 1977;41:244–53.
2. Rane A, Bertilsson L, Palmer L. Disposition of placentally transferred carbamazepine (Tegretol) in the newborn. Eur J Clin Pharmacol 1975;8:283–4.
3. Geigy Pharmaceuticals. Tegretol in epilepsy. In Monograph 319-80950, Ciba-Geigy, Ardsley, 1978:18–19.
4. McMullin GP. Teratogenic effects of anticonvulsants. Br Med J 1971;4:430.
5. Pynnonen S, Sillanpaa M. Carbamazepine and mothers milk. Lancet 1975;2:563.
6. Lander CM, Edwards VE, Endie MJ, Tyrer JH. Plasma anticonvulsant concentrations during pregnancy. Neurology 1977;27:128–31.
7. Nakane Y, Okuma T, Takahashi R, et al. Multi-institutional study on the teratogenicity and fetal toxicity to antiepileptic drugs: A report of a collaborative study group in Japan. Epilepsia 1980;21:633–80.
8. Janz D. The teratogenic risk of antiepileptic drugs. Epilepsia 1975;16:159–69.
9. Meyer JG. Teratogenic risk of anticonvulsants and the effects on pregnancy and birth. Eur Neurol 1979;10:179–90.
10. Niebly JR, Blake DA, Freeman JM, Luff RD. Carbamazepine levels in pregnancy and lactation. Obstet Gynecol 1979;53:130–40.
11. Hicks EP. Carbamazepine in two pregnancies. Clin Exp Neurol 1979;16:269–75.
12. Thomas D, Buchanan N. Teratogenic effects of anticonvulsants. J Pediatr 1981;99:163.
13. Paulson GW, Paulson RB. Teratogenic effects of anticonvulsants. Arch Neurol 1981;38:140–3.

Name: **CARBARSONE**

Class: **Amebicide**   Risk Factor: **D**

Fetal Risk Summary

No reports linking the use of carbarsone with congenital defects have been located. However, carbarsone contains approximately 29% arsenic, which has been associated with lesions of the central nervous system (1). In view of potential tissue accumulation and reported fetal fatalities secondary to arsenic poisonings, carbarsone is not recommended during pregnancy (1, 2).

Breast Feeding Summary

No data available.

References

1. Arnold W. Morphologic und pathogenese der Salvarsan-schadigungen des zentralnervensystems. Virchows Arch (Pathol Anat) 1944;311:1.
2. Lugo G, Cassady G, Palmisano P. Acute maternal arsenic intoxication with neonatal death. Am J Dis Child 1969;117:328.

Name: **CARBENICILLIN**

Class: **Antibiotic**   Risk Factor: **B**

Fetal Risk Summary

Carbenicillin is a penicillin antibiotic (see also Penicillin G). The drug crosses the placenta and distributes to most fetal tissues (1, 2). Following a 4-g intramuscular dose, mean peak concentrations in cord and maternal serums at 2 hours were similar. Amniotic fluid levels averaged 7 to 11% of maternal peak concentrations.

No reports linking the use of carbenicillin with congenital defects have been located. The Collaborative Perinatal Project monitored 50,282 mother-child pairs, 3,546 of which had documented 1st trimester exposure to penicillin derivatives (3). For use anytime during pregnancy, 7,171 exposures were recorded (4). In neither case was evidence found to suggest a relationship to large categories of major or minor malformations or to individual defects.

Breast Feeding Summary

No data available (see Penicillin G).

References

1. Biro L, Ivan E, Elek E, Arr M. Data on the tissue concentration of antibiotics in man. Tissue concentrations of semi-synthetic penicillins in the fetus. Int Z Pharmakol Ther Toxikol 1970;4:321–4.
2. Elek E, Ivan E, Arr M. Passage of penicillins from mother to foetus in humans. Int J Clin Pharmacol Ther Toxicol 1972;6:223–8.
3. Heinonen OP, Slone D, Shapiro S. *Birth Defects and Drugs in Pregnancy*. Littleton: Publishing Sciences Group, 1977:297–313.
4. *Ibid*, 435.

Name: **CARPHENAZINE**

Class: **Tranquilizer**   Risk Factor: **C**

Fetal Risk Summary

Carphenazine is a piperazine phenothiazine in the same group as prochlorperazine (see Prochlorperazine). Phenothiazines readily cross the placenta (1). No specific information on the use of carphenazine in pregnancy has been located. Although occasional reports have attempted to link various phenothiazine compounds with congenital malformations, the bulk of the evidence indicates these drugs are safe for the mother and fetus (see also Chlorpromazine).

Breast Feeding Summary

No data available.

Reference

1. Moya F, Thorndike V. Passage of drugs across the placenta. Am J Obstet Gynecol 1962;84:1778–98.

Name: **CASANTHRANOL**

Class: **Purgative**   Risk Factor: **C**

Fetal Risk Summary

Casanthranol is an anthraquinone purgative. In a large prospective study, 109 patients were exposed to this agent during pregnancy (1). No evidence of an increased risk for malformations was found (see also Cascara Sagrada).

Breast Feeding Summary

See Cascara Sagrada.

Reference

1. Heinonen OP, Slone D, Shapiro S. *Birth Defects and Drugs in Pregnancy.* Littleton: Publishing Sciences Group, 1977:442.

Name: **CASCARA SAGRADA**

Class: **Purgative**   Risk Factor **C**

Fetal Risk Summary

Cascara sagrada is an anthraquinone purgative. In a large prospective study, 188 patients were exposed to this agent during pregnancy (1). An increase in the expected frequency of malformations was found; however, specific data was not given. No other reports linking 1st trimester use of cascara sagrada with congenital defects have been located (see also Casanthranol).

Breast Feeding Summary

Most reviewers acknowledge the presence of anthraquinones in breast milk and warn of the consequences for the nursing infant (2–4). A comprehensive review that describes the excretion of laxatives into human milk has been published (5). The authors state that little is actually known about the presence of these agents in breast milk. Two reports suggest an increased incidence of diarrhea in infants when nursing mothers are given cascara sagrada or senna for postpartum constipation (6, 7).

References

1. Heinonen OP, Slone D, Shapiro S. *Birth Defects and Drugs in Pregnancy.* Littleton: Publishing Sciences Group, 1977:442.

2. Knowles JA. Breast milk: a source of more than nutrition for the neonate. Clin Toxicol 1974;7:69–82.
3. O'Brien TE. Excretion of drugs in human milk. Am J Hosp Pharm 1974;31:844–54.
4. Edwards A. Drugs in breast milk—a review of the recent literature. Aust J Hosp Pharm 1981;11:27–39.
5. Stewart JJ. Gastrointestinal drugs. In Wilson JT, ed. *Drugs in Breast Milk*. Australia: ADIS Press, 1981:65–71.
6. Tyson RM, Shrader EA, Perlman HH. Drugs transmitted through breast milk. Part I. Laxatives. J Pediatr 1937;11:824–32.
7. Greenleaf JO, Leonard HSD. Laxatives in the treatment of constipation in pregnant and breast-feeding mothers. Practitioner 1973;210:259–63.

Name: **CEFACLOR**

Class: **Antibiotic**   Risk Factor: **B**

Fetal Risk Summary

Cefaclor is a cephalosporin antibiotic (see also Cephalothin). No reports on its use in pregnancy have been located.

Breast Feeding Summary

Cefaclor is excreted into breast milk in low concentrations. Following a single 500-mg oral dose, average milk levels ranged from 0.16 to 0.21 μg/ml over a 5-hour period (1). Only trace amounts of the antibiotic could be measured at 1 and 6 hours. Although these levels are low, three potential problems exist for the nursing infant: modification of bowel flora, direct effects on the infant and interference with the interpretation of culture results if a fever work-up is required.

Reference

1. Takase Z. Clinical and laboratory studies of cefaclor in the field of obstetrics and gynecology. Chemotherapy (Tokyo) 1979;27(Suppl):668.

Name: **CEFADROXIL**

Class: **Antibiotic**   Risk Factor: **B**

Fetal Risk Summary

Cefadroxil is a cephalosporin antibiotic (see also Cephalothin). No controlled studies on its use in pregnancy have been located. At term, a 500-mg oral dose produced an average peak cord serum level of 4.6 μg/ml at 2.5 hours (about 40% of maternal serum) (1). Amniotic fluid levels achieved a peak of 4.4 μg/ml at 10 hours. No infant data was given.

Breast Feeding Summary

Cefadroxil is excreted into breast milk in low concentrations. Following a single 500-mg oral dose, peak milk levels of about 0.6 to 0.7 μg/ml occurred at 5 to 6 hours (1). A 1-g oral dose given to 6 mothers produced peak milk levels averaging 1.83 μg/ml (range 1.2 to 2.4 μg/ml) at 6 to 7 hours (2). In this latter group, milk:plasma ratios at 1, 2 and 3 hours were 0.009, 0.011 and 0.019, respectively. Although these levels are low, three potential problems exist for the nursing infant: modification of bowel flora, direct effects on the infant and interference with the interpretation of culture results if a fever work-up is required.

References

1. Takase Z, Shirafuji H, Uchida M. Experimental and clinical studies of cefadroxil in the treatment of infections in the field of obstetrics and gynecology. Chemotherapy (Tokyo) 1980;28(Suppl 2):424–31.
2. Kafetzi D, Siafas C, Georgakopoulos P, Papdatos C. Passage of cephalosporins and amoxicillin into the breast milk. Acta Paediatr Scand 1981;70:285–8.

Name: **CEFAMANDOLE**

Class: **Antibiotic**   Risk Factor: **B**

Fetal Risk Summary

Cefamandole is a cephalosporin antibiotic (see also Cephalothin). No controlled studies on its use in pregnancy have been located. Although pregnant patients were excluded from clinical trials of cefamandole, one patient did receive the drug in the 1st trimester (1). No apparent adverse effects were noted in the newborn.

Breast Feeding Summary

Cefamandole is excreted into breast milk in low concentrations. Following a 1-g intravenous dose, average milk levels in 4 patients ranged from 0.46 (1 hour) to 0.19 μg/ml (6 hours) (1). The milk:plasma ratio at 1 hour was 0.02. No neonate information was given. Although these levels are low, three potential problems exist for the nursing infant: modification of bowel flora, direct effects on the infant and interference with the interpretation of culture results if a fever work-up is required.

Reference

1. Personal communication. JT Anderson, Medical Research-Marketed Products, Clinical Investigation Division, Lilly Research Laboratories, May 12, 1981.

Name: CEFATRIZINE

Class: **Antibiotic**   Risk Factor: **B**

Fetal Risk Summary

Cefatrizine is a cephalosporin antibiotic (see also Cephalothin). No controlled studies on its use in pregnancy have been located. Transplacental passage of cefatrizine has been demonstrated in women undergoing elective therapeutic surgical abortion in the 1st and 2nd trimesters (1). None of the fetuses from prostaglandin F_{2a} abortions revealed evidence of cefatrizine.

Breast Feeding Summary

Most cephalosporins are excreted into breast milk in low concentrations but data for cefatrizine is lacking. For potential problems during breast feeding, see Cephalothin.

Reference

1. Bernard B, Thielen P, Garcia-Cazares SJ, Ballard CA. Maternal-fetal pharmacology of cefatrizine in the first 20 weeks of pregnancy. Antimicrob Agents Chemother 1977;12:231–6.

Name: CEFAZOLIN

Class: **Antibiotic**   Risk Factor: **B**

Fetal Risk Summary

Cefazolin is a cephalosporin antibiotic (see also Cephalothin). No controlled studies on its use in pregnancy have been located. Cefazolin crosses the placenta into the cord serum and amniotic fluid (1–4). In early pregnancy, distribution is limited to the body fluids and these concentrations are considerably lower than those found in the 2nd and 3rd trimesters (2). At term, 15 to 70 minutes after a 500-mg dose, cord serum levels range from 35 to 69% of maternal serum (3). The maximum concentration in amniotic fluid after 500 mg was 8 μg/ml at 2.5 hours (4). No data on the newborns was given.

Breast Feeding Summary

Cefazolin is excreted into breast milk in low concentrations. Following a 2-g intravenous dose, average milk levels ranged from 1.2 to 1.5 μg/ml over 4 hours (milk:plasma ratio 0.02) (5). When cefazolin is given as a 500-mg intramuscular dose, one to three times daily, the drug was not detectable (4). Although these levels are low, three potential problems exist for the nursing infant: modification of bowel flora, direct effects on the infant and interference with the interpretation of culture results if a fever work-up is required.

References

1. Dekel A, Elian I, Gibor Y, Goldman JA. Transplacental passage of cefazolin in the first trimester of pregnancy. Eur J Obstet Gynecol Reprod Biol 1980;10:303–7.
2. Bernard B, Barton L, Abate M, Ballard CA. Maternal-fetal transfer of cefazolin in the first twenty weeks of pregnancy. J Infect Dis 1977;136:377–82.
3. Cho N, Ito T, Saito T, et al. Clinical studies on cefazolin in the field of obstetrics and gynecology. Chemotherapy, (Tokyo) 1970;18:770–7.
4. von Kobyletzki D, Reither K, Gellen J, Kanyo A, Glocke M. Pharmacokinetic studies with cefazolin in obstetrics and gynecology. Infection 1974;2(Suppl):60–7.
5. Yoshioka H, Cho K, Takimato M, Maruyama S, Shimizu T. Transfer of cefazolin into human milk. J Pediatr 1979;94:151–2.

Name: **CEFOTAXIME**

Class: **Antibiotic** Risk Factor: **B**

Fetal Risk Summary

Cefotaxime is a cephalosporin antibiotic (see also Cephalothin). No controlled studies on its use in pregnancy have been located. During the 2nd trimester, the drug readily crosses the placenta (1). The half life of cefotaxime in fetal serum and in amniotic fluid was 2.3 and 2.8 hours, respectively.

Breast Feeding Summary

Cefotaxime is excreted into breast milk in low concentrations. Following a 1-g intravenous dose, mean peak milk levels of 0.33 μg/ml were measured at 2 to 3 hours (1, 2). The half-life in milk ranged from 2.36 to 3.89 hours (mean 2.93). The milk:plasma ratio at 1, 2 and 3 hours were 0.027, 0.09 and 0.16, respectively. Although these levels are low, three potential problems exist for the nursing infant: modification of bowel flora, direct effects on the infant and interference with the interpretation of culture results if a fever work-up is required.

References

1. Kafetzis DA, Lazarides CV, Siafas CA, Georgakopoulos PA, Papadatos CJ. Transfer of cefotaxime in human milk and from mother to foetus. J Antimicrob Chemother 1980;6 (Suppl A):135–41.
2. Kafetzis DA, Siafas CA, Georgakopoulos PA, Papadatos CJ. Passage of cephalosporins and amoxicillin into the breast milk. Acta Paediatr Scand 1981;70:285–8.

Name: **CEFOXITIN**

Class: **Antibiotic**   Risk Factor: **B**

Fetal Risk Summary

Cefoxitin is a cephalosporin antibiotic (see also Cephalothin). No controlled studies of its use in pregnancy have been located but multiple reports have described its transplacental passage (1–13). Two patients were given 1 g intravenously (IV) just prior to therapeutic abortion at 9 and 10 weeks gestation (9). At 55 minutes, the serum level in one woman was 10.5 µg/ml while none was found in the fetal tissues. At 4.25 hours in the second patient, the maternal serum was "nil" while the fetal tissue level was 35.7 µg/ml.

At term, following intramuscular or rapid IV doses of 1 or 2 g, cord serum levels up to 22 µg/ml (11–90%) of maternal levels have been measured (6–9). Amniotic fluid concentrations peak at 2 to 3 hours in the 3 to 15 µg/ml range (6, 7, 9, 10, 13). No apparent adverse effects were noted in any of the newborns.

Breast Feeding Summary

Cefoxitin is excreted into breast milk in low concentrations (5, 9, 11, 12). Up to 2 µg/ml have been detected in the milk of women receiving therapeutic doses (14). No data on the infants were given. Although these levels are low, three potential problems exist for the nursing infant: modification of bowel flora, direct effects on the infant and interference with the interpretation of culture results if a fever work-up is required.

References

1. Bergone-Berezin B, Kafe H, Berthelot G, Morel O, Benard Y. Pharmacokinetic study of cefoxitin in bronchial secretions. In *Current Chemotherapy: Proceedings of the 10th International Congress of Chemotherapy,* Zurich, Switzerland, September 18–23, 1977.
2. Aokawa H, Minagawa M, Yamamiohi K, Sugiyama A. Studies on cefoxitin. Chemotherapy (Tokyo) 1977;(Suppl):394.
3. Matsuda S, Tanno M, Kashiwakura S, Furuya H. Basic and clinical studies on cefoxitin. Chemotherapy (Tokyo) 1977;(Suppl):396.
4. Berthelot G, Bergogne-Berezin B, Morel O, Kafe H, Benard Y. Cefoxitin: pharmacokinetic study in bronchial secretions—transplacental diffusion. Paper presented at 10th International Congress of Chemotherapy, Zurich, Switzerland, September 18–23, 1977, program abstract No. 80.
5. Mashimo K, Mihashi S, Fukaya I, Okubo B, Ohgob M, Saito A. New drug symposium IV. Cefoxitin. Chemotherapy (Tokyo) 1978;26:114–9.
6. Matsuda S, Tanno M, Kashiwakura T, Furuya H. Laboratory and clinical studies on cefoxitin in the field of obstetrics and gynecology. Chemotherapy (Tokyo) 1978;26(Suppl 1):460–7.
7. Cho N, Ubhara K, Suigizaki K, et al. Clinical studies of cefoxitin in the field of obstetrics and gynecology. Chemotherapy (Tokyo) 1978;26(Suppl 1):468–75.
8. Seiga K, Minagawa M, Yamaji K, Sugiyama Y. Study on cefoxitin. Chemotherapy (Tokyo) 1978;26(Suppl 1):491–501.
9. Takase Z, Shirafuji H, Uchida M. Clinical and laboratory studies on cefoxitin in the field of obstetrics and gynecology. Chemotherapy (Tokyo) 1978;26(Suppl 1):502–5.
10. Bergogne-Berezin B, Lambert-Zeohovsky N, Rouvillois JL. Placental transfer of cefoxitin. Paper presented at the 18th Interscience Conference on Antimicrobial Agents and Chemo-

therapy, Atlanta, Georgia, October 1–4, 1978, program abstract No. 314.

1. Brogden RN, Heel RC, Speight TM, Avery GS. Cefoxitin: A review of its antibacterial activity, pharmacological properties and therapeutic use. Drugs 1979;17:1–37.
2. Dubois M, Delapierre D, Demonty J, Lambotte R, Dresse A. Transplacental and mammary transfer of cefoxitin. Paper presented at 11th International Congress of Chemotherapy and 19th Interscience Conference on Antimicrobial Agents and Chemotherapy, Boston, Massachusetts, October 1–5, 1979, program abstract No. 118.
3. Bergogne-Berezin B, Morel O, Kafe H, et al. Pharmacokinetic study of cefoxitin in man: diffusion into the bronchi and transfer across the placenta. Therapie 1979;34:345–54.
4. Personal communication. JJ Whalan, Merck, Sharpe & Dohme, May 13, 1981.

Name: **CEFUROXIME**

Class: **Antibiotic**   Risk Factor: **B**

Fetal Risk Summary

Cefuroxime is a cephalosporin antibiotic (see also Cephalothin). No controlled studies on its use in pregnancy have been located. Cefuroxime readily crosses the placenta in late pregnancy and labor achieving therapeutic concentrations in fetal serum and amniotic fluid (1–4). Following birth, antibiotic levels can be demonstrated up to 26 hours in the newborn. The pharmacokinetics of cefuroxime in pregnancy have been reported (5). Adverse effects in the newborn after *in utero* exposure have not been observed.

Breast Feeding Summary

Most cephalosporins are excreted into breast milk in low concentrations, but data for cefuroxime is lacking. For potential problems during breast feeding, see Cephalothin.

References

1. Craft I, Mullinger BM, Kennedy MRK. Placental transfer of cefuroxime. Br J Obstet Gynaecol 1981;88:141–5.
2. Brousfield P, Browning AK, Mullinger BM, Elstein M. Cefuroxime: potential use in pregnant women at term. Br J Obstet Gynaecol 1981;88:146–9.
3. Bergogne-Berezin E, Pierre J, Even P, Rouvillois JL, Dumez Y. Study of penetration of cefuroxime into bronchial secretions and of its placental transfer. Therapie 1980;35:677–84.
4. Tzingounis V, Makris N, Zolotas J, Michalas S, Aravantinos D. Cefuroxime prophylaxis in caesarean section. Pharmatherapeutica 1982;3:140–2.
5. Philipson A, Stiernstedt G. Pharmacokinetics of cefuroxime in pregnancy. Am J Obstet Gynecol 1982;142:823–8.

Name: CEPHALEXIN

Class: **Antibiotic**   Risk Factor: **B**

Fetal Risk Summary

Cephalexin is a cephalosporin antibiotic (see also Cephalothin). Several reports have described the administration of cephalexin to pregnant patients in various stages of gestation (1–7). None of these have linked the use of cephalexin with congenital defects or toxicity in the newborn.

Transplacental passage of cephalexin has been demonstrated only near term (1, 2). Following a 1-g oral dose, peak concentrations (μg/ml) for maternal serum, cord serum and amniotic fluid were about 34 (1 hour), 11 (4 hours), and 13 (6 hours) respectively (2). Patients in whom labor was induced were observed to have falling concentrations of cephalexin in all samples when labor was prolonged beyond 18 hours (3). In one report, all fetal blood samples gave a negative Coombs' reaction (1).

The manufacturer has unpublished information on 46 patients treated with cephalexin during pregnancy (8). Two of these patients received the drug from 1 to 2 months prior to conception to term. No effects on the fetus attributable to the antibiotic were observed. Follow-up examination on one infant at 2 months was normal.

Breast Feeding Summary

Cephalexin is excreted into breast milk in low concentrations. A 1-g oral dose given to 6 mothers produced peak milk levels at 4 to 5 hours averaging 0.51 μg/ml (range 0.24 to 0.85 μg/ml). Mean milk:plasma ratios at 1, 2 and 3 hours were 0.008, 0.021 and 0.14, respectively (9). Although these levels are low, three potential problems exist for the nursing infant: modification of bowel flora, direct effects on the infant and interference with the interpretation of culture results if a fever work-up is required.

References

1. Paterson ML, Henderson A, Lunan CB, McGurk S. Transplacental transfer of cephalexin. Clin Med 1972;79:23–4.
2. Creatsas G, Pavlatos M, Lolis D, Kaskarelis D. A study of the kinetics of cephapirin and cephalexin in pregnancy. Curr Med Res Opin 1980;7:43–6.
3. Hirsch HA. Behandlung von harnwegsinfektionen in gynakologic und geburtshilfe mit cephalexin. Int J Clin Pharmacol 1969;2(Suppl):121–3.
4. Brumfitt W, Pursell R. Double-blind trial to compare ampicillin, cephalexin, co-trimoxazole, and trimethoprim in treatment of urinary infection. Br Med J 1972;2:673–6.
5. Mizuno S, Metsuda S, Mori S. Clinical evaluation of cephalexin in obstetrics and gynaecology, Proceedings of a Symposium on the Clinical Evaluation of Cephalexin, Royal Society of Medicine, London, June 2 and 3, 1969.
6. Guttman D. Cephalexin in urinary tract infections—preliminary results, Proceedings of a Symposium on the Clinical Evaluation of Cephalexin, Royal Society of Medicine, London, June 2 and 3, 1969.
7. Soto RF, Fesbre F, Cordido A, et al. Ensayo con cefalexina en el tratamiento de infecciones urinarias en pacientes embarazadas. Rev Obst Gin Venezuela 1972;32:637–41.
8. Personal communication. CL Lynch, Medical Research—Marketed Products, Clinical Inves-

tigation Division, Dista Products, 1981.

9. Kafetzis D, Siafas C, Georgakopoulos P, Papadatos CJ. Passage of cephalosporins and amoxicillin into the breast milk. Acta Paediatr Scand 1981;70:285–8.

Name: **CEPHALOGLYCIN**

Class: **Antibiotic**   Risk Factor: **B**

Fetal Risk Summary

Cephaloglycin is a cephalosporin antibiotic (see also Cephalothin). No reports on its use in pregnancy have been located.

Breast Feeding Summary

Most cephalosporins are excreted into breast milk in low concentrations, but data concerning cephaloglycin is lacking. For potential problems during breast feeding, see Cephalothin.

Name: **CEPHALORIDINE**

Class: **Antibiotic**   Risk Factor: **B**

Fetal Risk Summary

Cephaloridine is a cephalosporin antibiotic (see also Cephalothin). No controlled studies of its use in pregnancy have been located. At term, following a 500-mg intramuscular (IM) dose, the drug readily crosses the placenta, achieving cord serum levels of approximately 20 μg/ml, almost 50% of the maternal serum concentration (1). Other investigators have reported lower peak cord serum levels at greater time intervals—about 10 μg/ml at 3 to 4 hours (2–4). Amniotic fluid concentrations greater than 8 μg/ml have been found (1–4). No effects attributable to the antibiotic were found in any of the infants.

Breast Feeding Summary

Cephaloridine is excreted into breast milk in low concentrations. Only trace amounts were found in the milk of 6 women given 500 mg IM (1). Although these levels are low for the nursing infant, three potential problems exist: modification of bowel flora, direct effects on the infant, and interference with the interpretation of culture results if a fever work-up is required.

References

1. Fukada M. Studies of chemotherapy during the perinatal period with special reference to such derivatives of Cephalosporin C as cefazolin, cephaloridine and cephalothin. Jap J

Antibiot 1973;26:197–212.
2. Barr W, Graham R. Placental transmission of cephaloridine. Postgrad Med J 1967;43(Suppl):101–4.
3. Barr W, Graham R. Placental transmission of cephaloridine. J Obstet Gynaecol Brit Commonw 1967;74:739–45.
4. Prakash A, Chalmers JA, Onojobi OIA, Henderson RJ, Cummings P. Transfer of limecycline and cephaloridine from mother to fetus—a comparative study. J Obstet Gynaecol Brit Commonw 1970;77:247–52.

Name: **CEPHALOTHIN**

Class: **Antibiotic**   Risk Factor: **B**

Fetal Risk Summary

Cephalothin, a cephalosporin antibiotic, has been used during all stages of gestation (1–3). No reports linking this use with congenital defects or toxcicity in the newborn have been located. The drug crosses the placenta and distributes in fetal tissues (4–10). Following a 1-g dose, average peak cord serum levels were found at 1 to 2 hours for the intramuscular route (2.8 μg/ml—16% of maternal peak), and at 10 minutes for intravenous (IV) administration (12.5 μg/ml—41% of maternal) (4–6). In amniotic fluid, cephalothin was slowly concentrated reaching an average level of 21 μg/ml at 4 to 5 hours (5).

Breast Feeding Summary

Cephalothin is excreted into breast milk in low concentrations. A 1-g IV bolus dose given to 6 mothers produced peak milk levels at 1 to 2 hours averaging 0.51 μg/ml (range 0.36 to 0.62 μg/ml) (11). Mean milk:plasma ratios at 1, 2 and 3 hours were 0.073, 0.26 and 0.50, respectively. Although these levels are low, three potential problems exist for the nursing infant: modification of bowel flora, direct effects on the infant and interference with the interpretation of culture results if a fever work-up is required.

References

1. Cunningham FG, Morris GB, Mickal A. Acute pyelonephritis of pregnancy: a clinical review. Obstet Gynecol 1973;42:112–7.
2. Harris RE, Gilstrap LC. Prevention of recurrent pyelonephritis during pregnancy. Obstet Gynecol 1974;44:637–41.
3. Moro M, Andrews M. Prophylactic antibiotics in cesarean section. Obstet Gynecol 1974;44:688–92.
4. MacAulay MA, Charles D. Placental transfer of cephalothin. Am J Obstet Gynecol 1968;100:940–5.
5. Sheng KT, Huang NN, Promadhattavedi V. Serum concentrations of cephalothin in infants and children and placental transmission of the antibiotic. Antimicrob Agents Chemother 1964:200–6.
6. Fukada M. Studies on chemotherapy during the perinatal period with special reference to such derivatives of Cephalosporin C as cefazolin, cephaloridine and cephalothin. Jap J Antibiot 1973;26:197–212.

7. Paterson L, Henderson A, Lunan CB, McGurk S. Transfer of cephalothin sodium to the fetus. J Obstet Gynaecol Br Commonw 1970;77:565–6.
8. Morrow S, Palmisano P, Cassady G. The placental transfer of cephalothin. J Pediatr 1968;73:262–4.
9. Stewart KS, Shafi M, Andrews J, Williams JD. Distribution of parenteral ampicillin and cephalosporins in late pregnancy. J Obstet Gynaecol Br Commonw 1973;80:902–8.
10. Corson SL, Bolognese RJ. The behavior of cephalothin in amniotic fluid. J Reprod Med 1970;4:105–8.
11. Kafetzis D, Siafas C, Georgakopoulos P, Papadatos CJ. Passage of cephalosporins and amoxicillin into the breast milk. Acta Paediatr Scand 1981;70:285–8.

Name: **CEPHAPIRIN**

Class: **Antibiotic**   Risk Factor: **B**

Fetal Risk Summary

Cephapirin is a cephalosporin antibiotic (see also Cephalothin). No controlled studies on its use in pregnancy have been located. At term, following a 1-g intramuscular dose, peak concentrations (μg/ml) for maternal serum, cord serum and amniotic fluid were about 17 (0.5 hours), 10 (4 hours) and 13 (6 hours), respectively (1). No data on the newborns was given.

Breast Feeding Summary

Cephapirin is excreted into breast milk in low concentrations. A 1-g intravenous bolus dose given to 6 mothers produced peak milk levels at 1 to 2 hours averaging 0.49 μg/ml (range 0.30 to 0.64 μg/ml) (2). Mean milk:plasma ratios at 1, 2, and 3 hours were 0.068, 0.250 and 0.480, respectively. Although these levels were low, three potential problems exist for the nursing infant: modification of bowel flora, direct effects on the infant and interference with the interpretation of culture results if a fever work-up is required.

References

1. Creatsas G, Pavlatos M, Lolis D, Kasharelis D. A study of the kinetics of cephapirin and cefalexin in pregnancy. Curr Med Res Opin 1980;7:43–6.
2. Kafetzis D, Siafas C, Georgakopoulos P, Papadatos CJ. Passage of cephalosporins and amoxicillin into the breast milk. Acta Paediatr Scand 1981;70:285–8.

Name: **CEPHRADINE**

Class: **Antibiotic**   Risk Factor: **B**

Fetal Risk Summary

Cephradine is a cephalosporin antibiotic (see also Cephalothin). No controlled studies on its use in pregnancy have been located. The drug rapidly crosses the placenta throughout gestation (1–3). In the 1st and 2nd trimesters, intravenous (IV) or oral doses produce amniotic fluid levels in the 1 μg/ml range or less. At term, oral doses of 2 g per day for 2 days or more allowed cephradine to concentrate in the amniotic fluid producing levels in the range of 3 to 15 μg/ml (1, 2). A 2-g IV dose 17 minutes prior to delivery produced high cord serum levels (29 μg/ml) but low amniotic fluid concentrations (1.1 μg/ml) (3). Serum samples taken from 2 of the newborns within 20 hours of birth indicated cephradine is excreted by the neonate (3). No other infant data was given in any of the studies.

Breast Feeding Summary

Cephradine is excreted into breast milk in low concentrations. After 500 mg orally every 6 hours for 48 hours, constant milk concentrations of 0.6 μg/ml were measured over 6 hours, a milk:plasma ratio of about 0.2 (1, 2). Although these levels are low, three potential problems exist for the nursing infant: modification of bowel flora, direct effects on the infant and interference with the interpretation of culture results if a fever work-up is required.

References

1. Mischler TW, Corson SL, Bolognese RJ, Letocha MJ, Neiss ES. Presence of cephradine in body fluids of lactating and pregnant women. Clin Pharmacol Ther 1974;15:214.
2. Mischler TW, Corson SL, Larranaga A, Bolognese RJ, Neiss ES, Vukovich RA. Cephradine and epicillin in body fluids of lactating and pregnant women. J Reprod Med 1978;21:130–6.
3. Craft I, Forster TC. Materno-fetal cephradine transfer in pregnancy. Antimicrob Agents Chemother 1978;14:924–6.

Name: **CHLORAL HYDRATE**

Class: **Sedative/Hypnotic**   Risk Factor: **C**

Fetal Risk Summary

No reports linking the use of chloral hydrate with congenital defects have been located. The drug has been given in labor and demonstrated in cord blood at concentrations similar to maternal levels (1). Sedative effects on the neonate have not been studied.

Breast Feeding Summary

Chloral hydrate and its active metabolite are excreted into breast milk. Peak concentrations of about 8 μg/ml were obtained about 45 minutes after a 1.3-g rectal dose (2). Only trace amounts are detectable after 10 hours.

References

1. Bernstine JB, Meyer AE, Hayman HB. Maternal and fetal blood estimation following the administration of chloral hydrate during labor. J Obstet Gynecol Br Emp 1954;61:683–5.
2. Berstine JB, Meyer AE, Berstine RL. Maternal blood and breast milk estimation following the administration of chloral hydrate during the puerperium. J Obstet Gynecol Br Emp 1956;63:228–31.

Name: **CHLORAMBUCIL**

Class: **Antineoplastic**   Risk Factor: **D**

Fetal Risk Summary

Chlorambucil has been used during pregnancy without causing congenital malformations (1, 2). However, there are two reports of unilateral agenesis of the left kidney and ureter in male fetuses following 1st trimester exposure to chlorambucil (see table below) (3, 4). Similar defects have been found in animals exposed to the drug (5). Chlorambucil is mutagenic as well as carcinogenic (6–10). These effects have not been reported in newborns following *in utero* exposure. Data from one review indicated that 40% of the infants exposed to anticancer drugs were of low birth weight (11). Long term studies of growth and mental development in offspring exposed to chlorambucil during the 2nd trimester, the period of neuroblast multiplication, have not been conducted (12). Amenorrhea and reversible azoospermia with high doses have been reported (13–16).

Author (ref)	No. Pts.	Indication	Gestational Age	Dose	Other Drugs	Fetal Effects	Comments
Shotton (3)	1	Hodgkin's	Through-out	6 mg/day	Not stated	Elective abortion of male fetus at 18 weeks gestation Agenesis left kidney and ureter	
Steege (4)	1	SLE Polymyositis Scleroderma	Through-out	4 mg/day	Predni-sone	Twin fetuses—1 male, 1 female; elective abortion at 20 weeks gestation Female—normal Male—agenesis left kidney and ureter	

Breast Feeding Summary

No data available.

References

1. Sokal JE, Lessmann EM. Effects of cancer chemotherapeutic agents on the human fetus. JAMA 1960;172:1765-71.
2. Jacobs C, Donaldson SS, Rosenberg SA, Kaplan HS. Management of the pregnant patient with Hodgkin's disease. Ann Intern Med 1981;95:669-75.
3. Shotton D, Monie IW. Possible teratogenic effect of chlorambucil on a human fetus. JAMA 1963;186:74-5.
4. Steege JF, Caldwell DS. Renal agenesis after first trimester exposure to chlorambucil. South Med J 1980;73:1414-5.
5. Monie IW. Chlorambucil-induced abnormalities of urogenital system of rat fetuses. Anat Rec 1961;139:145.
6. Lawler SD, Lele KP. Chromosomal damage induced by chlorambucil and chronic lymphocytic leukemia. Scand J Haematol 1972;9:603-12.
7. Westin J. Chromosome abnormalities after chlorambucil therapy of polycythemia vera. Scan J Haematol 1976;17:197-204.
8. Catovsky D, Galton DAG. Myelomonocytic leukaemia supervening on chronic lymphocytic leukaemia. Lancet 1971;1:478-9.
9. Rosner R. Acute leukemia as a delayed consequence of cancer chemotherapy. Cancer 1976;37:1033-6.
10. Reimer RR, Hoover R, Fraumeni JF, Young RC. Acute leukemia after alkylating-agent therapy of ovarian cancer. N Engl J Med 1977;297:177-81.
11. Nicholson HO. Cytotoxic drugs in pregnancy: review of reported cases. J Obstet Gynaecol Br Commonw 1968;75:307-12.
12. Dobbing J. Pregnancy and leukaemia. Lancet 1977;1:1155.
13. Freckman HA, Fry HL, Mendex FL, Maurer ER. Chlorambucil-prednisolone therapy for disseminated breast carcinoma. JAMA 1964;189:111-4.
14. Richter P, Calamera JC, Morganfeld MC, Kierszenbaum AL, Lavieri JC, Mancinni RE. Effect of chlorambucil on spermatogenesis in the human malignant lymphoma. Cancer 1970;25:1026-30.
15. Morgenfeld MC, Goldberg V, Parisier H, Bugnard SC, Bur GE. Ovarian lesions due to cytostatic agents during the treatment of Hodgkin's disease. Surg Gynecol Obstet 1972;134:826-8.
16. Schilsky RL, Lewis BJ, Sherins RJ, Young RC. Gonadal dysfunction in patients receiving chemotherapy for cancer. Ann Intern Med 1980;93:109-14.

Name: **CHLORAMPHENICOL**

Class: **Antibiotic**   Risk Factor: **C**

Fetal Risk Summary

No reports linking the use of chloramphenicol with congenital defects have been located. The drug crosses the placenta at term producing cord serum concentrations 30 to 106% of maternal levels (1, 2).

The Collaborative Perinatal Project monitored 50,282 mother-child pairs, 98 of which had 1st trimester exposure to chloramphenicol (3). For use anytime in pregnancy, 348 exposures were recorded (4). In neither case was evidence found to suggest a relationship to large categories of major or minor malformations or to individual defects. A 1977 case report described a 14-day course of intravenous chloramphenicol, 2 g daily, given to a patient with typhoid fever in the 2nd trimester (5). A normal infant was delivered at term. Twenty-two patients, in various stages of gestation, were treated with chloramphenicol for acute pyelonephritis (6). No difficulties in the newborn could be associated with the antibiotic. In a controlled study, 110 patients received 1 to 3 antibiotics during the 1st trimester for a total of 589 weeks (7). Chloramphenicol was given for a total of 205 weeks. The incidence of birth defects was similar to controls.

Although apparently non-toxic to the fetus, the use of chloramphenicol should be used with caution at term. Although specific details were not provided, one report claimed that cardiovascular collapse (gray syndrome) developed in babies delivered from mothers treated with chloramphenicol during the final stage of pregnancy (8). Additional reports of this severe adverse effect have not been located, although it is well known that newborns exposed directly to high doses of chloramphenicol may die from the gray syndrome (9–11). Because of this risk, some authors consider the drug to be contraindicated during pregnancy (12).

Breast Feeding Summary

Chloramphenicol should not be used in the lactating patient (13). Milk levels of this antibiotic are too low to precipitate the gray syndrome, but a theoretical risk exists for bone marrow depression. Two other potential problems exist for the nursing infant: modification of bowel flora and interference with the interpretation of culture results if a fever work-up is required. Several adverse effects were reported in 50 breast-fed infants exposed to chloramphenicol including refusal of the breast, falling asleep during feeding, intestinal gas and heavy vomiting after feeding (14).

Two milk samples, separated by 24 hours in the same patient, were reported as 16 and 25 μg/ml, representing milk:plasma ratios of 0.51 and 0.61, respectively (15). Both active drug and inactive metabolite were measured. No effect on the infant was mentioned. No infant toxicity was mentioned in a 1964 report that found peak levels occurring in milk 1 to 3 hours after a single oral dose of 1 g (16). In a similar study, continuous excretion of chloramphenicol into breast milk was established after the first day of therapy (17). Minimum and maximum milk concentrations were determined for 5 patients receiving 250 mg orally every 6 hours (0.54 and 2.84 μg/ml) and for 5 patients receiving 500 mg orally every 6 hours (1.75 and 6.10 μg/ml). No infant data was given.

References

1. Scott WC, Warner RF. Placental transfer of chloramphenicol (Chloromycetin). JAMA 1950;142:1331–2.
2. Ross S, Burke RG, Sites J, Rice EC, Washington JA. Placental transmission of chloramphenicol (Chloromycetin). JAMA 1950;142:1361.
3. Heinonen OP, Slone D, Shapiro S. Birth Defects and Drugs in Pregnancy. Littleton: Publishing Sciences Group, 1977:297–301.
4. Ibid, 435.
5. Schiffman P, Samet CM, Fox L, Neimand KM, Rosenberg ST. Typhoid fever in pregnancy— with probable typhoid hepatitis. NY State J Med 1977;77:1778–9.
6. Cunningham FG, Morris GB, Mickal A. Acute pyelonephritis of pregnancy: a clinical review.

Obstet Gynecol 1973;42:112-7.

7. Ravid R, Roaff R. On the possible teratogenicity of antibiotic drugs administered during pregnancy. In Klingberg MA, Abramovici, Chemke J, eds. Drugs and Fetal Development. New York: Plenum Press, 1972:505-10.

8. Oberheuser F. Praktische erfahrungen mit medikamenten in der schwangerschaft. Therapiewoche 1971;31:2200. (As reported in Manten A. Antibiotic drugs. In Dukes MNG, ed. Meyler's Side Effects of Drugs, Vol VIII. New York: American Elsevier, 1975:604.)

9. Sutherland JM. Fatal cardiovascular collapse of infants receiving large amounts of chloramphenicol. J Dis Child 1959;97:761-7.

10. Weiss CV, Glazko AJ, Weston JK. Chloramphenicol in the newborn infant. A physiologic explanation of its toxicity when given in excessive doses. N Engl J Med 1960;262:787-94.

11. Oberheuser F. Praktische erfahrungen mit medikamenten in der schwangerschaft. Therapiewoche 1971;31:2200.

12. Schwarz RH, Crombleholme WR. Antibiotics in pregnancy. South Med J 1979;72:1315-8.

13. Anonymous. Update: Drugs in breast milk. Med Lett Drugs Ther 1979;21:21-4.

14. Havelka J, Frankova A. Contribution to the question of side effects of chloramphenicol therapy in newborns. Cesk Pediatr 1972;21:31-3.

15. Smadel JE, Woodward TE, Ley HL Jr, Lewthwaite R. Chloramphenicol (Chloromycetin) in the treatment of Tsutsugamushi disease (Scrub Typhus). J Clin Invest 1949;28:1196-215.

16. Prochazka J, Havelka J, Hejzlar M. Excretion of chloramphenicol by human milk. Cas Lek Ces 1964;103:318-20.

17. Prochazka J, Hejzlar M, Popov V, Viktorinova D, Prochazka J. Excretion of chloramphenicol in human milk. Chemotherapy 1968;13:204-11.

Name: **CHLORDIAZEPOXIDE**

Class: **Sedative**   Risk Factor: **D**

Fetal Risk Summary

Chlordiazepoxide is a benzodiazepine (see also Diazepam). In a study evaluating 19,044 live births, the use of chlordiazepoxide was associated with a greater than four-fold increase in severe congenital anomalies (1). In 172 patients exposed to the drug during the first 42 days of gestation, the following defects were observed: mental deficiency; spastic diplegia and deafness; microcephaly and retardation; duodenal atresia and Meckel's diverticulum (1). Although not statistically significant, an increased fetal death rate was also found with maternal chlordiazepoxide ingestion (1). A survey of 390 infants with congenital heart disease matched with 1,254 normal infants found a higher rate of exposure to several drugs, including chlordiazepoxide, in the offspring with defects (2). Other studies have not confirmed a relationship with increased defects or mortality (3–6).

The Collaborative Perinatal Project monitored 50,282 mother-child pairs, 257 of which were exposed in the 1st trimester to chlordiazepoxide (4, 7). No association with large classes of malformations or to individual defects was found.

Neonatal withdrawal consisting of severe tremulousness and irritability has been attributed to maternal use of chlordiazepoxide (8). The onset of withdrawal symptoms occurred on the 26th day of life. Chlordiazepoxide readily crosses the placenta at term in an approximate 1:1 ratio (9–11). The drug has been used to reduce pain during labor but the maternal benefit was not significant (12, 13). Marked depression was observed in 3 infants whose mothers received chlordiazepoxide within a few hours of delivery (11). The infants were unresponsive, hypotonic, hypothermic, and fed poorly. Hypotonicity persisted for up to a week. Other studies have not seen depression (9, 10).

Breast Feeding Summary

No data available (see Diazepam).

References

1. Milkovich L, van den Berg BJ. Effects of prenatal meprobamate and chlordiazepoxide hydrochloride on human embryonic and fetal development. N Engl J Med 1974;291:1268–71.
2. Rothman KJ, Fyler DC, Golblatt A, Kreidberg MB. Exogenous hormones and other drug exposures of children with congenital heart disease. Am J Epidemiol 1979;109:433–9.
3. Crombie DL, Pinsent RJ, Fleming DM, Rumeau-Rouguette C, Goujard J, Huel G. Fetal effects of tranquilizers in pregnancy. N Engl J Med 1975;293:198–9.
4. Hartz SC, Heinonen OP, Shapiro S, Siskind V, Slone D. Antenatal exposure to meprobamate and chlordiazepoxide in relation to malformations, mental development, and childhood mortality. N Engl J Med 1975;292:726–8.
5. Bracken MB, Holford TR. Exposure to prescribed drugs in pregnancy and association with congenital malformations. Obstet Gynecol 1981;58:336–44.
6. Segal S, Pruitt AW, Anyan WR Jr, et al. Committee on drugs: psychotropic drugs in pregnancy and lactation. Pediatrics 1982;69:241–4.
7. Heinonen OP, Slone D, Shapiro S. *Birth Defects and Drugs in Pregnancy.* Littleton: Publishing Sciences Group, 1977:336–7.
8. Athinarayanan P, Pierog SH, Nigam SK, Glass L. Chlordiazepoxide withdrawal in the neonate. Am J Obstet Gynecol 1976;124:212–3.
9. Decancq HG Jr, Bosco JR, Townsend EH Jr. Chlordiazepoxide in labour: its effect on the newborn infant. J Pediatr 1965;67:836–40.
10. Mark PM, Hamel J. Librium for patients in labor. Obstet Gynecol 1968;32:188–94.
11. Stirrat GM, Edington PT, Berry DJ. Transplacental passage of chlordiazepoxide. Br Med J 1974;2:729.
12. Duckman S, Spina T, Attardi M, Meyer A. Double-blind study of chlordiazepoxide in obstetrics. Obstet Gynecol 1964;24:601–5.
13. Kanto JH. Use of benzodiazepines during pregnancy, labour and lactation, with particular reference to pharmacokinetic considerations. Drugs 1982;23:354–80.

Name: **CHLOROQUINE**

Class: **Antimalarial** Risk Factor: **D**

Fetal Risk Summary

Most reports of chloroquine usage during pregnancy fail to demonstrate fetal malformations although teratogenic effects on the vestibular apparatus have been suggested (1–3). Chloroquine should be considered the drug of choice for malaria, amebic hepatitis and discoid lupus erythematosus during pregnancy (4).

Author (ref)	No. Pts.	Indica- tion	Gestational Age	Dose	Other Drugs	Fetal Effects	Comment
Hart (1)	1	Discoid lupus	(6 pregnancies)				
			—	None	Not stated	Normal infant	
			1st trimester	500 mg/day	Not stated	Wilms' tumor, age 4; hemihypertrophy of left side	
			Throughout	500 mg/day	Not stated	Cochleovestibular pa- resis	
			—	None	Not stated	Normal infant	
			Throughout	250 mg/day	Not stated	Cochleovestibular pa- resis	
			Throughout	250 mg/day	Not stated	Normal infant	

Breast Feeding Summary

Chloroquine does not appear to be excreted in measurable amounts in the breast milk (5).

References

1. Hart CW, Naunton RF. The ototoxicity of chloroquine phosphate. Arch Otolaryngol 1964;80:407–12.
2. Ross JB, Garatsos S. Absence of chloroquine induced ototoxicity in a fetus. Arch Dermatol 1974;109:573.
3. Lewis R, Lauresen NJ, Birnbaum S. Malaria associated with pregnancy. Obstet Gynecol 1973;42:698–700.
4. Anonymous. Med Lett Drugs Ther 1965;7:9–10.
5. Anderson PO. Drugs and breast feeding. Drug Intel Clin Pharm 1977;11:210–1.

Name: **CHLOROTHIAZIDE**

Class: **Diuretic**   Risk Factor: **D**

Fetal Risk Summary

Chlorothiazide is a member of the thiazide group of diuretics. The information in this monograph applies to all members of the group, including the structurally related diuretics, Chlorthalidone, Metolazone, and Quinethazone. Thiazide and related diuretics are rarely administered during the 1st trimester. In the past, when these drugs were routinely given to prevent or treat toxemia, therapy was usually begun in the 2nd or 3rd trimesters and adverse effects in the fetus were rare (1–10). No increases in the incidence of congenital defects were discovered and thiazides were considered non-teratogenic (11–14). In contrast, the Collaborative Perinatal Project monitored 50,282 mother-child pairs, 233 of which were exposed in the 1st trimester to thiazide or related diuretics (15). All of the mothers had cardiovascular disorders, which makes interpretation of the data difficult. However, an increased risk for malformations was found for chlorthalidone (20 patients) and miscellaneous thiazide diuretics (35 patients, excluding chlorothiazide and hydrochlorothiazide). For use anytime during pregnancy, 17,492 exposures were recorded and only polythiazide showed a slight increase in risk (16).

Many investigators consider diuretics contraindicated in pregnancy, except for patients with heart disease, since they do not prevent or alter the course of toxemia and they may decrease placental perfusion (7, 17–21). In 4,035 patients treated for edema in the last half of the 3rd trimester (hypertensive patients were excluded), higher rates were found for induction of labor, stimulation of labor, uterine inertia, meconium staining, and perinatal mortality (20). All except perinatal mortality were statistically significant from 13,103 controls. Shoemaker found a decrease in endocrine function of the placenta as measured by placental clearance of estradiol in three patients treated with hydrochlorothiazide (22).

Chlorothiazide readily crosses the placenta at term and fetal serum levels may equal those of the mother (23). Chlorthalidone also crosses the placenta (24). Other diuretics probably cross to the fetus in similar amounts, although specific data is lacking. Thiazides are considered mildly diabetogenic since they can induce hyperglycemia (18). Several investigators have noted this effect in pregnant patients treated with thiazides (25–28). Other studies have failed to show maternal hyperglycemia (29, 30). Although apparently a low risk, newborns exposed to thiazide diuretics near term should be observed closely for symptoms of hypoglycemia resulting from maternal hyperglycemia (28).

Neonatal thrombocytopenia has been reported following the use near term of chlorothiazide, hydrochlorothiazide, and methyclothiazide (14, 25, 31–36). Other studies have not found a relationship between thiazide diuretics and platelet counts (37, 38). The positive reports involve only eleven patients and although the numbers are small, two of the affected infants died (25, 32). The mechanism of the thrombocytopenia is unknown, but the transfer of antiplatelet antibody from the mother to the fetus has been demonstrated (36). Thiazide-induced hemolytic anemia in two newborns was described in 1964 following the use of chlorothiazide and bendroflumethiazide at term (31). Thiazide diuretics may induce severe electrolyte imbalances in the mother's serum, amniotic fluid, and in the newborn (39–41). In one case, a stillborn fetus was attributed to electrolyte imbalance and/or maternal hypotension (39). Two hypotonic newborns were discovered to be hyponatremic, a condition believed to have resulted from maternal diuretic therapy (40). Finally, fetal bradycardia, 65 to 70 beats/minute, was shown to be secondary to chlorothiazide-induced maternal hypokalemia (41). In a 1963 study, no relationship was found between neonatal jaundice and chlorothiazide (42). Maternal and fetal death in two cases of acute hemorrhagic pancreatitis were attributed to the use of chlorothiazide in the 2nd and 3rd trimesters (43).

In summary, 1st trimester use of thiazide and related diuretics may cause an increased risk of congenital defects based on the results of one large study. Use in later trimesters does not seem to carry this risk. In addition to malformations, other risk to the fetus or newborn include hypoglycemia, thrombocytopenia, hyponatremia, hypokalemia, and death from maternal complications. Thiazide diuretics may have a direct effect on smooth muscle and inhibit labor. Use of diuretics during pregnancy should be discouraged except for patients with heart disease.

Breast Feeding Summary

Chlorothiazide is excreted into breast milk in low concentrations (44). Following a 500-mg single oral dose, milk levels were less than 1 μg/ml at 1, 2 and 3 hours. The authors speculated that the risks of pharmacological effects in nursing infants would be remote. However, it has been stated that thrombocytopenia can occur in the nursing infant if the mother was taking chlorothiazide (45). Documentation of this is needed (46). Chlorthalidone has a very low milk:plasma ratio of 0.05 (24). Data for other thiazide and related diuretics is lacking. However, thiazide diuretics have been used to suppress lactation (47, 48).

References

1. Finnerty FA Jr, Buchholz JH, Tuckman J. Evaluation of chlorothiazide (Diuril) in the toxemias of pregnancy. Analysis of 144 patients. JAMA 1958;166:141–4.
2. Zuspan FP, Bell JD, Barnes AC. Balance-ward and double-blind diuretic studies during pregnancy. Obstet Gynecol 1960;16:543–9.
3. Sears RT. Oral diuretics in pregnancy toxaemia. Br Med J 1960;2:148.
4. Assoli NS. Renal effects of hydrochlorothiazide in normal and toxemic pregnancy. Clin Pharmacol Ther 1960;1:48–52.
5. Tatum H, Waterman EA. The prophylactic and therapeutic use of the thiazides in pregnancy. GP 1961;24:101–5.
6. Flowers CE, Grizzle JE, Easterling WE, Bonner OB. Chlorothiazide as a prophylaxis against toxemia of pregnancy. Am J Obstet Gynecol 1962;84:919–29.
7. Weseley AC, Douglas GW. Continuous use of chlorothiazide for prevention of toxemia in pregnancy. Obstet Gynecol 1962;19:355–8.
8. Finnerty FA Jr. How to treat toxemia of pregnancy. GP 1963;27:116–21.
9. Fallis NE, Plauche WC, Mosey LM, Langford HG. Thiazide versus placebo in prophylaxis of toxemia of pregnancy in primagravid patients. Am J Obstet Gynecol 1964;88:502–4.
10. Landesman R, Aguero O, Wilson K, LaRussa R, Campbell W, Penaloza O. The prophylactic use of chlorthalidone, a sulfonamide diuretic, in pregnancy. J Obstet Gynaecol Br Commonw 1965;72:1004–10.
11. Cuadros A, Tatum H. The prophylactic and therapeutic use of bendroflumethiazide in pregnancy. Am J Obstet Gynecol 1964;89:891–7.
12. Finnerty FA Jr, Bepko FJ Jr. Lowering the perinatal mortality and the prematurity rate. The value of prophylactic thiazides in juveniles. JAMA 1966;195:429–32.
13. Kraus GW, Marchese JR, Yen SSC. Prophylactic use of hydrochlorothiazide in pregnancy. JAMA 1966;198:1150–4.
14. Gray MJ. Use and abuse of thiazides in pregnancy. Clin Obstet Gynecol 1968;11:568–78.
15. Heinonen OP, Slone D, Shapiro S. Birth Defects and Drugs in Pregnancy. Littleton: Publishing Sciences Group, 1977:371–3.
16. Ibid, 441.
17. Watt JD, Philipp EE. Oral diuretics in pregnancy toxemia. Br Med J 1960;1:1807.
18. Pitkin RM, Kaminetzky HA, Newton M, Pritchard JA. Maternal nutrition: a selective review of clinical topics. Obstet Gynecol 1972;40:773–85.
19. Lindheimer MD, Katz AI. Sodium and diuretics in pregnancy. N Engl J Med 1973;288:891–4.
20. Christianson R, Page EW. Diuretic drugs and pregnancy. Obstet Gynecol 1976;48:647–52.
21. Lammintausta R, Erkkola R, Eronen M. Effect of chlorothiazide treatment of renin-aldosterone system during pregnancy. Acta Obstet Gynecol Scand 1978;57:389–92.
22. Shoemaker ES, Grant NF, Madden JD, MacDonald PC. The effect of thiazide diuretics on

placental function. Tex Med 1973;69:109–15.
23. Garnet J. Placental transfer of chlorothiazide. Obstet Gynecol 1963;21:123–5.
24. Mulley BA, Parr GD, Pau WK, Rye RM, Mould JJ, Siddle NC. Placental transfer of chlorthalidone and its elimination in maternal milk. Eur J Clin Pharmacol 1978;13:129–31.
25. Menzies DN. Controlled trial of chlorothiazide in treatment of early pre-eclampsia. Br Med J 1964;1:739–42.
26. Ladner CN, Pearson JW, Herrick CN, Harrison HE. The effect of chlorothiazide on blood glucose in the third trimester of pregnancy. Obstet Gynecol 1964;23:555–60.
27. Goldman JA, Neri A, Ovadia J, Eckerling B, DeVries A. Effect of chlorothiazide on intravenous glucose tolerance in pregnancy. Am J Obstet Gynecol 1969;105:556–60.
28. Senior B, Slone D, Shapiro S, Mitchell AA, Heinonen OP. Benzothiadiazides and neonatal hypoglycaemia. Lancet 1976;2:377.
29. Lakin N, Zeytinoglu J, Younger M, White P. Effect of chlorothiazide on insulin requirements of pregnant diabetic women. JAMA 1960;173:353–4.
30. Esbenshade JH Jr, Smith RT. Thiazides and pregnancy: a study of carbohydrate tolerance. Am J Obstet Gynecol 1965;92:270–1.
31. Harley JD, Robin H, Robertson SEJ. Thiazide-induced neonatal haemolysis? Br Med J 1964;1:696–7.
32. Rodriguez SU, Leikin SL, Hiller MC. Neonatal thrombocytopenia associated with ante-partum administration of thiazide drugs. N Engl J Med 1964;270:881–4.
33. Leikin SL. Thiazide and neonatal thrombocytopenia. N Engl J Med 1964;271:161.
34. Prescott LF. Neonatal thrombocytopenia and thiazide drugs. Br Med J 1964;1:1438.
35. Jones JE, Reed JF Jr. Renal vein thrombosis and thrombocytopenia in the newborn infant. J Pediatr 1965;67:681–2.
36. Karpatkin S, Strick N, Karpatkin MB, Siskind GW. Cumulative experience in the detection of antiplatelet antibody in 234 patients with idiopathic thrombocytopenic purpura, systemic lupus erythematosus and other clinical disorders. Am J Med 1972;52:776–85.
37. Finnerty FA Jr, Assoli NS. Thiazide and neonatal thrombocytopenia. N Engl J Med 1964;271:160–1.
38. Jerkner K, Kutti J, Victoria L. Platelet counts in mothers and their newborn infants with respect to antepartum administration of oral diuretics. Acta Med Scand 1973;194:473–5.
39. Pritchard JA, Walley PJ. Severe hypokalemia due to prolonged administration of chlorothiazide during pregnancy. Am J Obstet Gynecol 1961;81:1241–4.
40. Alstatt LB. Transplacental hyponatremia in the newborn infant. J Pediatr 1965;66:985–8.
41. Anderson GG, Hanson TM. Chronic fetal bradycardia: possible association with hypokalemia. Obstet Gynecol 1974;44:896–8.
42. Crosland D, Flowers C. Chlorothiazide and its relationship to neonatal jaundice. Obstet Gynecol 1963;22:500–4.
43. Minkowitz S, Soloway HB, Hall JE, Yermakov V. Fatal hemorrhagic pancreatitis following chlorothiazide administration in pregnancy. Obstet Gynecol 1964;24:337–42.
44. Werthmann MW Jr, Krees SV. Excretion of chlorothiazide in human breast milk. J Pediatr 1972;81:781–3.
45. Anonymous. Drugs in breast milk. Med Lett Drugs Ther 1976;16:25–7.
46. Dailey JW. Anticoagulant and cardiovascular drugs. In Wilson JT, ed. Drugs in Breast Milk. Australia: ADIS Press, 1981:61–4.
47. Healy M. Suppressing lactation with oral diuretics. Lancet 1961;1:1353–4.
48. Catz CS, Giacoia GP. Drugs and breast milk. Pediatr Clin North Am 1972;19:151–66.

Name: **CHLOROTRIANISENE**

Class: **Estrogenic Hormone**   Risk Factor: **D**

Fetal Risk Summary

No data available. Use of estrogenic hormones during pregnancy is not recommended (see Oral Contraceptives).

Breast Feeding Summary

Chlorotrianisene is used to suppress postpartum breast engorgement in patients who do not desire to breast feed.

Name: **CHLORPHENIRAMINE**

Class: **Antihistamine/Antiemetic**   Risk Factor: **B**

Fetal Risk Summary

The Collaborative Perinatal Project monitored 50,282 mother-child pairs, 1,070 of which had 1st trimester exposure to chlorpheniramine (1). For use anytime during pregnancy, 3,931 exposures were recorded (2). In neither case was evidence found to suggest a relationship to large categories of major or minor malformations. Several possible associations with individual malformations were found but the statistical significance of these is unknown. Independent confirmation is required to determine the actual risk.

Polydactyly in Blacks (7 cases in 272 Blacks)

Hydrocephaly (8 cases)

Gastrointestinal defects (13 cases)

Congenital dislocation of hip (16 cases)

Eye and ear defects (7 cases)

Malformations of the female genitalia (6 cases)

Inguinal hernia (22 cases)

In a 1971 study, significantly fewer infants with malformations were exposed to antihistamines in the 1st trimester as compared to controls (3). Chlorpheniramine was the sixth most commonly used antihistamine.

A case of infantile malignant osteopetrosis was described in a 4-month-old boy exposed *in utero* on several occasions to Contac (chlorpheniramine, phenylpropranolamine and belladonna alkaloids) but this is a known genetic defect (4). The boy also had a continual "stuffy" nose.

Breast Feeding Summary

No data available.

References

1. Heinonen OP, Slone D, Shapiro S. *Birth Defects and Drugs in Pregnancy.* Littleton: Publishing Sciences Group, 1977:322–34.

2. *Ibid*, 437, 488.
3. Nelson MM, Forfar JO. Associations between drugs administered during pregnancy and congenital abnormalities of the fetus. Br Med J 1971;1:523–7.
4. Golbus MS, Koerper MA, Hall BD. Failure to diagnose osteopetrosis in utero. Lancet 1976;2:1246

Name: **CHLORPROMAZINE**

Class: **Tranquilizer** Risk Factor: **C**

Fetal Risk Summary

Chlorpromazine is a propylamino phenothiazine. The drug readily crosses the placenta (1–4). In animals, selective accumulation and retention occurs in the fetal pigment epithelium (5). Although delayed ocular damage from high prolonged doses in pregnancy has not been reported in humans, concern has been expressed for this potential toxicity (5, 6).

Chlorpromazine has been used for the treatment of nausea and vomiting of pregnancy during all stages of gestation, including labor, since the mid-1950's (7–9). The drug seems to be safe and effective for this indication. Its use in labor to promote analgesia and amnesia is usually safe but some patients, up to 18% in one series, have a marked unpredictable fall in blood pressure which could be dangerous to the mother and the fetus (10–14). Use of chlorpromazine during labor should be discouraged because of this adverse effect. An extrapyramidal syndrome (EPS), which may persist for months, has been observed in some infants whose mothers received chlorpromazine near term (15–19). This reaction is characterized by tremors, increased muscle tone with spasticity and hyperactive deep tendon reflexes. Hypotenicity has been observed in one newborn and paralytic ileus in two after exposure at term to chlorpromazine (4, 20). However, most reports describing the use chlorpromazine in pregnancy have concluded that it does not adversely affect the fetus or newborn (21–24). The Collaborative Perinatal Project monitored 50,282 mother-child pairs, 142 of which had 1st trimester exposure to chlorpromazine (25). For use anytime during pregnancy, 284 exposures were recorded. No evidence was found in either group to suggest a relationship to malformations, nor an effect on perinatal mortality rate, birth weight or intelligence quotient scores at 4 years of age. Opposite results were found in a prospective French study that compared 304 mothers exposed to phenothiazines during gestation with 10,921 non-exposed controls (26). Malformations were observed in 11 exposed infants (3.5%) and in 178 non-exposed infants (1.6%). This difference was statistically significant ($p < 0.01$). The association was significant ($p < 0.01$) for those phenothiazines with a 3-carbon aliphatic side chain of which chlorpromazine was the principal member. Other phenothiazine groups (2-carbon side chain, piperazine, and piperidine derivatives) were associated with lesser significance ($p < 0.05$). A single case of ectromelia/amphalocele was attributed to the combined use of chloropromazine and meclizine in the 1st trimester (27).

Chlorpromazine

In summary, although one survey found an increased incidence of defects and a report of ectromelia exists, most studies have found chlorpromazine to be safe for both mother and fetus if used occasionally in low doses. Other reviewers have also concluded that the phenothiazines are not teratogenic (24, 28). However, use near term should be avoided due to the danger of maternal hypotension and adverse effects in the newborn.

Author (ref)	No. Pts.	Indication	Gestational Age	Dose	Other Drugs	Fetal Effects	Comment
Hill (15)	1	Psychiatric	throughout	200 mg/day 50 mg/day	Thioridazine Trifluoperazine Hydrochlorthiazide	EPS for 10 months EPS for 6 months	2 pregnancies in same patient
Ayd (16)	22	Psychiatric	Throughout or 3rd trimester only	"large doses"	Other psychoactive drugs, alcohol, barbituates	EPS	EPS not observed if drug taken infrequently or only in first two trimesters
Tamer (17)	2	Psychiatric	2nd and 3rd trimesters	200–600 mg/day	Pb Phenytoin	EPS—onset 2nd day; retarded at 4 years EPS for 3 months— onset 2nd day	Mother had 2 seizures in 1st trimester
Levy (18)	1	Psychosis	2nd and 3rd trimesters	400–600 mg/day	Not stated	EPS for 6 months	
O'Connor (19)	1	Psychiatric	2nd and 3rd trimesters	1200 mg/day	Fluphenazine Heavy smoker	EPS for 9 months— onset 21st day	Normal development after 9 months
Rumeau-Roquette (26)	57	Various	Various	Various	Various	Malformations in 4 infants: 1 syndactyly 1 microcephaly, clubfoot/hand, muscular abdominal aplasia 1 endocardial fibroelastosis, brachymesophalangy, clinodactyly 1 microcephaly	2 siblings with microcephaly not exposed
O'Leary (27)	1	Nausea/ vomiting	1st trimester	50 mg/day	Meclizine	Stillborn at 28 weeks, with ectromelia and omphalocele	
Hammond (4)	1	Psychiatric	Term	8000 mg over 10 days	Amytal Haloperidol Amitryptiline Diperodon Lithium	Hypotonic, lethargic, depressed reflexes, jaundice, apathetic	Spontaneous return to normal within 3 weeks

| Falterman (20) | 2 | Psychia-tric | 2nd and 3rd trimes-ters | 400 mg/day | Benztropine Thiothixene Doxepin Pb Secobarbital | Abdominal disten-tion, hypoac-tive bowel sounds, bile-stained gastric aspirate | Spontaneous return to nor-mal within 3 days |

Breast Feeding Summary

Chlorpromazine is excreted into breast milk in very small concentrations. Following a 1200-mg oral dose (20 mg/kg), peak milk levels of 0.29 μg/ml were measured at 2 hours (29). This represented a milk:plasma ratio of less than 0.5. The drug could not be detected following a 600-mg oral dose. These amounts are probably insignificant and concur with the lack of reported adverse effects in breast-fed babies whose mothers were ingesting chlorpromazine (24).

References

1. Franchi G, Gianni AM. Chlorpromazine distribution in maternal and fetal tissues and biological fluids. Acta Anaesthesiol (Padava) 1957;8:197-207.
2. Moya F, Thorndike V. Passage of drugs across the placenta. Am J Obstet Gyencol 1962;84:1778-98.
3. O'Donoghue SEF. Distribution of pethidine and chlorpromazine in maternal, foetal and neonatal biological fluids. Nature 1971; 229:124-5.
4. Hammond JE, Toseland PA. Placental transfer of chlorpromazine. Arch Dis Child 1970;45:139-40.
5. Ullberg S, Lindquist NG, Sjostrand SE. Accumulation of chorio-retinotoxic drugs in the foetal eye. Nature 1970;227:1257-8.
6. Anonymous. Drugs and the fetal eye. Lancet 1971;1:122.
7. Karp M, Lamb VE, Benaron HBW. The use of chlorpromazine in the obstetric patient: a preliminary report. Am J Obstet Gynecol 1955;69:780-5.
8. Benaron HBW, Dorr EM, Roddick WJ, et al. Use of chlorpromazine in the obstetric patient: a preliminary report I. In the treatment of nausea and vomiting of pregnancy. Am J Obstet Gynecol 1955; 69:776-9.
9. Sullivan CL. Treatment of nausea and vomiting of pregnancy with chlorpromazine. A report of 100 cases. Postgrad Med 1957;22:429-32.
10. Harer WB. Chlorpromazine in normal labor. Obstet Gynecol 1956;8:1-9.
11. Lindley JE, Rogers SF, Moyer JH. Analgesic--potentiation effect of chlorpromazine during labor; a study of 2093 patients. Obstet Gynecol 1957;10:582-6.
12. Bryans CI Jr, Mulherin CM. The use of chlorpromazine in obstetrical analgesia. Am J Obstet Gynecol 1959;77:406-11.
13. Christhilf SM Jr, Monias MB, Riley RA Jr, Sheehan JC. Chlorpromazine in obstetric analgesia. Obstet Gynecol 1960;15:625-9.
14. Rodgers CD, Wickard CP, McCaskill MR. Labor and delivery without terminal anesthesia. A report of the use of chlorpromazine. Obstet Gynecol 1961;17:92-5.
15. Hill RM, Desmond MM, Kay JL. Extrapyramidal dysfunction in an infant of a schizophrenic mother. J Pediatr 1966;69:589-95.
16. Ayd FJ Jr, ed. Phenothiazine therapy during pregnancy—effects on the newborn infant. Inter Drug Ther Newslett 1968;3:39-40.
17. Tamer A, McKay R, Arias D, Worley L, Fogel BJ. Phenothiazine-induced extrapyramidal dysfunction in the neonate. J Pediatr 1969;75:479-80.
18. Levy W, Wisniewski K. Chlorpromazine causing extrapyramidal dysfunction in newborn infant of psychotic mother. N Y State J Med 1974;74:684-5.
19. O'Connor M, Johnson GH, James DI. Intrauterine effect of phenothiazines. Med J Aust 1981;1:416-7.

20. Falterman CG, Richardson J. Small left colon syndrome associated with maternal ingestion of psychotropic drugs. J Pediatr 1980;97:308–10.
21. Kris EB, Carmichael DM. Chlorpromazine maintenance therapy during pregnancy and confinement. Psychiatric Quart 1957;31:690–5.
22. Kris EB. Children born to mothers maintained on pharmacotherapy during pregnancy and postpartum. Recent Adv Biol Psychiat 1962;4:180–7.
23. Sobel DE. Fetal damage due to ECT, insulin coma, chlorpromazine, or reserpine. Arch Gen Psychiatry 1960;2:606–11.
24. Ayd FJ Jr. Children born of mothers treated with chlorpromazine during pregnancy. Clin Med 1964;71:1758–63.
25. Slone D, Siskind V, Heinonen OP, Monson RR, Kaufman DW, Shapiro S. Antenatal exposure to the pheothiazines in relation to congenital malformations, perinatal mortality rate, birth weight, and intelligence quotient score. Am J Obstet Gynecol 1977;128:486–8.
26. Rumeau-Rouquette C, Goujard J, Huel G. Possible teratogenic effect of phenothiazines in human beings. Teratology 1976;15:57–64.
27. O'Leary JL, O'Leary JA. Nonthalidomide ectromelia; report of a case. Obstet Gynecol 1964;23:17–20.
28. Ananth J. Congenital malformations with psychopharmacologic agents. Compr Psychiatry 1975;16:437–45.
29. Blacker KH, Weinstein BJ, Ellman GL. Mothers milk and chlorpromazine. Am J Psychol 1962;114:178–9.

Name: **CHLORPROPAMIDE**

Class: **Oral Hypoglycemic**   Risk Factor: **D**

Fetal Risk Summary

Chlorpropamide is a sulfonylurea used for the treatment of adult-onset diabetes mellitus. It is not indicated for the pregnant diabetic. When administered near term, the drug crosses the placenta and may persist in the neonatal serum for several days (1, 2). One mother, who took 500 mg per day throughout pregnancy, delivered an infant whose serum level was 15.4 mg/100 ml at 77 hours of life (1). Infants of three other mothers, who were consuming 100 to 250 mg per day at term, had serum levels varying between 1.8 to 2.8 mg/100 ml 8 to 35 hours post-delivery (2). All four infants had prolonged symptomatic hypoglycemia secondary to hyperinsulinism lasting for four to six days. In other reports, totaling 69 pregnancies, chlorpropamide in doses of 100 to 200 mg or more per day either gave no evidence of neonatal hypoglycemia/hyperinsulinism or no constant relationship between daily maternal dosage and neonatal complications (3, 4). However, chlorpropamide should be stopped at least 48 hours before delivery to avoid this potential complication (5).

Although teratogenic in animals, an increased incidence of congenital defects, other than that expected in diabetes mellitus, has not been found with chlorpropamide (6–15). Four malformed infants have been attributed to chlorpropamide but the relationship is unclear (6, 9). Maternal diabetes is known to increase the rate of malformations by two to four fold, but the mechanism(s) are not understood (see also Insulin). In spite of the lack of evidence for hlorpropamide teratogenicity, the drug should not be used in pregnancy ince it will not provide good control in patients who cannot be controlled by iet alone (5). The manufacturer recommends it not be used in pregnan-y (16).

Author (ref)	No. Pts.	Indication	Gestational Age	Dose	Other Drugs	Fetal Effects	Comment
ɔler (6)	3	Diabetes mellitus	Throughout	350–500 mg/ day	Metformin Insulin	Hands/fingers anomalies (1) Stricture lower ileum; died (1) Preauricular sinus (1)	
ɑmpbell (9)	1	Diabetes mellitus	Throughout	500 mg/day	Not stated	Microcephaly Spastic quadriplegia	

ɪreast Feeding Summary

ɔhlorpropamide is excreted into breast milk. Following a 500-mg oral dose, ɿe milk concentration in a composite of two samples obtained at 5 hours ʌas 5 μg/ml (17). The effects on a nursing infant from this amount of drug ɹre unknown.

ʁeferences

1. Zucker P, Simon G. Prolonged symptomatic neonatal hypoglycemia associated with maternal chlorpropamide therapy. Pediatrics 1968;42:824–5.
2. Kemball ML, McIver C, Milnar RDG, Nourse CH, Schiff D, Tiernan JR. Neonatal hypoglycaemia in infants of diabetic mothers given sulphonylurea drugs in pregnancy. Arch Dis Child 1970;45:696–701.
3. Sutherland HW, Stowers JM, Cormack JD, Bewsher PD. Evaluation of chlorpropamide in chemical diabetes diagnosed during pregnancy. Br Med J 1973;3:9–13.
4. Sutherland HW, Bewsher PD, Cormack JD, et al. Effect of moderate dosage of chlorpropamide in pregnancy on fetal outcome. Arch Dis Child 1974;49:283–91.
5. Friend JR. Diabetes. Clin Obstet Gynecol 1981;8:353–82.
6. Soler NG, Walsh CH, Malins JM. Congenital malformations in infants of diabetic mothers. Q J Med 1976;45:303–13.
7. Adam PAJ, Schwartz R. Diagnosis and treatment: should oral hypoglycemic agents be used in pediatric and pregnant patients? Pediatrics 1968;42:819–23.
8. Dignan PSJ. Teratogenic risk and counseling in diabetes. Clin Obstet Gynecol 1981;24:149–59.
9. Campbell GD. Chlorpropamide and foetal damage. Br Med J 1963;1:59–60.
0. Jackson WPU, Campbell GD, Notelovitz M, Blumsohn D. Tolbutamide and chlorpropamide during pregnancy in human diabetes. Diabetes 1962;11(Suppl):98–101.
1. Jackson WPU, Campbell GD. Chlorpropamide and perinatal mortality. Br Med J 1963;2:1652.
2. Macphail I. Chlorpropamide and foetal damage. Br Med J 1963;1:192.
3. Malins JM, Cooke AM, Pyke DA, Fitzgerald MG. Sulphonylurea drugs in pregnancy. Br Med J 1964;2:187.
4. Moss JM, Connor EJ. Pregnancy complicated by diabetes. Report of 102 pregnancies including eleven treated with oral hypoglycemic drugs. Med Ann Dist Columb 1965;34:253–60.
5. Douglas CP, Richards R. Use of chlorpropamide in the treatment of diabetes in pregnancy. Diabetes 1967;16:60–1.
6. Product information. Diabinese. Pfizer Incorporated, 1981.
7. Personal communication. D'Ambrosio GG, Pfizer Laboratories, Inc. 1982.

Name: **CHLORPROTHIXENE**

Class: **Tranquilizer**   Risk Factor: **C**

Fetal Risk Summary

Chlorprothixene is structurally and pharmacologically related to chlorproma-zine and thiothixene. No specific data on its use in pregnancy has been located (see also Chlorpromazine).

Breast Feeding Summary

No data available.

Name: **CHLORTETRACYCLINE**

Class: **Antibiotic**   Risk Factor: **D**

Fetal Risk Summary

See Tetracycline.

Breast Feeding Summary

Chlortetracycline is excreted into breast milk. Eight patients were given 2 to 3 g orally per day for 3 to 4 days (1). Average maternal and milk concentrations were 4.1 and 1.25 μg/ml respectively, producing a milk:plasma ratio of 0.4. Infant data was not given.

Theoretically, dental staining and inhibition of bone growth could occur in breast-fed infants whose mothers were consuming chlortetracycline. However, this theoretical possibility seems remote since in infants exposed to a closely related antibiotic, tetracycline, serum levels were undetectable (less than 0.05 μg/ml) (2). Three potential problems may exist for the nursing infant, even though there are no reports in this regard: modification of bowel flora, direct effects on the infant and interference with the interpretation of culture results if a fever work-up is required.

References

1. Guilbeau JA, Schoenbach EB, Schuab IG, Latham DV. Aureomycin in obstetrics; therapy and prophylaxis. JAMA 1950;143:520–6.
2. Posner AC, Prigot A, Konicoff NG. Further observations on the use of tetracycline hydrochloride in prophylaxis and treatment of obstetric infections. *Antibiotics Annual 1954–55*, New York: Medical Encyclopedia, 594–8.

ame: **CHLORTHALIDONE**

lass: **Diuretic**   Risk Factor: **D**

etal Risk Summary

hlorthalidone is structurally related to the thiazide diuretics. See Chlorothia-
de.

reast Feeding Summary

ee Chlorothiazide.

---

ame: **CHLORZOXAZONE**

lass: **Muscle Relaxant**   Risk Factor: **C**

etal Risk Summary

o data available.

reast Feeding Summary

o data available.

Name: **CHOLINE SALICYLATE**

lass: **Analgesic/Antipyretic**   Risk Factor: **C***

etal Risk Summary

ee Aspirin.

* Risk Factor D if used in the 3rd trimester.]

reast Feeding Summary

ee Aspirin.

Name: **CIMETIDINE**

lass: **Histamine (H₂) Receptor Antagonist**   Risk Factor: **B**

Fetal Risk Summary

No reports linking the use of cimetidine with congenital defects have been
ocated. Transient liver impairment has been described in a newborn exposed
to cimetidine at term (1). Other reports have not confirmed this toxicity (2–9).

The drug has been used at term with antacids to prevent maternal acid aspiration pneumonitis (Mendelson's syndrome) (4–9). No neonatal adverse effects were noted in these studies. At term, cimetidine crosses the placenta resulting in a peak mean fetal-maternal ratio of 0.84 at 1.5 to 2 hours (10).

Breast Feeding Summary

Cimetidine is excreted into breast milk and may accumulate in concentrations greater than that found in maternal plasma (11). Following a single 400-mg oral dose a theoretical milk:plasma ratio of 1.6 has been calculated (11). Multiple oral doses of 200 and 400 mg result in milk:plasma ratios of 4.6 to 7.44, respectively. An estimated 6 mg of cimetidine per liter of milk could be ingested by the nursing infant. The clinical significance of this ingestion is unknown.

References

1. Glade G, Saccar CL, Pereira GR. Cimetidine in pregnancy: apparent transient liver impairment in the newborn. Am J Dis Child 1980;134:87–8.
2. McGowan WAW. Safety of cimetidine treatment during pregnancy. J Royal Soc Med 1979;72:902–7.
3. Zulli P, DiNisio Q. Cimetidine treatment during pregnancy. Lancet 1978;2:945–6.
4. Husemeyer RP, Davenport HT. Prophylaxis for Mendelson's syndrome before elective caesarean sections. A comparison of cimetidine and magnesium trisilicate mixture regimens. Br J Obstet Gynaecol 1980;87:565–70.
5. Pickering BG,, Palahniuk RJ, Cumming M. Cimetidine premedication in elective caesarean section. Can Anaesth Soc J 1980;27:33–5.
6. Dundee JW, Moore J, Johnston JR, McCaughey W. Cimetidine and obstetric anaesthesia. Lancet 1981;2:252.
7. McCaughey W, Howe JP, Moore J, Dundee JW. Cimetidine in elective caesarean section. Effect on gastric acidity. Anaesthesia 1981;36:167–72.
8. Crawford JS. Cimetidine in elective caesarean section. Anaesthesia 1981;36:641–2.
9. McCaughey W, Howe JP, Moore J, Dundee JW. *Ibid*, 642.
10. Howe JP, McGowan WAW, Moore J, McCaughey W, Dundee JW. The placental transfer of cimetidine. Anaesthesia 1981;36:371–5.
11. Somogyi A, Gugler R. Cimetidine excretion into breast milk. Br J Clin Pharmacol 1979;7:627–9.

Name: **CINOXACIN**

Class: **Urinary Germicide**   Risk Factor: **B**

Fetal Risk Summary

No data available.

Breast Feeding Summary

No data available.

ame: CISPLATIN
lass: Antineoplastic   Risk Factor: **D**

etal Risk Summary

nly one case of cisplatin usage during pregnancy has been located (1). The
other at approximately 10 weeks gestation received a single intravenous
ose of 50 mg/kg for carcinoma of the uterine cervix. Two weeks later, a
adical hysterectomy was performed. The male fetus was morphologically
ormal for its developmental age.

reast Feeding Summary

o data available.

eference

1. Jacobs AJ, Marchevsky A, Gordon RE, Deppe G, Cohen CJ. Oat cell carcinoma of the uterine
   cervix in a pregnant woman treated with cis-diamminedichloroplatinum. Gynecol Oncol
   1980;9:405–10.

ame: CLIDINIUM
lass: Parasympatholytic   Risk Factor: **C**

etal Risk Summary

lidinium is an anticholinergic quaternary ammonium bromide. In a large
rospective study, 2,323 patients were exposed to this class of drugs during
he 1st trimester, 4 of whom took clidinium (1). A possible association was
ound between the total group and minor malformations.

reast Feeding Summary

o data available (see also Atropine).

eference

1. Heinonen OP, Slone D, Shapiro S. *Birth Defects and Drugs in Pregnancy*. Littleton: Publishing
   Sciences Group, 1977:346–53.

Name: CLINDAMYCIN
Class: Antibiotic   Risk Factor: **B**

Fetal Risk Summary

No reports linking the use of clindamycin with congenital defects have been
located. The drug crosses the placenta achieving maximum cord serum levels
of approximately 50% of the maternal serum (1, 2). Levels in the fetus were

considered therapeutic for susceptible pathogens. Fetal tissue levels increase following multiple dosing with the drug concentrating in the fetal liver (1). Maternal serum levels after dosing at various stages of pregnancy were similar to nonpregnant patients (2, 3). Clindamycin has been used for prophylactic therapy prior to cesarean section (4).

Breast Feeding Summary

Clindamycin is excreted into breast milk. In 2 patients receiving 600 mg intravenously every 6 hours, milk levels varied from 2.1 to 3.8 μg/ml (0.2 to 3.5 hours after drug) (5). When the patients were changed to 300 mg orally every 6 hours, levels varied from 0.7 to 1.8 μg/ml (2 to 7 hours after drug). Maternal serum levels were not given. Two grossly bloody stools were observed in a nursing infant whose mother was receiving clindamycin and gentamicin (6). No relationship to either drug could be established. However the condition cleared rapidly when breast feeding was stopped. Except for this one case, no other adverse effects in nursing infants have been reported. Three potential problems that may exist for the nursing infant are modification of bowel flora, direct effects on the infant and interference with the interpretation of culture results if a fever work-up is required.

References

1. Philipson A, Sabath LD, Charles D. Transplacental passage of erythromycin and clindamycin. N Engl J Med 1973;288:1219–21.
2. Weinstein AJ, Gibbs RS, Gallagher M. Placental transfer of clindamycin and gentamicin in term pregnancy. Am J Obstet Gynecol 1976;124:688–91.
3. Philipson A, Sabath LD, Charles D. Erythromycin and clindamycin absorption and elimination in pregnant women. Clin Pharmacol Ther 1976;19:68–77.
4. Rehu M, Jahkola M. Prophylactic antibiotics in caesarean section: effect of a short preoperative course of benzyl penicillin or clindamycin plus gentamicin on postoperative infectious morbidity. Ann Clin Res 1980;12:45–8.
5. Smith JA, Morgan JR, Rachlis AR, Papsin FR. Clindamycin in human breast milk. Can Med Assoc J 1975;112:806.
6. Mann CF. Clindamycin and breast-feeding. Pediatrics 1980;66:1030–1.

Name: **CLOFIBRATE**

Class: **Antilipemic Agent**   Risk Factor: **C**

Fetal Risk Summary

No reports linking the use of clofibrate with congenital defects have been located. There is pharmacological evidence that clofibrate crosses the rat placenta and reaches measurable levels, but data in humans is lacking (1). The drug is metaboilized by glucuronide conjugation and since this system is immature in the newborn, accumulation may occur. Consequently, the use of clofibrate near term is not recommended.

Breast Feeding Summary

No data available. Animal studies suggest that the drug is excreted into milk (1).

ference

. Chhabra S, Kurup CKR. Maternal transport of chlorophenoxyisobutyrate at the foetal and neonatal stages of development. Biochem Pharmacol 1978;27:2063–5.

---

ame: **CLOMIPHENE**

ass: **Fertility Agent (Nonhormonal)** Risk Factor: **C***

tal Risk Summary

omiphene is used to induce ovulation. It should not be used after conception as occurred. Several case reports of neural tube defects have been reported ter ovulation stimulation with clomiphene (1–5). However, an association etween the drug and these defects has not been established (6–10). Asch id Greenblatt reviewed the literature and found that the percentage of ongenital anomalies after clomiphene use is no greater than in the normal opulation (59 references) (6). The available studies have not been able to scriminate between a drug effect and the underlying subfertility state (8– 0). Other congenital malformations reported in patients who received clomi- nene prior to conception include (5, 6, 11–23):

Hydatidiform mole
Syndactyly
Pigmentation defects
Congenital heart defects
Down's syndrome
Hypospadias

Retinal aplasia
Clubfoot
Microcephaly
Cleft lip/palate
Ovarian dysplasia
Polydactyly
Hemangioma
Anencephaly

Inadvertent use of clomiphene early in the 1st trimester has been reported 2 patients (17, 23). A ruptured lumbosacral meningomyelocele was bserved in one infant exposed during the 4th week of gestation (17). There vas no evidence of neurological defect in the lower limbs or of ydrocephalus. The second infant was delivered with esophageal atresia vith fistula, congenital heart defects, hypospadius and absent left kidney 23). The mother also took methyldopa throughout pregnancy for mild ypertension.

Patients requiring the use of clomiphene should be cautioned that each ew course of the drug should be started only after pregnancy has been excluded.

* Risk factor X if used after conception has occurred.]

3reast Feeding Summary

Jo data available.

References

1. Barrett C, Hakim C. Anencephaly, ovulation stimulation, subfertility, and illegitimacy. Lancet 1973;2:916–7.
2. Dyson JL, Kohler HG, Anencephaly and ovulation stimulation. Lancet 1973;1:1256–7.
3. Field B, Kerr C. Ovulation stimulation and defects of neural tube closure. Lancet 1974;2;1511.

4. Sandler B. Anencephaly and ovulation stimulation. Lancet 1973;2:379.
5. Biale Y, Leventhal H, Altaras M, Ben-Aderet N. Anencephaly and clomiphene-induce pregnancy. Acta Obstet Gynecol Scand 1978;57:483-4.
6. Asch RH, Greenblatt RB. Update on the safety and efficacy of clomiphene citrate as therapeutic agent. J Reprod Med 1976;17:175-180.
7. Harlap S. Ovulation induction and congenital malformations. Lancet 1976;2:961.
8. James WH, Clomiphene, anencephaly, and spina bifida. Lancet 1977;1:603.
9. Ahlgren M, Kallen B, Rannevik G. Outcome of pregnancy after clomiphene therapy. Acta Obstet Gynecol Scand 1976;55:371-5.
10. Elwood JM. Clomiphene and anencephalic births. Lancet 1974;1:31.
11. Miles PA, Taylor HB, Hill WC. Hydatidiform mole in a clomiphene related pregnancy: a case report. Obstet Gynecol 1971;37:358-9.
12. Schneiderman CI, Waxman B. Clomid therapy and subsequent hydatidiform mole formation a case report. Obstet Gynecol 1972;39:787-8.
13. Wajntraub G, Kamar R, Pardo Y. Hydatidiform mole after treatment with clomiphene. Ferti Steril 1974;25:904.-5
14. Berman P. Congenital abnormalities associated with maternal clomiphene ingestion. Lancet 1975;2:878.
15. Drew AL. Letter to the editor. Dev Med Child Neurol 1974;16:276.
16. Hack M, Brish M, Serr DM, Insler V, Salomy M, Lunenfeld B. Outcome of pregnancy afte induced ovulation. Follow-up of pregnancies and children born after clomiphene therapy JAMA 1972;220:1329-33.
17. Ylikorkala O. Congenital anomalies and clomiphene. Lancet 1975;2:1262-3.
18. Laing IA, Steer CR, Dudgeon J, Brown JK. Clomiphene and congenital retinopathy. Lancet 1981;2:1107-8.
19. Ford WDA, Little KET. Fetal ovarian dysplasia possibly associated with clomiphene. Lancet 1981;2:1107.
20. Kistner RW. Induction of ovulation with clomiphene citrate. Obstet Gynecol Surv 1965;20:873-99.
21. Goldfarb AF, Morales A, Rakoff AE, Protos P. Critical review of 160 clomiphene-related pregnancies. Obstet Gynecol 1968;31:342-5.
22. Oakely GP, Flynt IW. Increased prevalence of Down's syndrome (Mongolism) among the offspring of women treated with ovulation-inducing agents. Teratology 1972;5:264.
23. Singhi M, Singhi S. Possible relationship between clomiphene and neural tube defects. J Pediatr 1978;93:152.

Name: **CLOMIPRAMINE**

Class: **Antidepressant**   Risk Factor: **D**

Fetal Risk Summary

No data available (see Imipramine).

Breast Feeding Summary

No data available (see Imipramine).

Name: **CLOMOCYLINE**

Class: **Antiobiotic**   Risk Factor: **D**

Fetal Risk Summary

See Tetracycline.

Breast Feeding Summary

See Tetracycline.

Name: **CLONAZEPAM**

Class: **Anticonvulsant** Risk Factor: **C**

Fetal Risk Summary

No reports linking the use of clonazepam with congenital defects have been located. Clonazepam is chemically and structurally similar to diazepam (see Diazepam)(1).

Breast Feeding Summary

No data available (see Diazepam).

Reference

1. Reith H, Schafer H. Antiepileptic drugs during pregnancy and the lactation period. Pharmacokinetic data. Dtsch Med Wochenschr 1979;104:818–23.

Name: **CLONIDINE**

Class: **Antihypertensive** Risk Factor: **C**

Fetal Risk Summary

No reports linking the use of clonidine with congenital defects have been located. The drug has been used in the 2nd and 3rd trimesters without adverse fetal effects being observed (1–3). Limited use of clonidine during 1st trimester makes assessment of its safety difficult (1).

Breast Feeding Summary

Animal data indicates clonidine enters breast milk in concentrations exceeding maternal blood (1). Following a 150-μg oral dose, human milk concentrations of 1.5 ng/ml may be achieved (milk:plasma ratio 1.5) (1). The significance of this amount is not known.

References

1. Personal communication, PA Bowers. Boehringer Ingelheim Ltd. 1981.
2. Turnbull AC, Ahmed S. Catapres in the treatment of hypertension in pregnancy, a preliminary study. In *Catapres In Hypertension.* Symposium of the Royal College of Surgeons. London, 1970:237–45.
3. Johnston CI, Aickin DR. The control of high blood pressure during labour with clonidine. Med J Aust 1971;2:132.

Name: **CLOTRIMAZOLE**

Class: **Antifungal Antibiotic**   Risk Factor: **B**

Fetal Risk Summary

No reports linking the use of clotrimazole with congenital defects have been located. The topical use of the drug in pregnancy has been studied (1–4). No adverse effects attributable to clotrimazole were observed.

Breast Feeding Summary

No data available.

References

1. Tan CG, Good CS, Milne LJR, Loudon JDO. A comparative trial of six day therapy with clotrimazole and nystatin in pregnant patients with vaginal candidiasis. Postgrad Med 1974;50(Suppl 1):102–5.
2. Frerich W, Gad A. The frequency of Candida infections in pregnancy and their treatment with clotrimazole. Curr Med Res Opin 1977;4:640–4.
3. Haram K, Digranes A. Vulvovaginal candidiasis in pregnancy treated with clotrimazole. Acta Obstet Gynecol Scand 1978;57:453–5.
4. Svendsen E, Lie S, Gunderson TH, Lyngstad-Vik I, Skuland J. Comparative evaluation of miconazole, clotrimazole and nystatin in the treatment of candidal vulvo-vaginitis. Curr Ther Res 1978;23:666–72.

Name: **CLOXACILLIN**

Class: **Antibiotic**   Risk Factor: **B**

Fetal Risk Summary

Cloxacillin is a penicillin antibiotic (see also Penicillin G). No reports linking its use with congenital defects have been located. The Collaborative Perinatal Project monitored 50,282 mother-child pairs, 3,546 of which had 1st trimester exposure to penicillin derivatives (1). For use anytime during pregnancy, 7,171 exposures were recorded (2). In neither case was evidence found to suggest a relationship to large categories of major or minor malformations or to individual defects.

Breast Feeding Summary

No data available (see Penicillin G).

References

1. Heinonen OP, Slone D, Shapiro S. *Birth Defects and Drugs in Pregnancy*. Littleton: Publishing Sciences Group, 1977;297–313.
2. *Ibid*, 435.

ame: **CODEINE**
lass: **Narcotic Analgesic/Antitussive**   Risk Factor: **C***

etal Risk Summary

he Collaborative Perinatal Project monitored 50,282 mother-child pairs, 563 f which had 1st trimester exposure to codeine (1). No evidence was found to uggest a relationship to large categories of major or minor malformations. ssociations were found with 6 individual defects (1, 2). Only the association ith respiratory malformation is statistically significant. The significance of the ther associations is unknown and independent confirmation is required.

Respiratory (8 cases)
Genitourinary (other than hypospadias) (7 cases)
Down's syndrome (1 case)
Tumors (4 cases)
Umbilical hernia (3 cases)
Inguinal hernia (12 cases)

For use anytime during pregnancy, 2,522 exposures were recorded (3). Vith the same qualifications, possible associations with 4 individual defects ere found (4):

Hydrocephaly (7 cases)
Pyloric stenosis (8 cases)
Umbilical hernia (7 cases)
Inguinal hernia (51 cases)

In an investigation of 1,427 malformed newborns compared to 3,001 ontrols, 1st trimester use of narcotic analgesics (codeine most common) was ssociated with inguinal hernias, cardiac and circulatory system defects, cleft p and palate, dislocated hip and other musculoskeletal defects (5). Second rimester use was associated with alimentary tract defects. In a large retro-pective Finnish study, the use of opiates (mainly codeine) during the 1st rimester was associated with an increased risk of cleft lip and palate (6, 7). inally, a survey of 390 infants with congenital heart disease matched with ,254 normal infants found a higher rate of exposure to several drugs, ncluding codeine, in the offspring with defects (8). Although all 4 of those tudies contain several possible biases that could have affected the results, he data serves a clear warning that indiscriminate use of codeine is not vithout risk to the fetus.

Use of codeine during labor produces neonatal respiratory depression to he same degree as other narcotic analgesics (9). The first known case of eonatal codeine addiction was described in 1965 (10). The mother had taken nalgesic tablets containing 360 to 480 mg of codeine per day for 8 weeks rior to delivery.

A second report described neonatal codeine withdrawal in 2 infants of onaddicted mothers (11). The mother of one infant began consuming a odeine cough medication 3 weeks prior to delivery. Approximately 2 weeks efore delivery, analgesic tablets with codeine were taken at a frequency of p to 6 tablets per day (48 mg of codeine per day). The second mother was treated with a codeine cough medication consuming 90 to 120 mg of codeine per day for the last 10 days of pregnancy. Apgar scores of both infants were 8 to 10 at 1 and 5 minutes. Typical symptoms of narcotic withdrawal were noted in the infants shortly after birth but not in the mothers.

[* Risk Factor D if used for prolonged periods or in high doses at term.]

Breast Feeding Summary

Codeine passes into breast milk in very small amounts (12, 13). This is probably insignificant (14).

References

1. Heinonen OP, Slone D, Shapiro S. *Birth Defects and Drugs in Pregnancy.* Littleton: Publishing Sciences Group, 1977:287–95.
2. *Ibid,* 471.
3. *Ibid,* 434.
4. *Ibid,* 484.
5. Bracken MB, Holford TR. Exposure to prescribed drugs in pregnancy and association with congenital malformations. Obstet Gynecol 1981;58:336–44.
6. Saxen I. Associations between oral clefts and drugs taken during pregnancy. Int J Epidemiol 1975;4;37–44.
7. Saxen I. Epidemiology of cleft lip and palate: an attempt to rule out chance correlations. Br J Prev Soc Med 1975;29:103–10.
8. Rothman KJ, Fyler DC, Goldblatt A, Kreidberg MB. Exogeneous hormones and other drug exposures of children with congenital heart disease. Am J Epidemiol 1979;109:433–9.
9. Bonica JJ. *Principles and Practice of Obstetric Analgesia and Anesthesia.* Philadelphia: FA Davis, 1967:245.
10. Van Leeuwen G, Guthrie R, Stange F. Narcotic withdrawal reaction in a newborn infant due to codeine. Pediatrics 1965;36;635–6.
11. Mangurten HH, Benawra R. Neonatal codeine withdrawal in infants of nonaddicted mothers. Pediatrics 1980;65:159–60.
12. Kwit NT, Hatcher RA. Excretion of drugs in milk. Am J Dis Child 1935;49:900–4.
13. Horning MG, Stillwell WG, Nowlin J, Lertratanangkoon K, Stillwell RN, Hill RM. Identification and quantification of drugs and drug metabolites in human breast milk using GC-MS-COM methods. Mod Probl Paediatr 1975;15:73–9.
14. Anonymous. Drugs in breast milk. Med Lett Drugs Ther 1974;16:25–7.

Name: **COLCHICINE**

Class: **Metaphase Inhibitor**   Risk Factor: **C**

Fetal Risk Summary

The original reports of colchicine cytogenetic effects have not been confirmed with recent studies (1, 2). Human lymphocytic cultures of cells have shown chromosomal damage when exposed to colchicine. No relationship between teratogenic effects and this damage has been established. Use of colchicine by the father prior to conception has been associated with teratogenicity (atypical Down's syndrome) (1). Other investigators were unable to find teratogenic or cytogenetic effects in 19 male and 19 female subjects (3).

Colchicine may or may not cause azoospermia (4, 5). Until colchicine safety is established, the drug should be avoided during the reproductive years.

Breast Feeding Summary

No data available.

References

1. Cestari AN, Vieira Filho JP, Yonenaga Y. A case of human reproductive abnormalities possibly induced by colchicine treatment. Rev Bras Biol 1965;25:253–6.
2. Serreira NR, Buoniconti A. Trisomy after colchicine therapy. Lancet 1968;2:1304.
3. Cohen MM, Levy M, Eliakim M. A cytogenetic evaluation of long-term colchicine therapy in the treatment of familial Mediterranean fever (FMF). Am J Med Sci 1977;274:147–52.
4. Merlin HE. Azoospermia caused by colchicine—a case report. Fertil Steril 1972;23:180–1.
5. Bremer WJ, Paulsen CA. Colchicine and testicular function in man. N Engl J Med 1976;294:1384–5.

Name: **COLISMETHATE**

Class: **Antibiotic**   Risk Factor: **B**

Fetal Risk Summary

No reports linking the use of colismethate with congenital defects have been located. The drug crosses the placenta at term (1).

Breast Feeding Summary

Colismethate is excreted into breast milk. The milk:plasma ratio is 0.17 to 0.18 (2). While this level is low, three potential problems exist for the nursing infant: modification of bowel flora, direct effects on the infant and interference with the interpretation of culture results if a fever work-up is required.

References

1. MacAulay MA, Charles D. Placental transmission of colistimethate. Clin Pharmacol Ther 1967;8:578–86.
2. Wilson JT. Milk/plasma ratios and contraindicated drugs. In Wilson JT, ed. *Drugs in Breast Milk*. Australia: ADIS Press, 1981:78–9.

Name: **CORTICOTROPIN/COSYNTROPIN**

Class: **Corticosteroid Stimulating Hormone**   Risk Factor: **C**

Fetal Risk Summary

Studies reporting the use of corticotropin in pregnancy have not demonstrated adverse fetal effects (1–4). However, corticosteroids have been suspected of causing malformations (see Cortisone). Since corticotropin stimulates the release of endogenous corticosteroids, this relationship should be considered when prescribing the drug to women in their reproductive years.

Breast Feeding Summary

No data available.

References

1. Johnstone FD, Cambell S. Adrenal response in pregnancy to long-acting tetracosactrin. J Obstet Gynaecol Br Commonw 1974;81:363–7.
2. Simmer HH, Tulchinsky D, Gold EM, et al. On the regulation of estrogen production by cortisol and ACTH in human pregnancy at term. Am J Obstet Gynecol 1974;119:283–96.
3. Arai K, Kuwabara Y, Okinaga S. The effect of adrenocorticotropic hormone and dexamethasone, administered to the fetus in utero, upon maternal and fetal estrogens. Am J Obstet Gynecol 1972;113:316–22.
4. Potert AJ. Pregnancy and adrenalcortical hormones. Br Med J 1962;2:967–72.

Name: **CORTISONE**

Class: **Corticosteroid**   Risk Factor: **D**

Fetal Risk Summary

Cortisone is often used during pregnancy; therefore reports of congenital defects are reflective of a much greater utilization of cortisone and not necessarily of a more potent teratogen than other glucocorticoids (see Prednisolone, Betamethasone, Dexamethasone, Corticotropin). The Collaborative Perinatal Project monitored 50,282 mother-child pairs, 34 of which had 1st trimester exposure to cortisone (1). No evidence of a relationship to congenital malformations was found. There have been 35 other reported cases of 1st trimester exposures in which congenital defects were observed in 9 infants (2–7). The congenital defects observed include: cataracts, cyclopia, interventricular septal defect, gastroschisis, hydrocephalus, cleft lip, coarctation of the aorta, clubfoot and undescended testicles. Concern has been expressed that neonatal adrenal hyperplasia or insufficiency may result from maternal corticosteroid administration (8, 9).

Breast Feeding Summary

No data available.

References

1. Heinonen OP, Slone D, Shapiro S. Birth Defects and Drugs in Pregnancy. Littleton: Publishing Sciences Group, 1977:389, 391.
2. Kraus AM. Congenital cataract and maternal steroid ingestion. J Pediatr Ophthal 1975;12:107.
3. Khudr G, Olding L. Cyclopia. Am J Dis Child 1973;125:102.
4. deVilliers DM. Kortisoon swangerskap en die ongebore kind. S Afr Med J 1967;41:781–2.
5. Malaps P. Foetal malformation and cortisone therapy. Br Med J 1965;1:795.
6. Harris JWS, Poss IP. Cortisone therapy in early pregnancy: Relation to cleft plate. Lancet 1956;1:1045–7.
7. Wells CN. Treatment of hyperemesis gravidarium with cortisone. I. Fetal results. Am J Obstet Gynecol 1953;66:598–601.

3. Unpublished data. Freeman RK, Women's Hospital, Memorial Medical Center, Long Beach, 1982.
9. Sidhu RK, Hawkins DF. Corticosteroids. Clin Obstet Gynecol 1981;8:383–404.

Name: **COUMARIN DERIVATIVES**

Class: **Anticoagulant**   Risk Factor: **D**

Fetal Risk Summary

Substantial evidence has accumulated that use of coumarin derivatives during pregnancy may result in significant problems for the fetus. Hall, Pauli and Wilson have recently reviewed this subject (167 references) (1). Since this review, two additional case reports have appeared (2, 3). The principal problems confronting the fetus are:

Embryopathy (fetal warfarin syndrome)
Central nervous system defects
Spontaneous abortion
Stillbirth
Prematurity
Hemorrhage

First trimester use of coumarin derivatives has resulted in 32 known cases of the fetal warfarin syndrome (FWS) (1–3). The common characteristics of the FWS are nasal hypoplasia due to failure of development of the nasal septum and strippled epiphyses. The bridge of the nose is depressed resulting in a flattened, upturned appearance. Other features which may be present are:

Birth weight less than 10th percentile for gestational age
Eye defects (blindness, optic atrophy, microphthalmia when drug used
in 2nd and/or 3rd trimesters as well)
Development retardation
Laryngeal calcification
Scoliosis
Deafness/hearing loss
Congenital heart disease
Death

The critical period of exposure, based on Hall's review, seems to be the 6th through the 9th weeks of gestation. All of the known cases of FWS were exposed during at least a portion of these weeks. Exposure outside of the 1st trimester carries the risk of central nervous system defects. No constant grouping of abnormalities were observed nor was there an apparent correlation between time of exposure and the defects, except that all fetuses were exposed in the 2nd and/or 3rd trimesters. Some of the malformations could be related to hemorrhage, but two nonbleeding related patterns were identified by Hall:

Dorsal midline dysplasia characterized by agenesis of corpus callosum,
Dandy-Walker malformations and midline cerebellar atrophy; enceph-
aloceles may be present
Ventral midline dysplasia characterized by optic atrophy (eye anomalies)
ies)
Other features of non-1st trimester exposure are:
Mental retardation

Spasticity
Seizures
Deafness
Scoliosis
Growth failure
Death

Long term effects in the child with central nervous system defects are more significant and debilitating than those from the fetal warfarin syndrome (1).

Fetal Outcome Following *In Utero* Exposure to Coumarin Derivatives (1–7)

Trimester Exposed	No. Pts.	Normal Terms	FWS Term	Premature Normal	Died	Bleed	Other Problems	Spont. Abort.	CNS Defects	Stillborn No Bleed	Bleed	FWS Plus CNS Defects	Term Bleed	G
1 1 + 3 1 +3	75	24 (32%)	4 (5%)	4 (5%)	2 (3%)	—	2 (3%)	33 (44%)	2 (3%)	2 (3%)	—	2 (3%)	—	
2 2 + 3 3	157	115 (73%)	—	1 (1%)	—	2 (1%)	7 (4%)	2 (1%)	2 (1%)	16 (10%)	3 (2%)	—	4 (3%)	
All trimesters	162	119 (73%)	10 (6%)	2 (1%)	3 (2%)	2 (1%)	2 (1%)	NA	3 (2%)	7 (4%)	4 (2%)	7 (4%)	3 (2%)	
Not specified	41	38 (93%)	—	1 (2%)	—	—	1 (2%)	1 (2%)	—	—	—	—	—	
Total	435	296 (68%) (68%)	14 (3%)	8 (2%)	5 (1%)	4 (1%)	12 (3%)	36 (8%)	7 (2%)	25 (6%)	7 (2%)	9 (2%)	7 (2%)	

* Length of gestation not specified.

Congenital abnormalities that do not fit the pattern of the FWS or central nervous system defects have been observed in 9 infants (2%) (1). Hall identifies these as incidental malformations that are probably not related to the use of coumarin derivatives.

Asplenia, 2-chambered heart, agenesis of pulmonary artery
Anencephaly, spina bifida, congenital absence of clavicles
Congenital heart disease, death
Fetal distress, focal motor seizures
Bilateral polydactyly
Congenital corneal leukoma
Nonspecified multiple defects
Asplenia, congenital heart disease, incomplete rotation of gut, short broad phalanges, hypoplastic nails
Single kidney, toe defects, other anomalies, death

In summary, the use of oral anticoagulants during pregnancy carries with it a significant risk to the fetus. For all cases, only about 70% will be expected to result in a normal, full term infant. If the maternal condition requires use of these agents, consideration should be given to the termination of the pregnancy.

Breast Feeding Summary

Excretion of coumarin derivatives into breast milk is dependent on the agent used. Two reports on warfarin have been located (8, 9). As shown in the table below, warfarin does not appear to pose a major risk to the breast-fed infant. Ethyl biscoumacetate and dicumarol also do not appear to pass into the breast milk in significant quantities (10, 11). However in one report, 5 of 42 infants had bleeding problems following maternal consumption of ethyl biscoumacetate (12). An unidentified metabolite was found in the milk which may have led to the high complication rate. In a 1970 case report, a massive scrotal hematoma in a baby shortly after herniotomy was concluded to be secondary to phenindione obtained from the mother's milk (13). The baby required blood transfusions and vitamin K. The passage of phenindione has also been demonstrated by assay (14).

Author (ref)	No. Pts.	Dose	Concentrations (μg/ml)		M:P Ratio	Effect on Infant
			Serum	Milk		
Orme (8)	13	2–12 mg/day	1.6–8.5 (μmol/l)	0	—	No warfarin detected in serum of 7 infants; no effect on bleeding time in 3 of 3 infants
de Swiet (9)	13	Not stated	—	—	—	No warfarin detected in infants' serum; no effect on bleeding time
Illingworth (10)	4	600–1200 mg/ day for 6–19 days	—	Peak 1.69 (0.09 to 1.69)	—	13 of 38 samples contained bis-coumacetate; no adverse effects in 22 babies
Brambel (11)	125	200 mg initially, then titrated to response	—	—	—	No adverse effect on infants' prothrombin time—mothers taking dicumarol
	1500	—	—	—	—	No adverse effects in infants—mothers taking dicumarol
Gostof (12)	42	Not stated	—	—	—	Bleeding in 5 infants—mothers taking ethyl biscoumacetate
Eckstein (13)	1	50 mg a.m., 25 or 50 mg in p.m.	—	—	—	Massive scrotal hematoma—mother taking phenindione
Goguel (14)	—	25, 50, or 75 mg × 1 (phenindione)	—	1–5 after 50- or 75-mg doses; 18 of 68 samples contained drug after 25 mg	—	—

References

1. Hall JG, Pauli RM, Wilson KM. Maternal and fetal sequelae of anticoagulation during pregnancy. Am J Med 1980;68:122–40.
2. Baillie M, Allen ED, Elkington AR. The congenital warfarin syndrome: a case report. Br J Ophthalmol 1980;64:633–5.
3. Harrod MJE, Sherrod PS. Warfarin embryopathy in siblings. Obstet Gynecol 1981;57:673–6.

4. Russo R, Bortolotti U, Schivazappa L, Girolami A. Warfarin treatment during pregnancy: a clinical note. Haemostasis 1979;8:96–8.
5. Biale Y, Cantor A, Lewenthal H, Gueron M. The course of pregnancy in patients with artificial heart valves treated with dipyridamole. Int J Gynaecol Obstet 1980;18:128–32.
6. Moe N. Anticoagulant therapy in the prevention of placental infarction and perinatal death. Obstet Gynecol 1981;59:481–3.
7. Kaplan LC, Anderson GG, Ring BA. Congenital hydrocephalus and Dandy-Walker malformation associated with warfarin use during pregnancy. Birth Defects 1982;18:79–83.
8. Orme ML'E, Lewis PJ, de Swiet M, et al. May mothers given warfarin breast-feed their infants? Br Med J 1977;1:1564–5.
9. de Swiet M, Lewis PJ. Excretion of anticoagulants in milk. N Engl J Med 1977;297:1471.
10. Illingworth RS, Finch E. Ethyl biscoumacetate (Tromexan) in human milk. J Obstet Gynaecol Br Commonw 1959;66:487–8.
11. Brambel CE, Hunter RE. Effect of dicumarol on the nursing infant. Am J Obstet Gynecol 1950;59:1153–9.
12. Gostof, Momolka, Zilenka. Les substances derivees du tromexane dans le lait maternel et leurs actions paradoxales sur la prothrombine. Schweiz Med Wochenschr 1952;30:764–5. In Daily JW. Anticoagulant and cardiovascular drugs. In Wilson JT, ed. Drugs in Breast Milk. Australia: ADIS Press, 1981: 63.
13. Eckstein HB, Jack B. Breas-feeding and anticoagulant therapy. Lancet 1970;1:672–3.
14. Goguel M, Noël G, Gillet JY. Therapeutique anticoagulante et allaitement: etude du passage de la phenyl-2-dioxo,1,3 indane dans le lait maternel. Rev Fr Gynecol Obstet 1970;65:409–12. In Anderson PO. Drugs and breast feeding—a review. Drug Intell Clin Pharmacol 1977;11:208–23.

Name: **CYCLACILLIN**

Class: **Antibiotic**   Risk Factor: **B**

Fetal Risk Summary

Cyclacillin is a penicillin antibiotic (see also Penicillin G). No reports linking its use with congenital defects have been located. The Collaborative Perinatal Project monitored 50,282 mother-child pairs, 3,546 of which had 1st trimester exposure to penicillin derivatives (1). For use anytime during pregnancy, 7,171 exposures were recorded (2). In neither case was evidence found to suggest a relationship to large categories of major or minor malformations or to individual defects.

Breast Feeding Summary

No data available (see Penicillin G).

References

1. Heinonen OP, Slone D, Shapiro S. Birth Defects and Drugs in Pregnancy. Littleton: Publishing Sciences Group, 1977:297–313.
2. Ibid, 435.

Name: **CYCLAMATE**

Class: **Sweetener** Risk Factor: **C**

Fetal Risk Summary

Controlled studies of the effects of cyclamate on the fetus are lacking. The drug crosses the placenta obtaining fetal blood levels about 25% of that found in the mother (1). Cyclamate has been suspected of producing cytogenetic effects in human lymphocytes (2). One group of investigators attempted to associate these effects with an increased incidence of malformations and behavioral problems, but a cause and effect relationship was not established (3).

Breast Feeding Summary

No data available.

References

1. Pitkin RM, Reynolds WA, Filer LJ. Placental transmission and fetal distribution of cyclamate in early human pregnancy. Am J Obstet Gynecol 1970;108:1043–50.
2. Bauchinger M. Cytogenetic effect of cyclamate on human peripheral lymphocytes in vivo. Dtsch Med Wochenschr 1970;95:2220–3.
3. Stone D, Matalka E, Pulaski B. Do artificial sweeteners ingested in pregnancy affect the offspring? Nature 1971;231:53.

Name: **CYCLANDELATE**

Class: **Vasodilator** Risk Factor: **C**

Fetal Risk Summary

No data available.

Breast Feeding Summary

No data available.

Name: **CYCLAZOCINE**

Class: **Narcotic Antagonist** Risk Factor: **D**

Fetal Risk Summary

Cyclazocine is not available in the United States. In addition to its ability to reverse narcotic overdose, it has been used in the treatment of narcotic dependence (1). Its actions are similar to nalorphine (see also Nalorphine).

Breast Feeding Summary

No data available.

References

1. Wade A. ed. *Martindale. The Extra Pharmacopoeia*, 27th ed. London:Pharmaceutical Press, 1977:985.

Name: **CYCLIZINE**

Class: **Antihistamine/Antiemetic**   Risk Factor: **B**

Fetal Risk Summary

Cyclizine is a piperazine antihistamine which is used as an antiemetic (see also Buclizine and Meclizine for closely related drugs). The drug is teratogenic in animals but apparently not in humans. In 111 patients given cyclizine during the 1st trimester, no increased malformation rate was observed (1). Similarly, the Collaborative Perinatal Project found no association between 1st trimester cyclizine use and congenital defects although the 15 exposed patients were small compared to the total sample (2). The FDA's OTC Laxative Panel acting on this data concluded that cyclizine is not teratogenic (3). In 1974, investigators searching for an association between antihistamines and oral clefts found no relationship between this defect and the cyclizine group (4). Finally, a retrospective study in 1971 found significantly fewer infants with malformations were exposed to antihistamines/antiemetics in the 1st trimester as compared to controls (5). Cyclizine was the fifth most commonly used antiemetic.

Breast Feeding Summary

No data available.

References

1. Milkovich L, Van den Berg BJ. An evaluation of the teratogenicity of certain antinauseant drugs. Am J Obstet Gynecol 1976;125:244–8.
2. Heinonen OP, Slone D, Shapiro S. *Birth Defects and Drugs in Pregnancy*. Littleton: Publishing Sciences Group, 1977:323.
3. Anonymous. Meclizine; cyclizine not teratogenic. Pink Sheets. F.D.C. Reports 1974:T&G-2.
4. Saxen I. Cleft palate and maternal diphenhydramine intake. Lancet 1974;1:407–8.
5. Nelson MM, Forfar JO. Associations between drugs administered during pregnancy and congenital abnormalities of the fetus. Br Med J 1971;1:523–7.

Name: **CYCLOPENTHIAZIDE**

Class: **Diuretic**   Risk Factor: **D**

Fetal Risk Summary

See Chlorothiazide.

Breast Feeding Summary

See Chlorothiazide.

Name: **CYCLOPHOSPHAMIDE**

Class: **Antineoplastic**   Risk Factor: **D**

Fetal Risk Summary

Cyclophosphamide is an alkylating antineoplastic agent. Both normal and malformed newborns have been reported following the use in pregnancy of cyclophosphamide (1–11). Six malformed infants have resulted from 1st trimester exposure (1–4). Data on 3 of these infants are shown in the table below. Pancytopenia occurred in a 1000-g male infant exposed to cyclophosphamide and 5 other antineoplastic agents in the 3rd trimester (10). Data from one review indicated that 40% of the infants exposed to anticancer drugs were of low birth weight (12). This finding was not related to the timing of exposure. Use of cyclophosphamide in the 2nd and 3rd trimesters does not seem to place the fetus at risk for congenital defects. However, long term studies of growth and mental development in offspring exposed to cyclophosphamide during the 2nd trimester, the period of neuroblast multiplication, have not been conducted (13).

The long term effects of cyclophosphamide on male and female germinal epithelium function are unknown (14, 15). Successful pregnancies have been reported following high dose therapy with this agent (16–18). Of interest, however, is a report associating paternal use of cyclophosphamide and 3 other antineoplastics prior to conception with congenital anomalies in an infant (see table below) (19). Cyclophosphamide is one of the most common causes of chemotherapy-induced irregular menses, amenorrhea, and azoospermia (14, 17, 18, 20–23). Azoospermia appears to be reversible when the drug is stopped (20–24). Chromosome abnormalities have been demonstrated in patients treated with cyclophosphamide for rheumatoid arthritis and scleroderma (25). Changes in chromosomal structure may lead to an increased incidence of malformations in future offspring.

Cyclophosphamide

Author (ref)	No. Pts.	Indica- tion	Gestational Age	Dose	Other Drugs	Fetal Effects	Comments
Greenberg (1)	1	Hodgkin's	Throughout	Various IV/PO*	Radiation	Four toes each foot Palate defect Flattened nasal bridge Skin tag Hypoplastic middle phalanx 5th finger Bilateral inguinal hernia sacs	
Toledo (2)	1	Hodgkin's	1st tri- mester	Various IV/PO	Radiation	Toes missing Single coronary ar- tery	
Coates (3)	1	Nephrotic syndrome	1st tri- mester	150 mg/day	Not stated	Hemangioma Umbilical hernia	
Russell (19)	1	Myelogenous leukemia in father	Father— prior to conception	Not stated	Cytarabine Daunorubicin Thioguanine	Fallot's tetralogy Syndactyly of 1st and 2nd digits right foot	A 2nd patient in this re- port ex- posed to other three agents but not cyclo- phospham- ide

* IV, intravenously, PO, orally.

Breast Feeding Summary

Cyclophosphamide is excreted into breast milk (26). Although the concentra- tions were not specified, the drug was found in milk up to 6 hours after a single 500-mg IV dose. The mother was not nursing.

References

1. Greenberg LH, Tanaka KR. Congenital anomalies probably induced by cyclophosphamide. JAMA 1964;188:423–6.
2. Toledo TM, Harper RC, Moser RH. Fetal effects during cyclophosphamide and irradiation therapy. Ann Intern Med 1971;74:87–91.
3. Coates A. Cyclophosphamide in pregnancy. Aust NZ J Obstet Gynaecol 1970;10:33–4.
4. Sweet DL, Kinzie J. Consequences of radiotherapy and antineoplastic therapy for the fetus. J Rep Med 1976;17:241–6.
5. Lasher MJ, Geller W. Cyclophosphamide and vinblastine sulfate in Hodgkin's disease during pregnancy. JAMA 1966;195:486–8.
6. Lergier JE, Jimenez E, Maldonado N, Veray F. Normal pregnancy in multiple myeloma treated with cyclophosphamide. Cancer 1974;34:1018–22.
7. Garcia V, San Miguel J, Borrasca AL. Doxorubicin in the first trimester of pregnancy. Ann Intern Med 1981;94:547.
8. Lowenthal RM, Funnell CF, Hope DM, Stewart IG, Humphrey DC. Normal infant after combination chemotherapy including teniposide for Burkitt's lymphoma in pregnancy. Med Pediatr Oncol 1982;10:165–9.
9. Daly H, McCann SR, Hanratty TD, Temperley IJ. Successful pregnancy during combination chemotherapy for Hodgkin's disease. Acta Haematol (Basel) 1980;64:154–6.
10. Pizzuto J, Aviles A, Noriega L, Niz J, Morales M, Romero F. Treatment of acute leukemia during pregnancy: presentation of nine cases. Cancer Treat Rep 1980;64:679–83.
11. Sears HF, Reid J. Granulocytic sarcoma: local presentation of a systemic disease. Cancer 1976;37:1808–13.

12. Nicholson HO. Cytotoxic drugs in pregnancy: review of reported cases. J Obstet Gynaecol Br Commonw 1968;75:307–12.
13. Dobbing J. Pregnancy and leukaemia. Lancet 1977:1:1155.
14. Schilsky RL, Lewis BJ, Sherins RJ, Young RC. Gonadal dysfunction in patients receiving chemotherapy for cancer. Ann Intern Med 1980;93:109–14.
15. Stewart BH. Drugs that cause and cure male infertility. Drug Ther 1975;5(No. 12):42–8.
16. Card RT, Holmes IH, Sugarman RG, Storb R, Thomas D. Successful pregnancy after high dose chemotherapy and marrow transplantation for treatment of aplastic anemia. Exp Hematol 1980;8:57–60.
17. Schwartz PE, Vidone RA. Pregnancy following combination chemotherapy for a mixed germ cell tumor of the ovary. Gynecol Oncol 1981;12:373–8.
18. Bacon C, Kernahan J. Successful pregnancy in acute leukaemia. Lancet 1975;2:515.
19. Russell JA, Powles RL, Oliver RTD. Conception and congenital abnormalities after chemotherapy of acute myelogenous leukaemia in two men. Br Med J 1976;1:1508.
20. Qureshji MA, Pennington JH, Goldsmith HJ, Cox PE. Cyclophosphamide therapy and sterility. Lancet 1972;2:1290–1.
21. George CRP, Evans RA. Cyclophosphamide and infertility. Lancet 1972;1:840–1.
22. Sherins RJ, DeVita VT Jr. Effect of drug treatment for lymphoma on male reproductive capacity. Ann Intern Med 1973;79:216–20.
23. Lendon M, Palmer MK, Hann IM, Shalet SM, Jones PHM. Testicular histology after combination chemotherapy in childhood for acute lymphoblastic leukaemia. Lancet 1978;2:439–41.
24. Hinkes E, Plotkin D. Reversible drug-induced sterility in a patient with acute leukemia. JAMA 1973;223:1490–1.
25. Tolchin SF, Winkelstein A, Rodnan GP, Pan SF, Nankin HR. Chromosome abnormalities from cyclophosphamide therapy in rheumatoid arthritis and progressive systemic sclerosis (scleroderma). Arthritis Rheum 1974;17:375–82.
26. Wiernik PH, Duncan JH. Cyclophosphamide in human milk. Lancet 1971;1:912.

Name: **CYCLOTHIAZIDE**

Class: **Diuretic**   Risk Factor: **D**

Fetal Risk Summary

See Chlorothiazide.

Breast Feeding Summary

See Chlorothiazide.

Name: **CYCRIMINE**

Class: **Parasympatholytic**   Risk Factor: **C**

Fetal Risk Summary

Cycrimine is an anticholinergic agent used in the treatment of parkinsonism. No reports of its use in pregnancy have been located (see also Atropine).

Breast Feeding Summary

No data available (see also Atropine).

Name: **CYPROHEPTADINE**

Class: **Antihistamine/Antiserotonin**   Risk Factor: **B**

Fetal Risk Summary

Cyproheptadine has been used as a serotonin antagonist to prevent habitual abortion in patients with increased serotonin production (1, 2). No congenital defects were observed when the drug was used in this manner. A 1980 case report described the use of cyproheptadine, 12 mg daily, to treat Cushing's syndrome in a 31-year-old patient (3). The drug was continued throughout a subsequent pregnancy. An apparently healthy 3010-g boy was delivered at 33 to 34 weeks gestation. After 4 months of normal development, the boy developed gastroenteritis and died. In a second patient with Cushing's syndrome, cyproheptadine was used for successful treatment (4). A normal pregnancy occurred approximately 2 years after treatment was stopped resulting in the birth of a healthy male infant.

Breast Feeding Summary

No data available.

References

1. Sadovsky E, Pfeifer Y, Polishuk WZ, Sulman FG. A trial of cyproheptadine in habitual abortion. Isr J Med Sci 1972;8:623–5.
2. Sadovsky E. Prevention of hypothalamic habitual abortion by Periactin. Harefuah 1970; 78:332–3, As reported in JAMA 1970;212:1253.
3. Kasperlik-Zaluska A, Migdaska B, Hartwig W, et al. Two pregnancies in a women with Cushing's syndrome treated with cyproheptadine. Br J Obstet Gynaecol 1980;87:1171–3.
4. Griffith DN, Ross EJ. Pregnancy after cyproheptadine treatment for Cushing's disease. N Engl J Med 1981;305:893–4.

Name: **CYTARABINE**

Class: **Antineoplastic**   Risk Factor: **D**

Fetal Risk Summary

Normal infants have resulted following *in utero* exposure to cytarabine during all stages of gestation (1–16). However, use during the 1st and 2nd trimesters has been associated with congenital and chromosomal abnormalities (see table below) (17–19). Congenital anomalies have also been associated with paternal use of cytarabine prior to conception by allegedly damaging the germ but without producing infertility (see table below) (20). Cytarabine may produce reversible azoospermia in males (21, 22). In addition, male fertility has been demonstrated during maintenance therapy with cytarabine (23). Pancytopenia was observed in a 1000-g male infant exposed to cytarabine and five other antineoplastic agents during the 3rd trimester (11). Data from one review indicated that 40% of the infants exposed to anticancer drugs were of low birth weight (24). This finding was not related to the timing of exposure. Long term studies of growth and mental development in offspring exposed to cytarabine during the 2nd trimester, the period of neuroblast multiplication, have not been conducted (25).

Author (ref)	No. Pts.	Indication	Gestational Age	Dose	Other Drugs	Fetal Effects	Comments
Maurer (17)	1	Myelogenous leukemia	2nd trimester	100 mg per M^2 IV*	Thioguanine	Elective abortion at 24 weeks Trisomy for group C autosomes without mosaicism	2nd pregnancy occurred on same therapy and no abnormal chromosomes
Wagner (18)	1	Lymphocytic leukemia	1st trimester	Not stated	Multiple antineoplastics prior to conception	Bilateral microtia Bilateral atresia of external auditory canals Right hand lobster claw; 3 digits Bilateral lower limb defects	
Schafer (19)	1	Myeloblastic leukemia	Throughout	160 mg/day for 5 days each month	Thioguanine	Two medial digits of both feet missing Distal phalanges of both thumbs missing with hypoplastic remnant of right thumb	Normal infants before and after case infant
Russell (20)	2	Myelogenous leukemia in 2 fathers	Fathers—prior to conception	Not stated	Daunorubicin Thioguanine Cyclophosphamide	1 Fallot's tetralogy Syndactyly of 1st and 2nd digits right foot 1 stillborn anencephalic	

*intravenously.

Breast Feeding Summary

No data available.

References

1. Pawliger DF, McLean FW, Noyes WD. Normal fetus after cytosine arabinoside therapy. Ann Intern Med 1971;74:1012.
2. Au-Yong R, Collins P, Young JA. Acute myeloblastic leukemia during pregnancy. Br Med J 1972;4:493–4.
3. Raich PC, Curet LB. Treatment of acute leukemia during pregnancy. Cancer 1975;36:861–2.
4. Gokal R, Durrant J, Baum JD, Bennett MJ. Successful pregnancy in acute monocytic leukaemia. Br J Cancer 1976;34:299–302.
5. Sears HF, Reid J. Granulocytic sarcoma: local presentation of a systemic disease. Cancer 1976;37:1808–13.
6. Durie BGM, Giles HR. Successful treatment of acute leukemia during pregnancy. Arch Intern Med 1977;137:90–1.

7. Lilleyman JS, Hill AS, Anderton KJ. Consequences of acute myelogenous leukemia in early pregnancy. Cancer 1977;40:1300–3.

8. Moreno H, Castleberry RP, McCann WP. Cytosine arabinoside and 6-thioguanine in the treatment of childhood acute myeloblastic leukemia. Cancer 1977;40:998–1004.

9. Newcomb M, Balducci L, Thigpen JT, Morrison FS. Acute leukemia in pregnancy: successful delivery after cytarabine and doxorubicin. JAMA 1978;239:2691–2.

10. Manoharan A, Leyden MJ. Acute non-lymphocytic leukaemia in the third trimester of pregnancy. Aust NZ J Med 1979;9:71–4.

11. Pizzuto J, Aviles A, Noriega L, Niz J, Morales M, Romero F. Treatment of acute leukemia during pregnancy: presentation of nine cases. Cancer Treat Rep 1980;64:679–83.

12. Colbert N, Najman A, Gorin NC, et al. Acute leukaemia during pregnancy: favourable course of pregnancy in two patients treated with cytosine arabinoside and anthracyclines. Nouv Presse Med 1980;9:175–8.

13. Tobias JS, Bloom HJG. Doxorubicin in pregnancy. Lancet 1980;1:776.

14. Taylor G, Blom J. Acute leukemia during pregnancy. South Med J 1980;73:1314–5.

15. Dara P, Slater LM, Armentrout SA. Successful pregnancy during chemotherapy for acute leukemia. Cancer 1981;47:845–6.

16. Plows CW. Acute myelomonocytic leukemia in pregnancy: report of a case. Am J Obstet Gynecol 1982;143:41–3.

17. Maurer LH, Forcier RJ, McIntyre OR, Benirschke K. Fetal group C trisomy after cytosine arabinoside and thioguanine. Ann Intern Med 1971;75:809–10.

18. Wagner VM, Hill JS, Weaver D, Baehner RL. Congenital abnormalities in baby born to cytarabine treated mother. Lancet 1980;2:98–9.

19. Schafer AI. Teratogenic effects of antileukemic chemotherapy. Arch Intern Med 1981;141:514–5.

20. Russell JA, Powles RL, Oliver RTD. Conception and congenital abnormalities after chemotherapy of acute myelogenous leukaemia in two men. Br Med J 1976;1:1508.

21. Lendon M, Palmer MK, Hann IM, Shalet SM, Jones PHM. Testicular histology after combination chemotherapy in childhood for acute lymphoblastic leukaemia. Lancet 1978;2:439–41.

22. Lilleyman JS. Male fertility after successful chemotherapy for lymphoblastic leukaemia. Lancet 1979;2:1125.

23. Matthews JH, Wood JK. Male fertility during chemotherapy for acute leukemia. N Engl J Med 1980;303:1235.

24. Nicholson HO. Cytotoxic drugs in pregnancy: review of reported cases. J Obstet Gynaecol Br Commonw 1968;75:307–12.

25. Dobbing J. Pregnancy and leukaemia. Lancet 1977;1:1155.

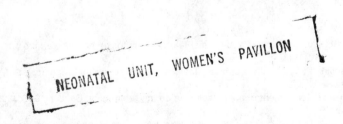

Name: **DACARBAZINE**
Class: **Antineoplastic**

Risk Factor: **D**

Fetal Risk Summary

No data available.

Breast Feeding Summary

No data available.

Reference

1. Personal communication. Lonergan RC. Miles Pharmaceuticals. 1981.

Name: **DACTINOMYCIN**
Class: **Antineoplastic**

Risk Factor: **D**

Fetal Risk Summary

Dactinomycin is an antimitotic antineoplastic agent. Normal pregnancies have followed the use of this drug prior to conception (1–4). Only one report of its use during pregnancy has been located (5). In this case, dactinomycin was administered during the 2nd trimester and apparently normal twins were delivered. Data from one review indicated that 40% of the infants exposed to anticancer drugs were of low birth weight (5). This finding was not related to the timing of exposure. Long term studies of growth and mental development in offspring exposed to dactinomycin and other antineoplastic drugs during the 2nd trimester, the period of neuroblast multiplication, have not been conducted (6).

Breast Feeding Summary

No data available.

References

1. Ross GT. Congenital anomalies among children born of mothers receiving chemotherapy for gestational trophoblastic neoplasms. Cancer 1976;37:1043–7.
2. Walden PAM, Bagshawe KD. Pregnancies after chemotherapy for gestational trophoblastic tumours. Lancet 1979;2:1241.

3. Schwartz PE, Vidone RA. Pregnancy following combination chemotherapy for a mixed germ cell tumor of the ovary. Gynecol Oncol 1981;12:373–8.
4. Pastorfide GB, Goldstein DP. Pregnancy after hydatidiform mole. Obstet Gynecol 1973;42:67–70.
5. Nicholson HO. Cytotoxic drugs in pregnancy: review of reported cases. J Obstet Gynaecol Br Commonw 1968;75:307–12.
6. Dobbing J. Pregnancy and leukaemia. Lancet 1977;1:1155.

Name: **DANTHRON**

Class: **Purgative**   Risk Factor: **C**

Fetal Risk Summary

Danthron is an anthraquinone purgative (see Cascara Sagrada).

Breast Feeding Summary

No data available (see Cascara Sagrada).

Name: **DAUNORUBICIN**

Class: **Antineoplastic**   Risk Factor: **D**

Fetal Risk Summary

The use of daunorubicin during pregnancy has been reported in 6 patients, 2 during the 1st trimester (1–5). No congenital defects were observed in the 5 liveborns and 1 electively aborted 20-week fetus. Data from one review indicated that 40% of the infants exposed to anticancer drugs were of low birth weight (6). This finding was not related to timing of the exposure. Long term studies of growth and mental development in offspring exposed to anticancer drugs during the 2nd trimester, the period of neuroblast multiplication, have not been conducted (7). Use of daunorubicin and other antineoplastic drugs in 2 males was associated with congenital defects in their offspring (see table below) (8). The authors speculated the drugs damaged the germ cells without producing infertility. In a third male, fertilization occurred during treatment with daunorubicin and resulted in the birth of a healthy infant (9). Successful pregnancies have also been reported in 2 women after treatment with daunorubicin (10).

Author (ref)	No. Pts.	Indication	Gestational Age	Dose	Other Drugs	Fetal Effects	Comments
Russell (8)	2	Myelogenous leukemia in 2 fathers	Fathers— Prior to conception	Not stated	Cytarabine Cyclophos- phamide Thioguanine	1 Fallot's tetralogy Syndactyly of 1st and 2nd digits, right foot 1 stillborn anencephalic	

Breast Feeding Summary

No data available.

References

1. Sears HF, Reid J. Granulocytic sarcoma: local presentation of a systemic disease. Cancer 1976;37:1808–13.
2. Lilleyman JS, Hill AS, Anderton KJ. Consequences of acute myelogenous leukemia in early pregnancy. Cancer 1977;40:1300–3.
3. Colbert N, Najman A, Gorin NC, et al. Acute leukaemia during pregnancy: favourable course of pregnancy in two patients treated with cytosine arabinoside and anthracyclines. Nouv Presse Med 1980;9:175–8.
4. Tobias JS, Bloom HJG. Doxorubicin in pregnancy. Lancet 1980;1:776.
5. Sanz MA, Rafecas FJ. Successful pregnancy during chemotherapy for acute promyelocytic leukemia. N Engl J Med 1982;306:939.
6. Nicholson HO. Cytotoxic drugs in pregnancy: review of reported cases. J Obstet Gynaecol Br Commonw 1968;75:307–12.
7. Dobbing J. Pregnancy and leukaemia. Lancet 1977;1:1155.
8. Russell JA, Powles RL, Oliver RTD. Conception and congenital abnormalities after chemotherapy of acute myelogenous leukaemia in two men. Br Med J 1976;1:1508.
9. Matthews JH, Wood JK. Male fertility during chemotherapy for acute leukemia. N Engl J Med 1980;303:1235.
10. Estiu M. Successful pregnancy in leukaemia. Lancet 1977;1:433.

Name: DECAMETHONIUM
Class: **Muscle Relaxant**   Risk Factor: **C**

Fetal Risk Summary

Decamethonium is no longer manufactured in the United States. No reports linking the use of decamethonium with congenital defects have been located. The drug has been used at term for maternal analgesia (1).

Breast Feeding Summary

No data available.

Reference

1. Moyn F, Thorndyke V. Passage of drugs across the placenta. Am J Obstet Gynecol 1962;84:1778–98.

Name: DEMECARIUM
Class: **Parasympathomimetic (Cholinergic)**   Risk Factor: **C**

Fetal Risk Summary

Demecarium is used in the eye. No reports of its use in pregnancy have been located. As a quaternary ammonium compound, it is ionized at physiologic pH and transplacental passage in significant amounts would not be expected (see also Neostigmine).

Breast Feeding Summary

No data available.

Name: **DEMECLOCYCLINE**

Class: **Antibiotic**   Risk Factor: **D**

Fetal Risk Summary

See Tetracycline.

Breast Feeding Summary

See Tetracycline.

Name: **DESIPRAMINE**

Class: **Antidepressant**   Risk Factor: **C**

Fetal Risk Summary

Desipramine is an active metabolite of imipramine (see also Imipramine). No reports linking the use of desipramine with congenital defects have been located. Neonatal withdrawal symptoms including cyanosis, tachycardia, diaphoresis and weight loss were observed after desipramine was taken throughout the pregnancy (1).

Breast Feeding Summary

Desipramine enters breast milk in low concentrations (2, 3). No reports of adverse effects have been located.

Author (ref)	No. Pts.	Dose	Concentrations (μg/ml)		M:P Ratio	Effect on Infant
			Serum	Milk		
Sovner (2)	1		41	17–35	0.4–0.9	Not stated

References:

1. Webster PA. Withdrawal symptoms in neonates associated with maternal antidepressant therapy. Lancet 1973;2:318–9.
2. Sovner R, Orsulak PJ. Excretion of imipramine and desipramine in human breast milk. Am J Psychiatry 1979;136:451–2.
3. Erickson SH, Smith GH, Heidrich F. Tricyclics and breast feeding. Am J Psychiatry 1979;136:1483.

Name: **DESLANOSIDE**
Class: **Cardiac Glycoside**   Risk Factor: **B**

Fetal Risk Summary
See Digitalis.

Breast Feeding Summary
See Digitalis.

Name: **DESMOPRESSIN**
Class: **Pituitary Hormone, Synthetic**   Risk Factor: **B**

Fetal Risk Summary
Desmopressin is a synthetic polypeptide structurally related to vasopressin.
See Vasopressin.

Breast Feeding Summary
See Vasopressin.

Name: **DEXAMETHASONE**
Class: **Corticosteroid**   Risk Factor: **C**

Fetal Risk Summary
No reports linking the use of dexamethasone with congenital defects have
been located. Other corticosteroids have been suspected of causing malformations (see Cortisone). Maternal free estriol and cortisol are significantly
depressed after dexamethasone therapy, but the effects of these changes on
the fetus have not been studied (1–3). Dexamethasone has been used in
patients with premature labor at about 26 to 34 weeks gestation to stimulate
fetal lung maturation (4–12). The benefits of this therapy are:
  Reduction in incidence of respiratory distress syndrome (RDS)
  Decreased severity of RDS if it occurs
  Decreased incidence of and mortality from intracranial hemorrhage
  Increased survival of premature infants
  Toxicity in the fetus and newborn following the use of dexamethasone is
rare. Leukocytosis was observed in a 840-g, 27-weeks' gestation male infant
whose mother received her last dose of dexamethasone (12 mg every 12
hours for 7 doses) 2.5 days before delivery (13). The WBC count returned to

normal in about one week. Although human studies have usually shown a benefit, the use of corticosteroids in animals has been associated with several toxic effects: (14, 15)

Reduced fetal head circumference
Reduced fetal adrenal weight
Increased fetal liver weight
Reduced fetal thymus weight
Reduced placental weight

Fortunately, none of these effects have been observed in human investigations. Long term follow-up of children exposed to dexamethasone in utero have not been conducted. Studies of children whose mothers were given betamethasone (a similar corticosteroid) have not shown an adverse effect on growth or mental development (see also Betamethasone) (16).

Breast Feeding Summary

No data available.

References

1. Reck G, Nowostawski, Bredwoldt M. Plasma levels of free estriol and cortisol under ACTH and dexamethasone during late pregnancy. Acta Endocrinol 1977;84:86–7.
2. Kauppilla A. ACTH levels in maternal, fetal and neonatal plasma after short term prenatal dexamethasone therapy. Br J Obstet Gynaecol 1977;84:128–34.
3. Warren JC, Cheatum SG. Maternal urinary estrogen excretion: effect of adrenal suppression. J Clin Endocrinol 1967;27:436–8.
4. Caspi I, Schreyer P, Weinraub Z, Reif R, Levi I, Mundel G. Changes in amniotic fluid lecithin-sphingomyelin ratio following maternal dexamethasone administration. Am J Obstet Gynecol 1975;122:327–31.
5. Spellacy WN, Buhi WC, Riggall FC, Holsinger KL. Human amniotic fluid lecithin/sphingo-myelin ratio changes with estrogen or glucocorticoid treatment. Am J Obstet Gynecol 1973;115:216–8.
6. Caspi E, Schreyer P, Weinraub Z, Reif R, Levi I, Mundel G. Prevention of the respiratory distress syndrome in premature infants by antepartum glucocorticoid therapy. Br J Obstet Gynaecol 1976;83:187–93.
7. Ballard RA, Ballard PL. Use of prenatal glucocorticoid therapy to prevent respiratory distress syndrome. Am J Dis Child 1976;130:982–7.
8. Thornfeldt RE, Franklin RW, Pickering NA, Thornfeldt CR, Amell G. The effect of glucocorti-coids on the maturation of premature lung membranes: preventing the respiratory distress syndrome by glucocorticoids. Am J Obstet Gynecol 1978;131:143–8.
9. Ballard PL, Ballard RA. Corticosteroids and respiratory distress syndrome: status 1979. Pediatrics 1979;63:163–5.
10. Taeusch HW Jr, Frigoletto F, Kitzmiller J, et al. Risk of respiratory distress syndrome after prenatal dexamethasone treatment. Pediatrics 1979;63:64–72.
11. Caspi E, Schreyer P, Weinraub Z, Lifshitz Y, Goldberg M. Dexamethasone for prevention of respiratory distress syndrome: multiple perinatal factors. Obstet Gynecol 1981;57:41–7.
12. Bishop EH. Acceleration of fetal pulmonary maturity. Obstet Gynecol 1981;58(Suppl):48S–51S.
13. Otero L, Conlon C, Reynolds P, Duval-Arnould B, Golden SM. Neonatal leukocytosis asso-ciated with prenatal administration of dexamethasone. Pediatrics 1981;68:778–80.
14. Taeusch HW Jr. Glucocorticoid prophylaxis for respiratory distress syndrome: a review of potential toxicity. J Pediatr 1975;87:617–23.
15. Johnson JWC, Mitzner W, London WT, Palmer AE, Scott R. Betamethasone and the rhesus fetus: multisystemic effects. Am J Obstet Gynecol 1979;133:677–84.

5. MacArthur BA, Howie RN, Dezoete JA, Elkins J. Cognitive and psychosocial development of 4-year-old children whose mothers were treated antenatally with betamethasone. Pediatrics 1981;68:638–43.

Name: DEXBROMPHENIRAMINE

Class: **Antihistamine**   Risk Factor:**C**

Fetal Risk Summary

Dexbrompheniramine is the *dextro-* isomer of brompheniramine (see Brompheniramine). No reports linking its use with congenital defects have been located.

Breast Feeding Summary

See Brompheniramine.

Name: DEXCHLORPHENIRAMINE

Class: **Antihistamine**   Risk Factor: **B$_M$**

Fetal Risk Summary

Dexchlorpheniramine is the *dextro-* isomer of chlorpheniramine (see also Chlorpheniramine). No reports linking its use with congenital defects have been located. One study recorded 14 exposures in the 1st trimester without evidence for an association with malformations (1). Animal studies for chlorpheniramine have not shown a teratogenic effect (2).

Breast Feeding Summary

No data available.

References

1. Heinonen OP, Slone D, Shapiro S. *Birth Defects and Drugs in Pregnancy.* Littleton: Publishing Sciences Group, 1977:323.
2. Product information. Polaramine. Schering Corporation, 1982.

Name: DEXTROAMPHETAMINE

Class: **Central Stimulant**   Risk Factor: **D**

Fetal Risk Summary

Contrasting reports on the safety of dextroamphetamine in pregnancy have appeared (1–7). Congenital defects that have been associated with dextro-

amphetamine include cardiac abnormalities, exencephaly, microcephaly and
biliar atresia. Amphetamine withdrawal syndrome has been described in a
neonate whose mother was self-administering excessive doses of intravenous
(IV) amphetamine (8). In contrast, another case report failed to demonstrate
any neonatal effects from the treatment of narcolepsy with large doses of
amphetamine (7). Except for the possible indication of narcolepsy, the use of
the drug during pregnancy is not recommended.

Author (ref)	No. Pts.	Indica-tion	Gestational Age	Dose	Other Drugs	Fetal Effects	Comment
Worsham (1)	184	Not stated	Not stated	Not stated	Not stated	Congenital heart disease 11% (controls 3%)	
Gilbert (2)	1	Appetite suppres-sant	Throughout	Not stated	Not stated	Atrial ventricular defect	
Malera (3)	1	Appetite suppres-sant	Throughout	20–30 mg/day	Chlorothiazide FeSO$_4$	Bifid exencephalia Hypotonia	
Levin (4)	5	Not stated	2nd tri-mester	Not stated	Phenobarbital ASA Oral contra-ceptive Diuretic	Biliary atresia	
Ramar (8)	1	Drug abuse	Throughout	250 mg IV every 6 hr	Not stated	Amphetamine with-drawal syn-drome	

Breast Feeding Summary

Data of the passage of dextroamphetamine into breast milk is lacking. Neonatal
insomnia or stimulation was not observed in 103 nursing infants whose
mothers were taking various amounts of the drug (9).

References

1. Nora JJ, Vargo T, Nora A. Dextroamphetamine: a possible environmental trigger of cardio-vascular malformations. Lancet 1970;1:1290–1.
2. Gilbert E, Khoury G. Dextroamphetamine and congenital cardiac malformations. J Pediatr 1970;76:638.
3. Matera R, Zablal H, Jimenez A. Bifid exencephalia: teratogen action of amphetamines. Int Surg 1968;50:79–85.
4. Levin J. Amphetamine ingestion with biliary atresia. J Pediatr 1971;79:130–1.
5. Nora JJ, McNamara DG, Frazer FC. Dextroamphetamine sulphate and human malformations. Lancet 1967;1:570–1.
6. Milkovich L, van den Berg BJ. Effects of antenatal exposure to anorectic drugs. Am J Obstet Gynecol 1977;129:637–42.
7. Briggs GG, Samson JH, Crawford DJ. Lack of abnormalities in a newborn exposed to amphetamine during gestation. Am J Dis Child 1975;129:249–50.
8. Ramer CM. The case of an infant born to an amphetamine addicted mother. Clin Pediatr (Phila) 1974;13:596–7.
9. Ayd FJ. Excretion of psychotropic drugs in human milk. Int Drug Ther News Bull 1973;8:33–40.

ame: **DIAZEPAM**

lass: **Sedative**   Risk Factor: **D**

etal Risk Summary

iazepam and its metabolite, *n*-demethyldiazepam, freely cross the placenta
nd accumulate in the fetal circulation (1–9). The plasma half-life in newborns
 significantly increased due to a decreased clearance of the drug. Because
ie transplacental passage is rapid, timing of the intravenous administration
ith uterine contractions will greatly reduce the amount of drug transferred to
ie fetus (6).

An association between diazepam and an increased risk of cleft lip and/or
alate has been suggested by three studies (10–12). The findings indicated
st or 2nd trimester use of diazepam, and selected other drugs, is significantly
reater among mothers of children born with oral clefts. Other studies have
ot found this association with diazepam (13). In an investigation of 1,427
ialformed newborns compared to 3,001 controls, 1st trimester use of tran-
uilizers (diazepam most common) was associated with inguinal hernia, car-
iac defects and pyloric stenosis (14). Second trimester exposure was asso-
iated with hemangiomas and cardiac and circulatory defects. The combina-
on of cigarette smoking and tranquilizer use increased the risk of delivering
 malformed infant by 3.7-fold as compared to those who smoked but did not
se tranquilizers (14). A survey of 390 infants with congenital heart disease
iatched with 1,254 normal infants found a higher rate of exposure to several
rugs, including diazepam, in the offspring with defects (15). Although these
tudies contained several possible biases that could have affected the results,
ie data serves as a clear warning against indiscriminate use of diazepam
uring gestation. Other congenital anomalies reported in infants exposed to
iazepam include (16–18):

    Absence of both thumbs (2 cases)
    Spina bifida (1 case)
    Absence of left forearm, syndactyly (1 case)

Many investigators have observed that the use of diazepam during labor is
ot harmful to the mother or her infant (19–26). A dose-response is likely as
ie frequency of newborn complications rises when doses exceed 30 to 40
ig or when diazepam is taken for extended periods allowing accumulation to
ccur (27–33).

Two major syndromes of neonatal complications have been observed:

    Floppy infant syndrome:
      hypotonia
      lethargy
      sucking difficulties
    Withdrawal syndrome:
      intrauterine growth retardation
      tremors

irritability
hypertonicity
diarrhea/vomiting
vigorous sucking

Under miscellaneous effects, diazepam may alter thermogenesis, cause loss of beat-to-beat variability in the fetal heart rate and decrease fetal movements (34–39).

Breast Feeding Summary

Diazepam and its metabolite, n-demethyldiazepam, enter breast milk (40–44). Lethargy and loss of weight have been reported (43). Milk: plasma ratios are varied. Diazepam may accumulate in breast-fed infants so its use in lactating women is not recommended.

Author (ref)	No. Pts.	Dose	Concentrations (μg/ml) Serum	Milk	M:P Ratio	Effect on Infant
van Geijn (40)	Not stated	15–60 mg/ 24 hr	0.5–2.0	0.03–0.5	—	Not stated
Cole (42)	9	Not stated	Varied	—	0.2–2.7	None observed
Patrick (43)	1	90 mg/ 24 hr	—	Not detected	—	Infant lethargic and lost 170 g weight during 24 hours Urine positive for diazepam and oxazepam Infant EEG showed bursts of rapid activity compatible with sedative medication
Catz (44)	Not stated		—	0.078	—	Infant serum contained 0.074 μg/ml of diazepam Asymptomatic

References

1. Erkkola R, Kanto J, Sellman R. Diazepam in early human pregnancy. Acta Obstet Gynecol Scand 1974;53:135–8.
2. Kanto J, Erkkola R, Sellman R. Accumulation of diazepam and n-demethyldiazepam in the fetal blood during labor. Ann Clin Res 1973;5:375–9.
3. Idanpaan-Heikkila JE, Jouppila PI, Puolakka JO, Vorne MS. Placental transfer and fetal metabolism of diazepam in early human pregnancy. Am J Obstet Gynecol 1971;109:1011–6.
4. Mandelli M, Morselli PL, Nordio S, Pardi G, Principi N. Sereni F, Tognoni G. Placental transfer of diazepam and its disposition in the newborn. Clin Pharmacol Ther 1975;17:564–72.
5. Gamble JAS, Moore J, Lamke H, Howard PJ. A study of plasma diazepam levels in mother and infant. Br J Obstet Gynaecol 1977;84:588–91.
6. Haram K, Bakke DM, Johannessen KH, Lund T. Transplacental passage of diazepam during labor: influence of uterine contractions. Clin Pharmacol Ther 1978;24:590–9.
7. Bakke OM, Haram K, Lygre T, Wallem G. Comparison of the placental transfer of thiopental and diazepam in caesarean section. Eur J Clin Pharmacol 1981;21:221–7.
8. Haram K, Bakke OM. Diazepam as an induction agent for caesarean section: a clinical and pharmacokinetic study of fetal drug exposure. Br J Obstet Gynaecol 1980;87:506–12.
9. Kanto JH. Use of benzodiazepines during pregnancy, labour and lactation, with particular reference to pharmacokinetic considerations. Drugs 1982;23:354–80.
10. Safra JM, Oakley GP. Association between cleft lip with or without cleft palate and neonatal exposure to diazepam. Lancet 1975;2:478–80.
11. Saxen I. Epidemiology of cleft lip and palate. Br J Prev Soc Med 1975;29:103–10.
12. Saxen I. Associations between oral clefts and drugs taken during pregnancy. Int J Epidemiol 1975;4:37–44.

3. Czeizel A. Diazepam, phenytoin, and etiology of cleft lip and/or cleft palate. Lancet 1976;1:810.

4. Bracken MB, Holford TR. Exposure to prescribed drugs in pregnancy and association with congenital malformations. Obstet Gynecol 1981;58:336–44.

5. Rothman KJ, Fyler DC, Goldblatt A, Kreidberg MB. Exogenous hormones and other drug exposures of children with congenital heart disease. Am J Epidemiol 1979;109:433–9.

6. Istvan EJ. Drug-associated congenital abnormalities. Can Med Assoc J 1970;103:1394.

7. Ringrose CAD. The hazard of neurotrophic drugs in the fertile years. Can Med Assoc J 1972;106:1058.

8. Fourth Annual Report of the New Zealand Committee on Adverse Drug Reactions. NZ Med J 1969;70:118–22.

9. Greenblatt DJ, Shader RI. Effect of benzodiazepines in neonates. N Engl J Med 1975;292:649.

0. Modif M, Brinkman CR, Assali NS. Effects of diazepam on uteroplacental and fetal hemodynamics and metabolism. Obstet Gynecol 1973;41:364–8.

1. Toaff ME, Hezroni J, Toaff R. Effect of diazepam on uterine activity during labor. Isr J Med Sci 1977;13:1007–9.

2. Shannon RW, Fraser GP, Aitken RG, Harper JR. Diazepam in preeclamptic toxaemia with special reference to its effect on the newborn infant. Br J Clin Pract 1972;26:271–5.

3. Yeh SY, Paul RIT, Cordero L, Hon EH. A study of diazepam during labor. Obstet Gynecol 1974;43:363–73.

4. Kasturilal, Shetti RN. Role of diazepam in the management of eclampsia. Curr Ther Res 1975;18:627–30.

5. Eliot BW, Hill JG, Cole AP, Hailey DM. Continuous pethidine/diazepam infusion during labor and its effects on the newborn. Br J Obstet Gynaecol 1975;82:126–31.

6. Lean TH, Retnam SS, Sivasamboo R. Use of benzodiazepines in the management of eclampsia. J Obstet Gynaecol Br Commonw 1968;75:856–62.

7. Scanlon JW. Effect of benzodiazepines in neonates. N Engl J Med 1975;292:649.

8. Gillberg C. "Floppy infant syndrome" and maternal diazepam. Lancet 1977;2:244.

9. Haram K. "Floppy infant syndrome" and maternal diazepam. Lancet 1977;2:612–3.

0. Speight AN. Floppy-infant syndrome and maternal diazepam and/or nitrazepam. Lancet 1977;1:878.

1. Rementeria JL, Bhatt K. Withdrawal symptoms in neonates from intrauterine exposure to diazepam. J Pediatr 1977;90:123–6.

2. Thearle MJ, Dunn PM. Exchange transfusions for diazepam intoxication at birth followed by jejunal stenosis. Proc R Soc Med 1973;66:13–4.

3. Backes CR, Cordero L. Withdrawal symptoms in the neonate from presumptive intrauterine exposure to diazepam: report of case. JAOA 1980;79:584–5.

4. Cree JE, Meyer J, Hailey DM. Diazepam in labour: its metabolism and effect on the clinical condition and thermogenesis of the newborn. Br Med J 1973;4:251–5.

5. McAllister CB. Placental transfer and neonatal effects of diazepam when administered to women just before delivery. Br J Anaesth 1980;52:423–7.

6. Owen JR, Irani SF, Blair AW. Effect of diazepam administered to mothers during labour on temperature regulation of neonate. Arch Dis Child 1972;47:107–10.

7. Scher J, Hailey DM, Beard RW. The effects of diazepam on the fetus. J Obstet Gynaecol Br Commonw 1972;79:635–8.

8. van Geijn HP, Jongsma HW, Doesburg WH, Lemmens WA, deHaan J, Eskes TK. The effect of diazepam administration during pregnancy or labor on the heart rate variability of the newborn infant. Eur J Obstet Gynaecol Reprod Biol 1980;10:187–201.

9. Birger M, Homberg R, Insler V. Clinical evaluation of fetal movements. Int J Gynaecol Obstet 1980;18:377–82.

0. van Geijn HP, Kenemans P, Vise T, Vanderkleijn E, Eskes TK. Pharamcokinetics of diazepam and occurrence in breast milk. Proceedings of the Sixth International Congress of Pharmacology, Helsinki 1975:514.

1. Hill RM, Nowlin J, Lertratanangkoon K, Stillwell WG, Stillwell RN, Horning MG. The identification and quantification of drugs in human breast milk. Clin Res 1974;22:77A.

42. Cole AP, Hailey DM. Diazepam and active metabolite in breast milk and their transfer to the neonate. Arch Dis Child 1975; 50:741–2.
43. Patrick MJ, Tilstone WJ, Reavey P. Diazepam and breast-feeding. Br Med J 1972;1:542–3.
44. Catz CS. Diazepam in breast milk. Drug Ther 1973;3:72–3.

Name: **DIAZOXIDE**

Class: **Antihypertensive**   Risk Factor: **C**

Fetal Risk Summary

Diazoxide readily crosses the placenta and reaches fetal plasma concentrations similar to maternal levels (1). The drug has been used for the treatment of severe hypertension associated with pregnancy (1–11). Some investigators have cautioned against the use of diazoxide in pregnancy (12, 13). In one study, the decrease in maternal blood pressure was sufficient to produce a state of clinical shock and endanger placental perfusion (12). Transient fetal bradycardia has been reported in other studies following a rapid, marked decrease in maternal blood pressure (7, 14). Fatal maternal hypotension has been reported in one patient after diazoxide therapy (15). Thien has recommended the infusion technique for administering diazoxide rather than rapid boluses to prevent maternal and fetal complications (16).

Diazoxide is a potent relaxant of uterine smooth muscle and may inhibit uterine contractions if given during labor (2, 3, 5–7, 17–19). The degree and duration of uterine inhibition are dose-dependent (18). Augmentation of labor with oxytocin may be required in patients receiving diazoxide.

Hyperglycemia in the newborn (glucose 500–700 mg/dl) secondary to intravenous diazoxide therapy in a mother just prior to delivery has been observed to persist up to 3 days (20). Neuman found hyperglycemia, without ketoacidosis, in all of the mothers and newborns in his series (12). The glucose levels returned to near normal within 24 hours. The use of oral diazoxide for the last 19 to 69 days of pregnancy has been associated with alopecia, hypertrichosis lanuginosa and decreased ossification of the wrist (1). However, long term oral therapy has not caused similar problems in other newborns exposed *in utero* (4).

Since other anithypertensive drugs are available for severe maternal hypertension, and the long term effects on the infant have not been evaluated, diazoxide should be used with caution, if at all, during pregnancy. If diazoxide is needed after other therapies have failed, small doses, preferably by continuous infusion, are recommended.

Breast Feeding Summary

No data available.

References

1. Milner RDG, Chouksey SK. Effects of fetal exposure to diazoxide in man. Arch Dis Child 1972;47:537–43.
2. Finnerty FA JR, Kakaviatos N, Tuckman J, Magill J. Clinical evaluation of diazoxide: a new treatment for acute hypertension. Circulation 1963;28:203–8.
3. Finnerty FA Jr. Advantages and disadvantages of furosemide in the edematous states of pregnancy. Am J Obstet Gynecol 1969;105:1022–7.
4. Pohl JEF, Thurston H, Davis D, Morgan MY. Successful use of oral diazoxide in the treatment of severe toxaemia of pregnancy. Br Med J 1972;2:568–70.
5. Pennington JC, Picker RH. Diazoxide and the treatment of the acute hypertensive emergency in obstetrics. Med J Aust 1972;2:1051–4.
6. Koch-Weser J. Diazoxide. N Engl J Med 1976;294:1271–4.
7. Morris JA, Arce JJ, Hamilton CJ, et al. The management of severe preeclampsia and eclampsia with intravenous diazoxide. Obstet Gynecol 1977;49:675–80.
8. Keith TA III. Hypertension crisis: recognition and management. JAMA 1977;237:1570–7.
9. MacLean AB, Doig JR, Aickin DR. Hypovolaemia, pre-eclampsia and diuretics. Br J Obstet Gynaecol 1978;85:597–601.
10. Barr PA, Gallery ED. Effect of diazoxide on the antepartum cardiotocograph in severe pregnancy-associated hypertension. Aust NZ J Obstet Gynaecol 1981;21:11–5.
11. MacLean AB, Doig JR, Chatfield WR, Aickin DR. Small-dose diazoxide administration in pregnancy. Aust NZ J Obstet Gynaecol 1981;21:7–10.
12. Neuman J, Weiss B, Rabello Y, Cabal L, Freeman RK. Diazoxide for the acute control of severe hypertension complicating pregnancy: a pilot study. Obstet Gynecol 1979;53(Suppl):50S–5S.
13. Perkins RP. Treatment of toxemia of pregnancy. JAMA 1977;238:2143–4.
14. Michael CA. Intravenous diazoxide in the treatment of severe preeclamptic toxaemia and eclampsia. Aust NZ J Obstet Gynaecol 1973;13:143–6.
15. Henrich WL, Cronin R, Miller PD, Anderson RJ. Hypotensive sequelae of diazoxide and hydralazine therapy. JAMA 1977;237:264–5.
16. Thien T, Koene RAP, Schijf C, Pieters GFFM, Eskes TKAB, Wijdeveld PGAB. Infusion of diazoxide in severe hypertension during pregnancy. Eur J Obstet Gynaecol Reprod Biol 1980;10:367–74.
17. Barden TP, Keenan WJ. Effects of diazoxide in human labor and the fetus-neonate. (Abstract) Obstet Gynecol 1971;37:631–2.
18. Landesman R, Adeodato de Souza FJ, Countinho EM, Wilson KH, Bomfim de Sousa FM. The inhibitory effect of diazoxide in normal term labor. Am J Obstet Gynecol 1969;103:430–3.
19. Paulissian R. Diazoxide. Int Anesthesiol Clin 1978;16:201–36.
20. Milsap RL, Auld PAM. Neonatal hyperglycemia following maternal diazoxide administration. JAMA 1980;243:144–5.

Name: **DIBENZEPIN**

Class: **Antidepressant**   Risk Factor: **D**

Fetal Risk Summary

No data available (see Imipramine).

Breast Feeding Summary

No data available (see Imipramine).

Name: **DICLOXACILLIN**

Class: **Antibiotic**   Risk Factor: **B**

Fetal Risk Summary

Dicloxacillin is a penicillin antibiotic (see also Penicillin G). The drug crosses the placenta into the fetal circulation and amniotic fluid. Levels are low compared to other penicillins due to the high degree of maternal protein binding (1, 2). Following a 500-mg intravenous dose, the fetal peak serum level of 3.4 μg/ml occurred at 2 hours (8% of maternal peak) (2). A peak of 1.8 μg/ml was obtained at 6 hours in the amniotic fluid.

No reports linking the use of dicloxacillin with congenital defects have been located. The Collaborative Perinatal Project monitored 50,282 mother-child pairs, 3,546 of which had 1st trimester exposure to penicillin derivatives (3). For use anytime in pregnancy, 7,171 exposures were recorded (4). In neither case was evidence found to suggest a relationship to large categories of major or minor malformations or to individual defects.

Breast Feeding Summary

No data available (see Penicillin G).

References

1. MacAulay M, Berg S, Charles D. Placental transfer of dicloxacillin at term. Am J Obstet Gynecol 1968;102:1162–8.
2. Depp R, Kind A, Kirby W, Johnson W. Transplacental passage of methicillin and dicloxacillin into the fetus and amniotic fluid. Am J Obstet Gynecol 1970;107:1054–7.
3. Heinonen OP, Slone D, Shapiro S. Birth Defects and Drugs in Pregnancy. Littleton: Publishing Sciences Group, 1977;297–313.
4. Ibid, 435.

Name: **DICUMAROL**

Class: **Anticoagulant**   Risk Factor: **D**

Fetal Risk Summary

See Coumarin Derivatives.

Breast Feeding Summary

See Coumarin Derivatives.

Name: **DICYCLOMINE**
Class: **Parasympatholytic**   Risk Factor: **B**

Fetal Risk Summary

See Doxylamine.

Breast Feeding Summary

See Doxylamine.

Name: **DIENESTROL**
Class: **Estrogenic Hormone**   Risk Factor: **D**

Fetal Risk Summary

Dienestrol is used topically. Estrogens are readily absorbed and intravaginal use can lead to significant concentrations of estrogen in the blood (1, 2). The Collaborative Perinatal Project monitored 614 mother-child pairs with 1st trimester exposure to estrogenic agents, including 36 with exposure to dienestrol (3). An increase in the expected frequency of cardiovascular, eye and ear, and Down's syndrome was found (4). An increased risk of malformations due to 1st trimester exposure to dienestrol was not found. Use of estrogenic hormones during pregnancy is not recommended (see Oral Contraceptives).

Breast Feeding Summary

No reports of adverse effects of dienestrol on the nursing infant have been located. It is theoretically possible that systemic effects of decreased milk volume and decreased nitrogen and protein content could occur (see Mestranol, Ethinylestradiol).

References:

1. Gilman AG, Goodman LS, Gilman A. *The Pharmacological Basis of Therapeutics.* New York: MacMillan, 1980:1428.
2. Rigg LA, Hermann H, Yen SSC. Absorption of estrogens from vaginal creams. N Engl J Med 1978;298:195–7.
3. Heinonen OP, Slone D, Shapiro S. *Birth Defects and Drugs in Pregnancy.* Littleton: Publishing Sciences Group, 1977:389, 391.
4. *Ibid*, 395.

Name: **DIETHYLPROPION**

Class: **Central Stimulant/Anorectant**   Risk Factor: **B**

Fetal Risk Summary

No reports linking the use of diethylpropion with congenital defects have been located. The drug has been studied as an appetite suppressant in 28 pregnant patients and although adverse effects were common in the women, no problems were observed in their offspring (1). A retrospective survey of 1,232 patients exposed to diethylpropion during pregnancy found no difference in the incidence of defects (0.9%) when compared to a matched control group (1.1%) (2). Animal studies have not revealed a teratogenic potential (3).

Breast Feeding Summary

No data available.

References

1. Silverman M, Okun R. The use of an appetitie suppressant (diethylpropion hydrochloride) during pregnancy. Curr Ther Res 1971;13:648–53.
2. Bunde CA, Leyland HM. A controlled retrospective survey in evaluation of teratogenicity. J New Drugs 1965;5:193–8.
3. Schardein JL. Drugs as Teratogens. Cleveland: CRC Press, 1976:73–5.

Name: **DIETHYLSTILBESTROL**

Class: **Estrogenic Hormone**   Risk Factor: **X**

Fetal Risk Summary

Substantial evidence has accumulated that the use of diethylstilbestrol (DES) during pregnancy may result in significant problems for both male and female offspring. Several authors have recently reviewed this subject (125 references) (1–5). Approximately 4 to 6 million women were treated with DES to prevent reproductive problems such as miscarriage, premature delivery, intrauterine fetal death and toxemia (1, 2, 6).

Controlled studies have sinced proven that DES was not successful in preventing these disorders (5). The problems identified with in utero exposure to DES are:

Female Offspring
　　Anatomic abnormalities
　　　　Lower mullerian tract
　　　　　　Adenosis and clear cell adenocarcinoma
　　　　　　Cervicovaginal structure defects
　　　　　　　　Collars, hoods, septa and cockscombs
　　　　　　　　Cervical mucus effects
　　　　　　　　Cervical stenosis
　　　　　　　　Cervical incompetence

Upper mullerian tract
  Uterine structural defects
  Fallopian tube structural defects
Male Offspring
  Anatomic abnormalities
  Reproductive dysfunction
  Altered semen analysis
  Infertility

A registry to study the epidemiological, clinical and pathological aspects of clear cell adenocarcinoma of the vagina and cervix in DES-exposed women was established in 1971 (2). Over 400 cases of clear cell adenocarcinoma have been reported to the registry. Analysis of these cases has suggested that the risk of carcinoma may be higher when DES treatment was given before the 12th week of pregnancy (2). The risk of developing clear cell adenocarcinoma in a DES-exposed female is between 0.14 and 1.4 per 1,000 (about 4.5 to 14 times greater than in non-exposed women).

Reports linking the use of DES with major dysmorphogenic defects have not been located. The Collaborative Perinatal Project monitored 614 mother-child pairs with 1st trimester exposure to estrogenics, including 164 with exposure to DES (7). Evidence for an increase in the expected frequency for cardiovascular defects, eye and ear anomalies, and Down's syndrome was found (8). However, no evidence was discovered for an increased risk with DES. A number of authors have discussed the epithelial and structural genital alterations in DES-exposed female offspring (2, 3, 5, 6, 9–12). Gross abnormalities of the cervix and vagina have been reported in 22% to 58% of DES-exposed women (5). These epithelial changes as well as alterations of the body of the uterus have led to concern regarding the possibility of increased pregnancy wastage and premature births (4, 10, 13–16). Increased rates of spontaneous abortions, premature births and ectopic pregnancies are well established by these latter reports, although the relationship to the abnormal changes of the cervix and/or vagina is still unclear (4). Serial observations of cervicovaginal adenosis in 173 DES-exposed women have been described (12). The evidence suggests that the adenosis is a dynamic lesion that may disappear with time.

Adverse effects of *in utero* exposure to DES for the male offspring have been reported (1, 5, 17–22). Abnormalities noted to occur at greater frequencies in DES-exposed males include:
  Epididymal cysts
  Hypotrophic testis
  Microphallus
  Variococele
  Capsular induration
  Altered semen (decreased count, concentration, motility and morphology)

An increase in problems with passing urine and urogenital tract infections has also been observed (17). Recent data have suggested that *in utero* DES exposure may adversely affect male fertility (1). It is not known if the decreased fertility is a transient phenomenon. Changes in the psychosexual performance of boys has been attributed to *in utero* exposure to DES and progesterone

(23, 24). The mothers received estrogen/progestogen regimens for diabetes. A trend to less heterosexual experience and fewer masculine interests than controls was shown. Use of DES during pregnancy is contraindicated.

Breast Feeding Summary

No data available. It is theoretically possible that decreased milk volume and decreased nitrogen and protein content could occur (see Mestranol, Ethinyl Estradiol).

References

1. Stenchever MA, Williamson RA, Leonard J, Karp LE, Ley B, Shy K, Smith D. Possible relationship between in utero diethylstilbestrol exposure and male fertility. Am J Obstet Gynecol 1981;140:186-93.
2. Herbst AL. Diethylstilbestrol and other sex hormones during pregnancy. Obstet Gynecol 1981;58(Suppl):35s-40s.
3. Prins RP, Morrow P, Townsend DE, Disaia PJ. Vaginal embryogenesis, estrogens, and adenosis. Obstet Gynecol 1976;48:246-50.
4. Sandberg EC, Riffle NL, Higdon JV, Getman CE. Pregnancy outcome in women exposed to diethylstilbestrol in utero. Am J Obstet Gynecol 1981;140:194-205.
5. Stillman RJ. In utero exposure to diethylstilbestrol: adverse effects on the reproductive tract and reproductive performance in male and female offspring. Am J Obstet Gynecol 1982; 142:905-21
6. Nordquist SAB, Medhat IA, Ng AB. Teratogenic effects of intrauterine exposure to DES in female offspring. Comp Ther 1979;5:69-74.
7. Heinonen OP, Slone D, Shapiro S. *Birth Defects and Drugs in Pregnancy.* Littleton: Publishing Sciences Group, 1977:389,91.
8. *Ibid*, 395.
9. Ben-Baruch G, Menczer J, Mashiach S, Serr DM. Uterine anomalies in diethylstilbestrol-exposed women with fertility disorders. Acta Obstet Gynecol Scand 1981;60:395-7.
10. Pillsbury SG. Jr. Reproductive significance of changes in the endometrial cavity associated with exposure in utero in diethylstilbestrol. Am J Obstet Gynecol 1980;137:178-82.
11. Professional and Public Relations Committee of the diethylstilbestrol and adenosis project of the Division of Cancer Control and Rehabilitation. Exposure in utero to diethylstilbestrol and related synthetic hormones. Association with vaginal and cervical cancers and other abnormalities. JAMA 1976;236:1107-9.
12. Burke L, Antonioli D, Friedman EA. Evolution of diethylstilbestrol-associated genital tract lesions. Obstet Gynecol 1981;57:79-84.
13. Herbst AL, Hubby MM, Blough RR, Azizi F. A comparison of pregnancy experience in DES-exposed daughters. J Reprod Med 1980;24:62-9.
14. Barnes AB, Colton T, Gundersen J, et al. Fertility and outcome of pregnancy in women exposed in utero to diethylstilbestrol. N Engl J Med 1980;302:609-13.
15. Veridiano NP, Dilke I, Rogers J, Tancer ML. Reproductive performance of DES-exposed female progeny. Obstet Gynecol 1981;58:58-61.
16. Mangan CE, Borow L, Burnett-Rubin MM, et al. Pregnancy outcome in 98 women exposed to diethylstilbestrol in utero, their mothers, and unexposed siblings. Obstet Gynecol 1982; 59:315-9.
17. Henderson BE, Benton B, Cosgrove M, et al. Urogenital tract abnormalities in sons of women treated with diethylstilbestrol. Pediatrics 1976;58:505-7.
18. Gill WB, Schumacher GFB, Bibbo M. Pathological semen and anatomical abnormalities of the genital tract in human male subjects exposed to diethylstilbestrol in utero. J Urol 1977;117:477-80.
19. Gill WB, Schumacher GFB, Bibbo M, Strous FH, Schoenberh HW. Association of diethylstilbestrol exposure in utero with cryptorchidism, testicular hypoplasia and semen abnormalities. J Urol 1979;122:36-9.

20. Gill WB, Schumacher GFB, Bibbo M. Structural and functional abnormalities in the sex organs of male offspring of mothers treated with diethylstilbestrol (DES). J Reprod Med 1976;16:147–53.
21. Driscoll SG, Taylor SM. Effects of prenatal maternal estrogen on the male urogenital system. Obstet Gynecol 1980;56:537–42.
22. Bibbo M, Gill WB, Azizi F, et al. Follow-up study of male and female offspring of DES-exposed mothers. Obstet Gynecol 1977;49:1–8.
23. Yalom ID, Green R, Fisk N. Prenatal exposure to female hormones. Effect on psychosexual development in boys. Arch Gen Psychiatry 1973;28:554–61.
24. Burke L, Apfel RJ, Fischer S, Shaw J. Observations on the psychological impact of diethylstilbestrol exposureand suggestions on management J. Reprod Med 1980;24:99–102.

Name: **DIGITALIS**

Class: **Cardiac Glycoside**   Risk Factor: **B**

Fetal Risk Summary

No reports linking digitalis or the various digitalis glycosides with congenital defects have been located. Animal studies have failed to show a teratogenic effect (1). Rapid passage to the fetus has been observed after digoxin and digitoxin (2–9). Okita found the amount of digitoxin recovered from the fetus was dependent on the length of gestation (2). In the late 1st trimester, only 0.05 to 0.10% of the injected dose was recovered from 3 fetuses. Digitoxin metabolites accounted for 0.18 to 0.33%. At 34 weeks of gestation, digitoxin recovery was 0.85% and metabolites 3.49% from one fetus. Average cord concentrations of digoxin in 3 reports were 50, 81 and 83% of the maternal serum (3, 4, 9). Highest fetal concentrations of digoxin in the 2nd half of pregnancy were found in the heart (5). The fetal heart has only a limited binding capacity for digoxin in the 1st half of pregnancy (5). In animals, amniotic fluid acts as a reservoir for digoxin, but no data is available in humans after prolonged treatment (5). The pharmacokinetics of digoxin in pregnant women have been reported (10). Digoxin has been used to treat fetal tachycardia and congestive heart failure by administering the drug to the mother (11–13). Fetal toxicity resulting in neonatal death has been reported after maternal overdose (14). The mother, in her 8th month of pregnancy, took an estimated 8.9 mg of digitoxin as a single dose. Delivery occurred 4 days later. The baby demonstrated digitalis cardiac effects until death at age 3 days from prolonged intrauterine anoxia. In a series of 22 multiparous patients maintained on digitalis, spontaneous labor occurred more than 1 week earlier than in 64 matched controls (15). The 1st stage of labor in the treated patients averaged 4.3 hours versus 8 hours in the control group. Ho and co-workers found no effect on duration of pregnancy or labor in 122 patients with heart disease (16).

Breast Feeding Summary

Digoxin is excreted into breast milk. Data for other cardiac glycosides has not been located. Digoxin milk:plasma ratios have varied from 0.6 to 0.9 (4, 7, 17,

18). Although these amounts seem high, they represent very small amounts of digoxin due to significant maternal protein binding. No adverse effects in the nursing infant have been reported.

Author (ref)	No. Pts.	Dose	Concentrations (μg/ml)		M:P Ratio	Effect on Infant
			Serum	Milk		
Chan (4)	11	0.25 mg/day	1.4 nmol/l	0.8 nmol/l	0.6	Half-life in infant: 36 hours
Finley (7)	1	0.75 mg/day	2.1	1.9	0.9	Infant serum level: 0.2 ng/ml
Levy (17)	5	Not stated	0.9	0.6	0.7	Calculated infant daily dose: 1-2 μg
Loughnan (18)	2	0.25 mg/day	1.1	0.96 (peak)	0.9	
			0.8	0.61 (peak)	0.8	

References

1. Shepard TH. *Catalog of Teratogenic Agents*, ed. 3. Baltimore: Johns Hopkins University Press, 1980:116-7.
2. Okita GT, Plotz EF, Davis ME. Placental transfer of radioactive digitoxin in pregnant women and its fetal distribution. Circ Res 1956;4:376-80.
3. Rogers MC, Willserson JT, Goldblatt A, Smith TW. Serum digoxin concentrations in the human fetus, neonate and infant. N Engl J Med 1972;287:1010-3.
4. Chan V, Tse TF, Wong V. Transfer of digoxin across the placenta and into breast milk. Br J Obstet Gynaecol 1978;85:605-9.
5. Saarikoski S. Placental transfer and fetal uptake of ^{3}H-Digoxin in humans. Br J Obstet Gynaecol 1976;83:879-84.
6. Allonen H, Kanto J, Lisalo E. The foeto-maternal distribution of digoxin in early human pregnancy. Acta Pharmacol Toxicol 1976;39:477-80.
7. Finley JP, Waxman MB, Wong PY, Lickrish GM. Digoxin excretion in human milk. J Pediatr 1979;94:339-40.
8. Soyka LF. Digoxin: placental transfer, effects on the fetus, and therapeutic use in the newborn. Clin Perinatol 1975;2:23-35.
9. Padeletti L, Porciani MC, Scimone G. Placental transfer of digoxin (beta-methyl-digoxin) in man. Int J Clin Pharmacol Biopharm 1979;17:82-3.
10. Marzo A, Lo Cicero G, Brina A, Zuliani G, Ghirardi P, Pardi G. Preliminary data on the pharmacokinetics of digoxin in pregnancy. Boll Soc Ital Biol Sper 1980;56:219-23.
11. Lingman G, Ohrlander S, Ohlin P. Intrauterine digoxin treatment of fetal paroxysmal tachycardia: case report. Br J Obstet Gynaecol 1980;87:340-2.
12. Kerenyi TD, Gleicher N, Meller J, et al. Transplacental cardioversion of intrauterine supraventricular tachycardia with digitalis. Lancet 1980;2:393-4.
13. Harrigan JT, Kangos JJ, Sikka A, et al. Successful treatment of fetal congestive heart failure secondary to tachycardia. N Engl J Med 1981;304:1527-9.
14. Sherman JL Jr, Locke RV. Transplacental neonatal digitalis intoxication. Am J Cardiol 1960;6:834-7.
15. Weaver JB, Pearson JF. Influence of digitalis on time of onset and duration of labour in women with cardiac disease. Br Med J 1973;3:519-20.
16. Ho PC, Chen TY, Wong V. The effect of maternal cardiac disease and digoxin administration on labour, fetal weight and maturity at birth. Aust NZ J Obstet Gynaecol 1980;20:24-7.
17. Levy M, Granit L, Laufer N. Excretion of drugs in human milk. N Engl J Med 1977;297:789.
18. Loughnan PM. Digoxin excretion in human breast milk. J Pediatr 1978;92:1019-20.

Name: **DIGITOXIN**
Class: **Cardiac Glycoside**   Risk Factor: **B**

Fetal Risk Summary
See Digitalis.

Breast Feeding Summary
See Digitalis.

Name: **DIGOXIN**
Class: **Cardiac Glycoside**   Risk Factor: **B**

Fetal Risk Summary
See Digitalis.

Breast Feeding Summary
See Digitalis.

Name: **DIHYDROCODEINE BITARTRATE**
Class: **Narcotic Analgesic**   Risk Factor: **B***

Fetal Risk Summary
No reports linking the use of dihydrocodeine with congenital defects have been located. Usage in pregnancy is primarily confined to labor. Respiratory depression in the newborn has been reported to be less than with meperidine, but depression is probably similar when equianalgesic doses are compared (1–3).

* Risk Factor D if used for prolonged periods or if high doses given at term.]

Breast Feeding Summary
No data available.

References

1. Ruch WA, Ruch RM. A preliminary report on dihydrocodeine-scopolamine in obstetrics. Am J Obstet Gynecol 1957;74:1125–7.
2. Myers JD. A preliminary clinical evaluation of dihydrocodeine bitartrate in normal parturition. Am J Obstet Gynecol 1958;75:1096–100.
3. Bonica JJ. Principles and Practice of Obstetric Analgesia and Anesthesia. Philadelphia: FA Davis, 1967: 245.

Name: **DIIODOHYDROXYQUIN**

Class: **Amebicide**   Risk Factor: **C**

Fetal Risk Summary

No data available.

Breast Feeding Summary

No data available.

Name: **DIMENHYDRINATE**

Class: **Antiemetic**   Risk Factor: **B**

Fetal Risk Summary

Dimenhydrinate is the clorotheophylline salt of the antihistamine diphenhydramine. A prospective study in 1963 compared dimenhydrinate usage in 3 groups of patients: 266 with malformed infants and 2 groups of 266 each without malformed infants (1). No difference in usage of the drug was found between the 3 groups. The Collaborative Perinatal Project monitored 50,282 mother-child pairs, 319 of which had 1st trimester exposure to dimenhydrinate (2). For use anytime in pregnancy, 697 exposures were recorded (3). In neither case was evidence found to suggest a relationship to large categories of major or minor malformations. Two possible associations with individual malformations were found, but the statistical significance of these are unknown. Independent confirmation is required to determine the actual risk.

Cardiovascular defects (5 cases)

Inguinal hernia (8 cases)

Two reports have described the oxytocic effect of intravenous dimenhydrinate on the full-term uterus (4, 5). When used either alone or with oxytocin, the result was a smoother, shorter labor.

Breast Feeding Summary

No data available.

References

1. Mellin GW, Katzenstein M. Meclozine and fetal abnormalities. Lancet 1963;1:222–3.
2. Heinonen OP, Slone D, Shapiro S. *Birth Defects and Drugs in Pregnancy.* Littleton: Publishing Sciences Group, 1977:367–70.
3. *Ibid*, 440.
4. Watt LO. Oxytocic effects of dimenhydrinate in obstetrics. Can Med Assoc J 1961;84:533–4.
5. Rotter CW, Whitaker JL, Yared J. The use of intravenous Dramamine to shorten the time of labor and potentiate analgesia. Am J Obstet Gynecol 1958:75:1101–4.

Name: **DIOCTYL CALCIUM SULFOSUCCINATE**
Class: **Laxative**   Risk Factor: **C**

Fetal Risk Summary
See Dioctyl Sodium Sulfosuccinate.

Breast Feeding Summary
No data available.

Name: **DIOCTYL POTASSIUM SULFOSUCCINATE**
Class: **Laxative**   Risk Factor: **C**

Fetal Risk Summary
See Dioctyl Sodium Sulfosuccinate.

Breast Feeding Summary
No data available.

Name: **DIOCTYL SODIUM SULFOSUCCINATE**
Class: **Laxative**   Risk Factor: **C**

Fetal Risk Summary
No reports linking the use of dioctyl sodium sulfosuccinate (DSS) with congenital defects have been located. DSS is a common ingredient in many laxative preparations available to the public. In a large prospective study, 116 patients were exposed to this drug during pregnancy (1). No evidence for an association with malformations was found.

Breast Feeding Summary
No data available.

References
1. Heinonen OP, Slone D, Shapiro S. *Birth Defects and Drugs in Pregnancy*. Littleton: Publishing Sciences Group, 1977:442.

Name: **DIOXYLINE**

Class: **Vasodilator**   Risk Factor: **C**

Fetal Risk Summary

No data available.

Breast Feeding Summary

No data available.

Name: **DIPHEMANIL**

Class: **Parasympatholytic**   Risk Factor: **C**

Fetal Risk Summary

Diphemanil is an anticholinergic quarternary ammonium methylsulfate. No reports of its use in pregnancy have been located (see also Atropine).

Breast Feeding Summary

No data available (see also Atropine).

Name: **DIPHENADIONE**

Class: **Anticoagulant**   Risk Factor: **D**

Fetal Risk Summary

See Coumarin Derivatives.

Breast Feeding Summary

See Coumarin Derivatives.

Name: **DIPHENHYDRAMINE**

Class: **Antihistamine**   Risk Factor: **C**

Fetal Risk Summary

The Collaborative Perinatal Project monitored 50,282 mother-child pairs, 595 of which had 1st trimester exposure to diphenhydramine (1). For use anytime during pregnancy, 2,948 exposures were recorded (2). In neither case was evidence found to suggest a relationship to large categories of major or minor malformations. Several possible associations with individual malformations were found, but the statistical significance of these are unknown (1–3). Independent confirmation is required to determine the actual risk.

    Genitourinary (other than hypospadias) (5 cases)
    Hypospadias (3 cases)
    Eye and ear defects (3 cases)
    Syndromes (other than Down's syndrome) (3 cases)
    Inguinal hernia (13 cases)
    Clubfoot (5 cases)
    Any ventricular septal defect (open or closing) (5 cases)
    Malformations of diaphragm (3 cases)

Cleft palate and diphenhydramine usage in the 1st trimester were statistically associated in a 1974 study (4). A group of 599 children with oral clefts were compared to 590 controls without clefts. In utero exposures to diphenhydramine in the groups were 20 and 6, respectively, a significant difference. However, in a 1971 report significantly fewer infants with malformations were exposed to antihistamines in the 1st trimester as compared to controls (5). Diphenhydramine was the second most commonly used antihistamine.

Diphenhydramine withdrawal was reported in a newborn infant whose mother had taken 150 mg per day during pregnancy (6). Generalized tremulousness and diarrhea began on the 5th day of life. Treatment with phenobarbital resulted in the gradual disappearance of the symptoms.

Breast Feeding Summary

Diphenhydramine is excreted into human breast milk but levels have not been reported (7). Although the levels are not thought to be sufficiently significant in therapeutic doses to affect the infant, the manufacturer considers the drug contraindicated in nursing mothers. The reason given for this is the increased sensitivity of newborn or premature infants to antihistamines.

References

1. Heinonen OP, Sloan D, Shapiro S. Birth Defects and Drugs in Pregnancy. Littleton: Publishing Sciences Group, 1977:323–37.
2. Idib, 437.
3. Ibid, 475.
4. Saxen I. Cleft palate and maternal diphenydramine intake. Lancet 1974;1:407–8.
5. Nelson MM, Forfar JO. Associations between drugs administered during pregnancy and congenital abnormalities of the fetus. Br Med J 1971;1:523–7.
6. Parkin DE. Probable Benadryl withdrawal manifestations in a newborn infant. J Pediatr 1974;85:580.
7. O'Brien TE. Excretion of drugs in human milk. Am J Hosp Pharm 1974;31:844–54.

Name: **DIPHENOXYLATE**

Class: **Antidiarrheal**   Risk Factor: **C**

Fetal Risk Summary

Diphenoxylate is a narcotic related to meperidine. It is available only in combination with atropine (to discourage overdosage) for the treatment of diarrhea. No reports linking it with congenital defects have been located. In one study, no malformed infants were observed after 1st trimester exposure in 7 patients (1).

Breast Feeding Summary

The manufacturer reports that diphenoxylate is excreted into breast milk and the effects of that drug and atropine may be evident in the nursing infant (2). One source recommends the drug should not be used in lactating mothers (3).

References

1. Heinonen OP, Slone D, Shapiro S. *Birth Defects and Drugs in Pregnancy*. Littleton: Publishing Sciences Group, 1977:287.
2. Product information. Lomotil. Searle and Company, 1982.
3. Stewart JJ. Gastrointestinal drugs. In Wilston JT, ed. *Drugs in Breast Milk*. Australia: ADIS Press, 1981:71.

Name: **DIPYRIDAMOLE**

Class: **Vasodilator**   Risk Factor: **C**

Fetal Risk Summary

No reports linking the use of dipyridamole with congenital defects have been located. The drug has been used in pregnancy as a vasodilator and to prevent thrombus formation in patients with prosthetic heart valves (1–8). A single intravenous 30-mg dose of dipyridamole was shown to increase uterine perfusion in the 3rd trimester in 10 patients (9). In one report, a malformed infant was produced, but other drugs, one known to be a teratogen, were also taken by the mother (1). In another report, the only complication was a maternal blood loss of 700 ml, about twice normal, after vaginal delivery (6). These have been the only problems mentioned in 26 patients and their offspring.

Author (ref)	No. Pts.	Indica- tion	Gestational Age	Dose	Other Drugs	Fetal Effects	Comment
Tejani (1)	1	Prevent thrombus formation	Through- out	Not stated	Coumadin Digoxin Quinidine	Occipital meningocele Microphthalmia Hydrocephalus Bulge—suboccipital region	Defects consist- ent with fetal warfarin syn- drome

Author (ref)	No. Pts.	Indica- tion	Gestational Age	Dose	Other Drugs	Fetal Effects	Comment
						Encephalocele (possible) Occipital bone defects Low set ears High arched palate Hypoplastic nasal bones and cartilages Blind Persistent truncus arteriosus	

Breast Feeding Summary

Dipyridamole is excreted into breast milk but in levels too low to measure with current techniques (7). The manufacturer knows of no problems in breast-fed infants whose mothers were taking this drug (7).

References

1. Tejani N. Anticoagulant therapy with cardiac valve prosthesis during pregnancy. Obstet Gynecol 1973;42:785–93.
2. Del Bosque MR. Dipiridamol and anticoagulants in the management of pregnant women with cardiac valvular prosthesis. Ginecol Obstet Mex 1973;33:191–8.
3. Littler WA, Bonnar J, Redman CWG, Beilin LJ, Lee GD. Reduced pulmonary arterial compliance in hypertensive patients. Lancet 1973;1:1274–8.
4. Biale Y, Lewenthal H, Gueron M, Beu-Aderath N. Caesarean section in patient with mitral-valve prosthesis. Lancet 1977;1:907.
5. Taguchi K. Pregnancy in patients with a prosthetic heart valve. Surg Gynecol Obstet 1977;145:206–8.
6. Ahmad R, Rajah SM, Mearns AJ, Deverall PB. Dipyridamole in successful management of pregnant women with prosthetic heart valve. Lancet 1976;2:1414–5.
7. Personal communication. Bowers PA. Boehringer Engelheim Ltd, 1981.
8. Biale Y, Cantor A, Lewenthal H, Gueron M. The course of pregnancy in patients with artificial heart valves treated with dipyridamole. Int J Gynaecol Obstet 1980;18:128–32.
9. Lauchkner W, Schwarz R, Retzke U. Cardiovascular action of dipyridamole in advanced pregnancy. Zentralbl Gynaekol 1981;103:220–7.

Name: **DISOPYRAMIDE**

Class: **Antiarrhythmic**   Risk Factor: **C**

Fetal Risk Summary

No reports linking the use of disopyramide with congenital defects in humans or animals have been located. At term, a cord blood level of 0.9 μg/ml (39% of maternal serum) was measured 6 hours after a maternal 200-mg dose (1). Disopyramide has been used throughout pregnancy without evidence of congenital abnormality or growth retardation (1, 2). Early onset of labor has been reported in one patient (3). The mother, in her 32nd week of gestation, was given 300 mg orally, followed by 100 or 150 mg every 6 hours for posterior-mitral-leaflet prolapse. Uterine contractions, without vaginal bleeding or cervical changes, and abdominal pain occurred 1 to 2 hours after each dose. When disopyramide was stopped, symptoms subsided over the next 4 hours. Oxytocin induction 1 week later resulted in the delivery of a healthy infant.

Breast Feeding Summary

Disopyramide is excreted into breast milk at levels not exceeding the maternal serum (4). The manufacturer recommends against breast feeding if the mother is taking this drug.

References

1. Shaxted EJ, Milton PJ. Disopyramide in pregnancy: a case report. Curr Med Res Opin 1979;6:70–2.
2. Personal communication. Anderson MS, GD Searle and Company, 1981.
3. Leonard RF, Braun TE, Levy AM. Initiation of uterine contractions by disopyramide during pregnancy. N Engl J Med 1978;299:84–5.
4. Product information. Norpace. GD Searle and Company, 1981.

Name: **DISULFIRAM**

Class: **(Unclassified)**   Risk Factor: **X**

Fetal Risk Summary

Disulfiram is used to prevent alcohol consumption in patients with a history of alcohol abuse. The use of disulfiram in pregnancy has been described in 7 pregnancies (1, 2). Four of the eight fetuses exposed (1 set of twins) had congenital defects. Although controversial, heavy alcohol intake prior to conception has been suspected of producing the fetal alcohol syndrome (FAS) (3–5). However, the anomalies described in the four infants exposed to disulfiram do not fit the pattern seen with the FAS. Based on the above data, termination of pregnancy is recommended if disulfiram is used during the 1st trimester.

Author (ref)	No. Pts.	Indica- tion	Gestational Age	Dose	Other Drugs	Fetal Effects	Comment
Favre- Tissot (1)	5	Not stated	Not stated	Not stated	"Tranquil- izers"	2 with clubfoot 1 spontaneous abortion 2 normal	
Nora (2)	3	Alcohol- ism	1st tri- mester	Not stated	Not stated	1 multiple anomalies in male including VACTERL syn- drome (radial aplasia, ver- tebral fusion, tracheo- esophageal fistula) 1 normal female (twin of above male) 1 phocomelia of lower ex- tremities in male	Alcohol and other teratogens excluded

Breast Feeding Summary

No data available.

References

1. Favre-Tissot M, Delatour P. Psychopharmacologie et teratogenese a propos du sulfirame: essal experimental. Annales Medico-psychogiques 1965;1:735–40. (As cited in Shepard TH. *Catalog of Teratogenic Agents*, ed. 3. Baltimore:Johns Hopkins University Press, 1980:127.
2. Nora AH, Nora JJ, Blu J. Limb-reduction anomalies in infants born to disulfiram-treated alcoholic mothers. Lancet 1977;2:664.
3. Scheiner AP, Donovan CM, Bartoshesky LE. Fetal alcohol syndrome in child whose parents had stopped drinking. Lancet 1979;1:1077–8.
4. Scheiner AP. Fetal alcohol syndrome in a child whose parents had stopped drinking. Lancet 1979;2:858.
5. Smith DW, Graham JM Jr. Fetal alcohol syndrome in child whose parents had stopped drinking. Lancet 1979;2:527.

Name: **DOBUTAMINE**

Class: **Sympathomimetic (Adrenergic)**   Risk Factor: **C**

Fetal Risk Summary

Dobutamine is structurally related to dopamine. It has not been studied in human pregnancy (see also Dopamine).

Breast Feeding Summary

No data available.

Name: **DOPAMINE**

Class: **Sympathomimetic (Adrenergic)**   Risk Factor: **C**

Fetal Risk Summary

Experience with dopamine in human pregnancy is limited. Dopamine has been used to prevent renal failure in 9 oligoanuric eclamptic patients by re-establishing diuresis (1). The drug has also been used to treat hypotension in 26 patients undergoing cesarean section (2). No newborn adverse effects attributable to dopamine administration were observed in either study. Since dopamine is indicated only for life-threatening situations, chronic use would not be expected. Animal studies have shown both increases and decreases in uterine blood flow (2). Human studies on uterine perfusion have not been conducted.

Breast Feeding Summary

No data available.

References

1. Gerstner G, Grunberger W. Dopamine treatment for prevention of renal failure in patients with severe eclampsia. Clin Exp Obstet Gynecol 1980;7:219–22.
2. Clark RB, Brunner JA III. Dopamine for the treatment of spinal hypotension during cesarean section. Anesthesiology 1980;53:514–7.

Name: **DOTHIEPIN**

Class: **Antidepressant**   Risk Factor: **D**

Fetal Risk Summary

No data available (see Imipramine).

Breast Feeding Summary

No data available (see Imipramine).

Name: **DOXEPIN**

Class: **Antidepressant**   Risk Factor: **C**

Fetal Risk Summary

No reports linking the use of doxepin with congenital defects have been located (see also Imipramine). Paralytic ileus has been observed in an infant exposed to doxepin at term (1). The condition was thought to be primarily due to chlorpromazine, but the authors speculated that the anticholinergic effects of doxepin worked synergistically with the phenothiazine.

Breast Feeding Summary

No data available (see Imipramine).

References

1. Falterman CG, Richardson CJ. Small left colon syndrome associated with maternal ingestion of psychotropic drugs. J Pediatr 1980;97:308–10.

Name: **DOXORUBICIN**

Class: **Antineoplastic** Risk Factor: **D**

Fetal Risk Summary

Several reports have described the use of doxorubicin in pregnancy, including during the 1st trimester (1–11). Except for one infant with transient polycythemia and hyperbilirubinemia, no adverse effects were observed. Congenital defects have not been reported with doxorubicin. The drug was not detected in the amniotic fluid at 20 weeks of gestation, which suggests that the drug is not transferred in measurable amounts to the fetus (1). However, long term studies of growth and mental development of offspring exposed to doxorubicin and other antineoplastic agents in the 2nd trimester, the period of neuroblast multiplication, have not been conducted (12). Doxorubicin may cause reversible testicular dysfunction (13, 14). Effects on ovarian function have not been reported.

Breast Feeding Summary

No data available.

References

1. Roboz J, Gleicher N, Wu K, Kerenyi T, Holland J. Does doxorubicin cross the placenta? Lancet 1979;2:1382–3.
2. Khursid M, Saleem M. Acute leukaemia in pregnancy. Lancet 1978;2:534–5.
3. Newcomb M, Balducci L, Thigpen JT, Morrison FS. Acute leukemia in pregnancy: successful delivery after cytarabine and doxorubicin. JAMA 1978;239:2691–2.
4. Hassenstein E, Riedel H. Zur teratogenitat von Adriamycin ein fallbericht. Geburtshilfe Frauenheilkd 1978;38:131–3.
5. Cervantes F, Rozman C. Adriamycina y embarazo. Sangre (Barc) 1980;25:627.
6. Pizzuto J, Aviles A, Noriega L, Niz J, Morales M, Romero F. Treatment of acute leukemia during pregnancy: presentation of nine cases. Cancer Treat Rep 1980;64:679–83.
7. Tobias JS, Bloom HJG. Doxorubicin in pregnancy. Lancet 1980;1:776.
8. Garcia V, San Miguel J, Borrasca AL. Doxorubicin in the first trimester of pregnancy. Ann Intern Med 1981;94:547.
9. Garcia V, San Miguel IJ, Borrasca AL. Adriamycin and pregnancy. Sangre (Barc) 1981;26:129.
10. Dara P, Slater LM, Armentrout SA. Successful pregnancy during chemotherapy for acute leukemia. Cancer 1981;47:845–6.
11. Lowenthal RM, Funnell CF, Hope DM, Stewart IG, Humphrey DC. Normal infant after combination chemotherapy including teniposide for Burkitt's lymphoma in pregnancy. Med Pediatr Oncol 1982;10:165–9.
12. Dobbing J. Pregnancy and leukaemia. Lancet 1977;1:1155.
13. Lendon M, Palmer MK, Hann IM, Shalet SM, Jones PHM. Testicular histology after combination chemotherapy in childhood for acute lymphoblastic leukaemia. Lancet 1978;2:439–41.
14. Schilsky RL, Lewis BJ, Sherins RJ, Young RC. Gonadal dysfunction in patients receiving chemotherapy for cancer. Ann Intern Med 1980;93:109–14.

Name: **DOXYCYCLINE**

Class: **Antibiotic**   Risk Factor: **D**

Fetal Risk Summary

See Tetracycline.

Breast Feeding Summary

Doxycycline is excreted into breast milk. Oral doxycycline, 200 mg followed after 24 hours by 100 mg, was given to 15 nursing mothers (1). Milk:plasma ratios determined at 3 and 24 hours after the second dose were 0.3 and 0.4, respectively. Mean milk concentrations were 0.77 and 0.38 μg/ml.

Theoretically, dental staining and inhibition of bone growth could occur in breast-fed infants whose mothers were consuming doxycycline. However, this theoretical possibility seems remote, since in infants exposed to a closely related antibiotic, tetracycline, serum levels were undetectable (less than 0.05 μg/ml) (2). Three potential problems may exist for the nursing infant even though there are no reports in this regard: modification of bowel flora, direct effects on the infant and interference with the interpretation of culture results if a fever work-up is required.

References

1. Morganti G, Ceccarelli G, Ciaffi EG. Comparative concentrations of a tetracycline antibiotic in serum and maternal milk. Antibiotica 1968;6:216–23.
2. Posner AC, Prigot A, Konicoff NG. Further observations on the use of tetracycline hydrochloride in prophylaxis and treatment of obstetric infections. *Antibiotics Annual 1954–55*. New York: Medical Encyclopedia, 594–8.

Name: **DOXYLAMINE**

Class: **Antiemetic**   Risk Factor: **B**

Fetal Risk Summary

The combination of doxylamine, pyridoxine and dicyclomine (Bendectin, others) was originally marketed in 1956. The drug was reformulated (USA and Canada) in 1976 to eliminate dicyclomine because that component was not found to contribute to its effectiveness as an antiemetic. The drug is available without prescription outside the United States. Over 30 million women have taken this product during pregnancy (1). Several studies have appeared which support the safe use of the combination in pregnancy (2–14). Arrayed against this experience are an estimated 160 cases of congenital defects reported to the FDA as being "Bendectin-induced" (15). Two additional reports have described anomalies in three infants exposed to this antiemetic early in pregnancy (16, 17). A theoretical mechanism for the proposed toxicity has also appeared (18). Critics have decried the lack of controls in the studies supporting the safety of Bendectin (15, 19). However, a recent prospective study examined 1,690 mother-child pairs, 375 of whom reported exposure to Bendectin during pregnancy (11). An infant was considered to have a Bendectin-induced defect if skeletal, limb, cleft lip or palate or cardiac defects were present. Statistical analysis of birth weight, length, head circumference, gestational age and congenital defects failed to demonstrate a relationship between Bendectin and adverse fetal outcome.

Although the literature supports the relative safety of this product when compared to the normal background of malformations, it is not possible to state that it is completely without risk to the fetus (20). The combination antiemetic should be reserved for the treatment of pregnancy-induced nausea and vomiting only when dietary measures have failed (21).

Breast Feeding Summary
No data available.

References

1. Combs CD. Personal communication. Merrell Dow Pharmaceutical Inc. 1981.
2. Milkovich L, van den Berg BJ. An evaluation of the teratogenicity of certain antinauseant drugs. Am J Obstet Gynecol 1976;125:244–8.
3. Shapiro S, Heinonen OP, Siskind V, Kaufman DW, Monson RR, Slone D. Antenatal exposure to doxylamine succinate and dicyclomine hydrochloride (Bendectin) in relation to congenital malformations, perinatal mortality rate, birth weight, intelligence quotient score. Am J Obstet Gynecol 1977;128:480–5.
4. Rothman KJ, Flyer DC, Goldblatt A, Kreidberg MB. Exogenous hormones and other drug exposures of children with congenital heart disease. Am J Epidemiol 1979;109:433–9.
5. Bunde CA, Bowles DM. A technique for controlled survey of case records. Curr Ther Res 1963;5:245–8.
6. Gibson GT, Collen DP, McMichael AJ, Hartshorne JM. Congenital anomalies in relation to the use of doxylamine/dicyclomine and other antenatal factors. An ongoing prospective study. Med J Aust 1981;1:410–4.
7. Correy JF, Newman NM. Debendox and limb reduction deformities. Med J Aust 1981;1:417–8.
8. Clarke M, Clayton DG. Safety of debendox. Lancet 1981;2:659–60.
9. Harron DWG, Griffiths K, Shanks RG. Debendox and congenital malformations in Northern Ireland. Br Med J 1980;4:1379–81.
10. Smithells RW, Sheppard S. Teratogenicity testing in humans: a method demonstrating safety of Bendectin. Teratology 1978;17:31–5.
11. Morelock S, Hingson R, Kayne H, et al. Bendectin and fetal development: a study at Boston City Hospital. Am J Obstet Gynecol 1982;142:209–13.
12. Cordero JF, Oakley GP, Greenberg F, James LM. Is Bendectin a teratogen? JAMA 1981;245:2307–10.
13. Mitchell AA, Rosenberg L, Shapiro S, Slone D. Birth defects related to Bendectin use in pregnancy: I. Oral clefts and cardiac defects. JAMA 1981;245:2311–4.
14. Fleming DM, Knox JDE, Crombie DL. Debendox in early pregnancy and fetal malformation. Br Med J 1981;283:99–101.
15. Korcok M. The Bendectin debate. Can Med Assoc J 1980;123:922–8.
16. Soverchia G, Perri PF. Two cases of malformations of a limb in infants of mothers treated with an antiemetic in a very early phase of pregnancy. Pediatr Med Chir 1981;3:97–9.
17. Donaldson GL, Bury RG. Multiple congenital abnormalities in a newborn boy associated with maternal use of fluphenazine enanthate and other drugs during pregnancy. Acta Paediatr Scand 1982;71:335–8.
18. Pearson RD. Bendectin and fetal malformations. Can Med Assoc J 1981;124:259.
19. Hall JB. Debendox in pregnancy. Lancet 1981;2:154–5.
20. Anonymous. FDA's position on Bendectin. Am Coll Obstet Gynecol Nwsltr 1979;23:2–3.
21. Anonymous. F-D-C Reports. The Pink Sheets. September 22, 1980:1–8.

Name: **DROPERIDOL**

Class: **Tranquilizer**   Risk Factor: **C**

Fetal Risk Summary

Droperidol is a butyrophenone derivative structurally related to haloperidol (see also Haloperidol). The drug has been used to promote analgesia for cesarean section patients without affecting the respiration of the newborn (1, 2). The placental transfer of droperidol is slow (2).

Breast Feeding Summary

No data avaiable.

References

1. Smith AM, McNeil WT. Awareness during anesthesia. Br Med J 1969;1:572–3.
2. Zhdanov GG, Ponomarev GM. The concentration of droperidol in the venous blood of the parturients and in the blood of the umbilical cord of neonates. Anesteziol Reanimatol 1980;4:14–6.

Name: **DYPHYLLINE**

Class: **Spasmolytic/Vasodilator**   Risk Factor: **C**

Fetal Risk Summary

No data available (see also Theophylline).

Breast Feeding Summary

Dyphylline is excreted into breast milk. In 20 normal lactating women a single 5 mg/kg intramuscular dose produced an average milk:plasma ratio of 2.08 (1). The milk and serum elimination rates were equivalent.

References

1. Jarboe CH, Cook LN, Malesic I, Fleischaker J. Dyphylline elimination kinetics in lactating women: blood to milk transfer. J Clin Pharmacol 1981;21:405–10.

Name: **ECHOTHIOPHATE**
Class: **Parasympathomimetic (Cholinergic)**   Risk Factor: **C**

Fetal Risk Summary

Echothiophate is used in the eye. No reports of its use in pregnancy have been located. As a quaternary ammonium compound, it is ionized at physiologic pH and transplacental passage in significant amounts would not be expected (see also Neostigmine).

Breast Feeding Summary

No data available.

Name: **EDROPHONIUM**
Class: **Parasympathomimetic (Cholinergic)**   Risk Factor: **C**

Fetal Risk Summary

Edrophonium is a quaternary ammonium chloride with anticholinesterase activity used in the diagnosis of myasthenia gravis. The drug has been used in pregnancy without producing fetal malformations (1–7). Because it is ionized at physiologic pH, edrophonium would not be expected to cross the placenta in significant amounts. Caution has been advised against the use in pregnancy of intravenous anticholinesterases since thay may cause premature labor (1, 3). This effect on the pregnant uterus increases near term. Intramuscular neostigmine should be used in place of intravenous edrophonium if diagnosis of myasthenia gravis is required in a pregnant patient (3). In one report, however, intravenous edrophonium was given to a woman in the 2nd trimester in an unsuccessful attempt to treat tachycardia secondary to Wolff-Parkinson-White syndrome (6). No effect on the uterus was mentioned and she continued with an uneventful full term pregnancy. Although apparently safe for the fetus, cholinesterase inhibitors may affect the condition of the newborn (2). Transient muscular weakness has been observed in about 20% of newborns whose mothers were treated for myasthenia gravis during pregnancy. While the exact cause of the neonatal myasthenia is unknown, anticholinesterases may contribute to the condition (7).

Breast Feeding Summary

Because it is ionized at physiologic pH, edrophonium would not be expected to be excreted into breast milk (8).

References

1. Foldes FF, McNall PG. Myasthenia gravis: a guide for anesthesiologists. Anesthesiology 1962;23:837–72.
2. Plauche WG. Myasthenia gravis in pregnancy. Am J Obstet Gynecol 1964;88:404–9.
3. McNall PG, Jafarnia MR. Management of myasthenia gravis in the obstetrical patient. Am J Obstet Gynecol 1965;92:518–25.
4. Hay DM. Myasthenia gravis in pregnancy. J Obstet Gynaecol Br Commonw 1969;76:323–9.
5. Heinonen OP, Slone D, Shapiro S. *Birth Defects and Drugs in Pregnancy*. Littleton: Publishing Sciences Group, 1977:345–56.
6. Gleicher N, Meller J, Sandler RZ, Sullum S. Wolff-Parkinson-White syndrome in pregnancy. Obstet Gynecol 1981;58:748–52.
7. Blackhall MI, Buckley GA, Roberts DV, Roberts JB, Thomas BH, Wilson A. Drug-induced neonatal myasthenia. J Obstet Gynaecol Br Commonw 1969;76:157–62.
8. Wilson JT. Pharmacokinetics of drug excretion. In Wilson JT, ed. *Drugs in Breast Milk.* Australia: ADIS Press, 1981:17.

Name: **EPHEDRINE**

Class: **Sympathomimetic (Adrenergic)**   Risk Factor: **C**

Fetal Risk Summary

Ephedrine is a sympathomimetic used widely for bronchial asthma, allergic disorders, hypotension and the alleviation of symptoms caused by upper respiratory infections. It is a common component of proprietary mixtures containing antihistamines, bronchodilators and other ingredients. Thus it is difficult to separate the effects of ephedrine on the fetus from other drugs, disease states and viruses. Ephedrine-like drugs are teratogenic in some animal species, but human teratogenicity has not been suspected (1, 2). Recent data may require a reappraisal of this opinion. The Collaborative Perinatal Project monitored 50,282 mother-child pairs, 373 of which had 1st trimester exposure to ephedrine (3). For use anytime during pregnancy, 873 exposures were recorded (4). No evidence for a relationship to large categories of major or minor malformations or to individual defects was found. However, an association in the 1st trimester was found between the sympathomimetic class of drugs as a whole and minor malformations (not life-threatening or major cosmetic defects), inguinal hernia and clubfoot (3). This data is presented as a warning that indiscriminate use of ephedrine, especially in the 1st trimester, is not without risk.

Ephedrine is routinely used to treat or prevent maternal hypotension following spinal anesthesia (5–7). Significant increases in fetal heart rate and beat-to-beat variability may occur (5). These effects are not due to decreases in uterine blood flow and subsequent asphyxia.

Breast Feeding Summary

No data available.

References

1. Nishimura H, Tanimura T. *Clinical Aspects of the Teratogenity of Drugs*. Amsterdam: Excerpta Medica, 1976:231.
2. Shepard TH. *Catalog of Teratogenic Agents*, ed. 3. Baltimore: Johns Hopkins University Press, 1980:134–5.
3. Heinonen OP, Slone D, Shapiro S. *Birth Defects and Drugs in Pregnancy*. Littleton: Publishing Sciences Group, 1977:345–56.
4. *Ibid*, 439.
5. Wright RG, Shnider SM, Levinson G, Rolbin SH, Parer JT. The effect of maternal administration of ephedrine on fetal heart rate and variability. Obstet Gynecol 1981;57:734–8.
6. Antoine C, Young BK. Fetal lactic acidosis with epidural anesthesia. Am J Obstet Gynecol 1982;142:55–9.
7. Datta S, Alper MH, Ostheimer GW, Weiss JB. Method of ephedrine administration and nausea and hypotension during spinal anesthesia for cesarean section. Anesthesiology 1982;56:68–70.

Name: **EPINEPHRINE**

Class: **Sympathomimetic (Adrenergic)**   Risk Factor: **C**

Fetal Risk Summary

Epinephrine is a sympathomimetic that is widely used for conditions such as shock, glaucoma, allergic reactions, bronchial asthma and nasal congestion. Since it occurs naturally in all humans, it is difficult to separate the effects of its administration from effects on the fetus induced by endogenous epinephrine, other drugs, disease states and viruses. The drug readily crosses the placenta (1). Epinephrine is teratogenic in some animal species, but human teratogenicity has not been suspected (2, 3). Recent data may require a reappraisal of this opinion. The Collaborative Perinatal Project monitored 50,282 mother-child pairs, 189 of which had 1st trimester exposure to epinephrine (4). For use anytime during pregnancy, 508 exposures were recorded (5). A statistically significant association was found between 1st trimester use of epinephrine and major and minor malformations. An association was also found with inguinal hernia after both 1st trimester and anytime use (6). Although not specified, this data may reflect the potentially severe maternal status for which epinephrine administration is indicated. Caution is advised, however, against the indiscriminate use of epinephrine in pregnancy.

Breast Feeding Summary

No data available.

References

1. Morgan CD, Sandler M, Panigel M. Placental transfer of catecholamines in vitro and in vivo. Am J Obstet Gynecol 1972;112:1068–75.

2. Nishimura H, Tanimura T. *Clinical Aspects of the Teratogenicity of Drugs.* Amsterdam: Excerpta Medica, 1976:231.
3. Shepard TH. *Catalog of Teratogenic Agents*, ed. 3. Baltimore: Johns Hopkins University Press, 1980:134–5.
4. Heinonen OP, Slone D, Shapiro S. *Birth Defects and Drugs in Pregnancy.* Littleton: Publishing Sciences Group, 1977:345–56.
5. *Ibid*, 439.
6. *Ibid*, 477, 492.

Name: **ERYTHRITYL TETRANITRATE**

Class: **Vasodilator**   Risk Factor: **C**

Fetal Risk Summary

See Nitroglycerin or Amyl Nitrite.

Breast Feeding Summary

No data available.

Name: **ERYTHROMYCIN**

Class: **Antibiotic**   Risk Factor: **B**

Fetal Risk Summary

No reports linking the use of erythromycin with congenital defects have been located. The drug crosses the placenta but in concentrations too low to treat most pathogens (1–3). Fetal tissue levels increase after multiple doses (3). However, a case has been described in which erythromycin was used successfully to treat maternal syphilis but failed to adequately treat the fetus (4). During pregnancy, erythromycin serum concentrations vary greatly as compared to normal men and nonpregnant women, which might account for the low levels observed in the fetus (5).

The estolate salt of erythromycin has been observed to induce hepatotoxicity in pregnant patients (6). Approximately 10% of 161 women treated with the estolate form in the 2nd trimester had abnormally elevated levels of SGOT, which returned to normal after therapy was discontinued.

The use of erythromycin in the 1st trimester was reported in a mother who delivered an infant with left absence-of-tibia syndrome (7). The mother was also exposed to other drugs which makes a relationship to the antibiotic unlikely.

The Collaborative Perinatal Project monitored 50,282 mother-child pairs, 79 of which had 1st trimester exposure to erythromycin (8). For use anytime during pregnancy, 230 exposures were recorded (9). No evidence was found

) suggest a relationship to large categories of major and minor malformations
r to individual defects. Erythromycin, like many other antibiotics, lowers urine
striol concentrations (see also Ampicillin for mechanism and significance)
11). The antibiotic has been used during the 3rd trimester to reduce maternal
nd infant colonization with group B β-hemolytic streptococcus (12). No
dverse effects were observed in the newborns.

Breast Feeding Summary

Erythromycin is excreted into breast milk (8). Following oral doses of 400 mg
every 8 hours, milk levels ranged from 0.4 to 1.6 μg/ml. Oral doses of 2 g per
day produced milk concentrations of 1.6 to 3.2 μg/ml. The milk:plasma ratio
n both groups was 0.5. No reports of adverse effects in infants exposed to
erythromycin in breast milk have been located. However, three potential
problems exist for the nursing infant: modification of bowel flora, direct effects
on the infant and interference with the interpretations of culture results if a
ever work-up is required.

References

1. Heilman FR, Herrell WE, Wellman WE, Geraci JE. Some laboratory and clinical observations on a new antibiotic, erythromycin (Ilotycin). Proc Staff Meet Mayo Clin 1952;27:285–304.
2. Kiefer L, Rubin A, McCoy JB, Foltz EL. The placental transfer of erythromycin. Am J Obstet Gynecol 1955;69:174–7.
3. Philipson A, Sabath LD, Charles D. Transplacental passage of erythromycin and clindamycin. N Engl J Med 1973;288:1219–20.
4. Fenton LJ, Light LJ. Congenital syphilis after maternal treatment with erythromycin. Obstet Gynecol 1976;47:492–4.
5. Philipson A, Sabath LD, Charles D. Erythromycin and clindamycin absorption and elimination in pregnant women. Clin Pharmacoal Ther 1976;19:68–77.
6. McCormack WM, George H, Donner A, et al. Hepatotoxicity of erythromycin estolate during pregnancy. Antimicrob Agents Chemother 1977;12:630–5.
7. Jaffe P, Liberman MM, McFadyen I, Valman HB. Incidence of congenital limb-reduction deformities. Lancet 1975;1:526–7.
8. Heinonen OP, Slone D, Shapiro S. *Birth Defects and Drugs in Pregnancy.* Littleton: Publishing Sciences Group, 1977:297–313.
9. *Ibid*, 435.
0. Knowles JA. Drugs in milk. Ped Currents 1972;21:28–32.
11. Gallagher JC, Ismail MA, Aladjem S. Reduced urinary estriol levels with erythromycin therapy. Obstet Gynecol 1980;56:381–2.
12. Merenstein GB, Todd WA, Brown G, Yost CC, Luzier T. Group B β-hemolytic streptococcus: randomized controlled treatment study at term. Obstet Gynecol 1980;55:315–8.

Name: **ESTRADIOL**

Class: **Estrogenic Hormone**　　　　　　　　　　Risk Factor: **D**

Fetal Risk Summary

Estradiol and its salts (cypionate, valerate) are used for treatment of meno-
pausal symptoms, female hypogonadism and primary ovarian failure. The
Collaborative Perinatal Project monitored 614 mother-child pairs with 1st

trimester exposure to estrogenic agents (including 48 with exposure to estradiol) (1). An increase in the expected frequency of cardiovascular defects. eye and ear anomalies, and Down's syndrome was found (2). Evidence of an increase in risk of malformations due to 1st trimester exposure with estradiol was not observed.

Developmental changes in the psychosexual performance of boys has been attributed to *in utero* exposure to estradiol and progesterone (3). The mothers received estrogen/progestogen regimen for their diabetes. Hormone-exposed males demonstrated a trend to have less heterosexual experience and fewer masculine interests than controls. Use of estrogenic hormones during pregnancy is not recommended (see Oral Contraceptives).

Breast Feeding Summary

Estradiol is used to suppress postpartum breast engorgement in patients who do not desire to breast feed.

References

1. Heinonen OP, Slone D, Shapiro S. *Birth Defects and Drugs in Pregnancy.* Littleton: Publishing Sciences Group, 1977:389,391.
2. *Ibid*, 395.
3. Yalom ID, Green R, Fisk N. Prenatal exposure to female hormones. Effect of psychosexual development in boys. Arch Gen Psychiatry 1973;28:554–61.

Name: **ESTROGENS, CONJUGATED**

Class: **Estrogenic Hormone**   Risk Factor: **D**

Fetal Risk Summary

Conjugated estrogens are a mixture of estrogenic substances (primarily estrone). The Collaborative Perinatal Project monitored 13 mother-child pairs who were exposed to conjugated estrogens during the 1st trimester (1). An increased risk for malformations was found, although identification of the malformations was not provided. Estrogenic agents as a group were monitored in 614 mother-child pairs. An increase in the expected frequency of cardiovascular defects, eye and ear anomalies, and Down's syndrome was reported (2). No adverse effects were observed in one infant exposed during the 1st trimester to conjugated estrogens (3). However, in a second infant exposed during the 4th to 7th weeks of gestation, multiple anomalies were found (see table) (4).

Conjugated estrogens have been used to induce ovulation in anovulatory women (5). They have also been used as partially successful contraceptives when given within 72 hours of unprotected, midcycle coitus (6). No fetal adverse effects were mentioned in either of these reports.

Author (ref)	No. Pts.	Indication	Gestational Age	Dose	Other Drugs	Fetal Effects	Comment
4)	1	Induce menstruation	4–7 weeks	1.25 mg times 20 doses	Prochlorperazine Bendectin Aspirin Vitamins	Cleft palate Wormian bones Heart defect Dislocated hips Absent tibiae Polydactyly Abnormal dermal pattern	Relationship to estrogens unclear

Breast Feeding Summary

No reports of adverse effects from conjugated estrogens in the nursing infant have been located. It is theoretically possible that decreased milk volume and decreased nitrogen and protein content could occur (see Mestranol, Ethinyl Estradiol).

References

1. Heinonen OP, Slone D, Shapiro S. *Birth Defects and Drugs in Pregnancy*. Littleton: Publishing Sciences Group, 1977:389,391.
2. *Ibid*, 395.
3. Hagler S, Schultz A, Hankin H, Kunstadter RH. Fetal effects of steroid therapy during pregnancy. Am J Dis Child 1963;106:586–90.
4. Ho CK, Kaufman RL, McAlister WH. Congenital malformations. Am J Dis Child 1975;129:714–6.
5. Price R. Pregnancies using conjugated oestrogen therapy. Med J Aust 1980;2:341–2.
6. Dixon GW, Schlesselman JJ, Ory HW, Blye RP. Ethinyl estradiol and conjugated estrogens as postcoital contraceptives. JAMA 1980;244:1336–9.

Name: **ESTRONE**

Class: **Estrogenic Hormone**   Risk Factor: **D**

Fetal Risk Summary

See Estrogens, Conjugated.

Breast Feeding Summary

See Estrogens, Conjugated.

Name: **ETHACRYNIC ACID**

Class: **Diuretic**   Risk Factor: **[**

Fetal Risk Summary

Ethacrynic acid is a potent diuretic. It has been used for toxemia, pulmonar
edema and diabetes insipidus during pregnancy (1–10). Although it is not a
animal teratogen, and limited 1st trimester human experience has not show
an increased incidence of malformations, ethacrynic acid is not recommende
for use in pregnant women (11, 12). Diuretics do not prevent or alter th
course of toxemia and they may decrease placental perfusion (13–15). Oto
toxicity has been observed in a mother and her newborn following the use o
ethacrynic acid and kanamycin during the 3rd trimester (16).

Breast Feeding Summary

No data available (see also Chlorothiazide).

References

1. Delgado Urdapilleta J, Dominguez Robles H, Villalobos Roman M, Perez Diaz A. Ethacryni
   acid in the treatment of toxemia of pregnancy. Ginecol Obstet Mex 1968;23:271–80.
2. Felman D, Theoleyre J, Dupoizat H. Investigation of ethacrynic acid in the treatment o
   excessive gain in weight and pregnancy arterial hypertension. Lyon Med 1967;217:1421–8
3. Sands RX, Vita F. Ethacrynic acid (a new diuretic), pregnancy, and excessive fluid retention
   Am J Obstet Gynecol 1968;101:603–9.
4. Kittaka S, Aizawa M, Tokue I, Shimizu M. Clinical results in edecril tablet in the treatment o
   toxemia of late pregnancy. Obstet Gynecol (Japan) 1968;36:934–7.
5. Mahon R, Dubecq JP, Baudet E, Coqueran J. Use of edecrin in obstetrics. Bull Fed So
   Gynecol Obstet Lang Fr 1968;20:440–2.
6. Imaizumi S, Suzuoki Y, Torri M, et al. Clinical trial of ethacrynic acid (Edecril) for toxemia o
   pregnancy. Jpn J Med Consult New Remedies 1969;6:2364–8.
7. Young BK, Haft JI. Treatment of pulmonary edema with ethacrynic acid during labor. Am
   Obstet Gynecol 1970;107:330–1.
8. Harrison KA, Ajabor LN, Lawson JB. Ethacrynic acid and packed-blood-cell transfusion ir
   treatment of severe anaemia in pregnancy. Lancet 1971;1:11–4.
9. Fort AT, Morrison JC, Fisk SA. Iatrogenic hypokalemia of pregnancy by furosemide anc
   ethacrynic acid: two case reports. J Reprod Med 1971;6:21–2.
10. Pico I, Greenblatt RB. Endocrinopathies and infertility. IV. Diabetes insipidus and pregnancy
    Fertil Steril 1969;20:384–92.
11. Product information. Edecrin. Merck Sharpe & Dohme, 1980.
12. Wilson AL, Matzke GR. The treatment of hypertension in pregnancy. Drug Intell Clin Pharm
    1981;15:21–6.
13. Pitkin RM, Kaminetzky HA, Newton M, Pritchard JA. Maternal nutrition: a selective review o
    clinical topics. Obstet Gynecol 1972;40:773–85.
14. Lindheimer MD, Katz AI. Sodium and diuretics in pregnancy. N Engl J Med 1973;288:891–
    4.
15. Christianson R, Page EW. Diuretic drugs and pregnancy. Obstet Gynecol 1976;48:647–52.
16. Jones HC. Intrauterine ototoxicity: a case report and review of literature. J Natl Med Assoc
    1973;65:201–3.

ame: **ETHAMBUTOL**

ass: **Antituberculosis Agent**   Risk Factor: **B**

tal Risk Summary

) reports linking the use of ethambutol with congenital defects have been cated. The literature supports the safety of ethambutol in combination with niazid during pregnancy (1–3). Bobrowitz studied 38 patients (42 pregnanes) receiving antitubercular therapy of 2 to 5 drug regimens (1). The minor normalities noted were within the expected frequency of occurrence. Lewit served six aborted fetuses at 5 to 12 weeks old (2). Embryonic optic stems were specifically examined and were found normal.

east Feeding Summary

data available.

ferences

. Bobrowitz ID. Ethambutol in pregnancy. Chest 1974;66:20–4.
. Lewit T, Nebel L, Terracina S, Karman S. Ethambutol in pregnancy: observations on embryogenesis. Chest 1974;66:25–6.
. Snider DE, Layde PM, Johnson MW, Lyle MA. Treatment of tuberculosis during pregnancy. Am Rev Respir Dis 1980;122:65–79.

---

ame: **ETHANOL**

ass: **Sedative**   Risk Factor: **D***

etal Risk Summary

he teratogenic effects of alcohol have been recognized since antiquity, but is knowledge gradually fell into disfavor and was actually dismissed as perstition in the 1940's (1). Approximately 3 decades later, the characterstic pattern of anomalies which came to be known as the fetal alcohol yndrome (FAS) were rediscovered, first in France and then in the United tates (2–5). Mild FAS (low birthweight) has been induced by the daily onsumption of as little as 2 drinks (1 ounce absolute alcohol) in early regnancy, but the complete syndrome is usually seen when maternal conumption is 4 to 5 drinks (2–2.5 ounces absolute alcohol) per day or more. eavy alcohol intake by both the mother and father prior to conception has lso been suspected of producing the FAS (6, 7). However, this association as been challenged (8). The features of the FAS involve craniofacial, limb, rowth and central nervous system anomalies. Other problems occurring in bout one-half of the cases are cardiac septal and urogenital defects and emangiomas (3–5, 9). Liver abnormalities have also been reported (10, 11). ehavioral problems, including minimal brain dysfunction, are long-term efects of the FAS (1).

A strong association between moderate drinking (>1 ounce absolute alcohol
twice per week) and 2nd trimester (15–27 weeks) spontaneous abortions has
been found (12, 13). Alcohol consumption at this level may increase the risk
of miscarriage by 2 to 4 fold, apparently by acting as an acute fetal toxin
Sandor described cardiac malformations in 43 patients (57%) in a series of 76
children with the FAS evaluated for 0 to 6 years (age: birth to 18 years) (14)
Functional murmurs (12 cases, 16%) and ventricular septal defects (VSD) (20
patients, 26%) accounted for the majority of anomalies. Other cardiac lesions
present, in descending order of frequency, were: double outlet right ventricle
and pulmonary atresia, dextrocardia (with VSD), patent ductus arteriosus with
secondary pulmonary hypertension, and cor pulmonale.

Fetal Alcohol Syndrome

Craniofacial
> Eyes: short palpebral fissures, ptosis, strabismus, epicanthal folds, my-
> opia, microphthalmia, blepharophimosis
> Ears: poorly formed concha, posterior rotation
> Nose: short, upturned hypoplastic philtrum
> Mouth: prominent lateral palatine ridges, thinned upper vermilion, retrog-
> nathia in infancy, micrognathia or relative prognathia in adolescence
> cleft lip or palate, small teeth with faulty enamel
> Maxilla: hypoplastic

Central nervous system
> Dysfunction is demonstrated by mild to moderate retardation, microceph-
> aly, poor coordination, hypotonia, irritability in infancy and hyperactivity
> in childhood

Growth
> Prenatal (affecting body length more than weight) and postnatal deficiency

Cardiac
> Murmurs, atrial septal defect, ventricular septal defect, great vessel
> anomalies, tetralogy of Fallot

Renogenital
> Labial hypoplasia, hypospadias, renal defect

Cutaneous
> Hemangiomas, hirsutism in infancy

Skeletal
> Abnormal palmar creases, pectus excavatum, restriction of joint move-
> ment, nail hypoplasia, radioulnar synostosis, pectus carinatum, bifid
> xiphoid, Klippel-Feil anomaly, scoliosis

Muscular
> Hernias of diaphragm, umbilicus or groin, diastasis recti

Author (ref)	No. Pts.	Indication	Gestational Age	Dose	Other Drugs	Fetal Effects	Comment
son 5)	41	Maternal alcoholism	Through-out	Not stated	Not stated	40 FAS	Data includes original 8 patients reported by Jones in 1973 (4)
tzman 6)	3	Maternal alcoholism	Through-out	Not stated	Not stated	3 FAS 3 withdrawal symptoms beginning in 1st 24 hr of life 2 renal anomalies 2 eye anomalies	
eukelaer 7)	1	Maternal alcoholism	Through-out	Not stated	Not stated	1 FAS 1 renal anomalies	
i 8)	6	Maternal alcoholism Paternal alcoholism	Through-out	Not stated	Not stated	6 FAS 6 renal anomalies	
bick 10)	3	Maternal alcoholism	Through-out	Not stated	Not stated	3 FAS 3 liver anomalies 2 thick, sclerotic central veins 1 congenital hepatic fibrosis 1 renal anomalies	First report of liver anomalies associated with FAS
n 11)	1	Maternal alcoholism	Through-out	Not stated	Not stated	1 Hepatoblastoma at age 27 months (infant treated with azathioprine and prednisone)	Infant received renal transplant at 7 months; association between FAS and liver disease unclear
eg 19)	2	Maternal alcoholism	Through-out	Not stated	Heroin Other abuse drugs likely	2 FAS 2 cardiovascular anomalies VSD 2 pulmonary artery dysplasia	

Risk Factor X if used in large amounts or for prolonged periods.]

reast Feeding Summary

lthough alcohol passes freely into breast milk reaching concentrations approximating maternal serum levels, the effect on the infant is probably insignificant except in rare cases or at very high concentrations (20). The toxic metabolite of ethanol, acetaldehyde, apparently does not pass into milk even though considerable levels can be measured in the mother's blood (21). One report calculated the amount of alcohol received in a single feeding from a other with a blood concentration of 100 mg/dl (equivalent to a heavy, abitual drinker) as 164 mg, an insignificant amount (22). Maternal blood lcohol levels have to reach 300 mg/dl before mild sedation might be seen in e baby.

Potentiation of severe hypoprothrombic bleeding, a pseudo-Cushing syndrome and an effect on the milk-ejecting reflex have been reported (23–25).

Author (ref)	No. Pts.	Dose	Milk Concentration	Comment
Hoh (23)	23	Maternal alcoholism	Assumed equivalent to maternal serum levels	Severe hypoprothrombinemic bleeding; alcohol may have potentiated bleeding by depressing hepatic prothrombin synthesis
Binkiewicz (24)	1	Maternal alcoholism	100 mg/dl	Pseudo-Cushing syndrome
Cobo (25)	40	<1 g/kg	—	No significant response effect on milk-ejecting response
		1-2 g/kg	—	Significant reduction in milk-ejecting response probably due to inhibition of oxytocin release

References

1. Shaywitz BA. Fetal alcohol syndrome: an ancient problem rediscovered. Drug Ther 1978;8:95-108.
2. Lemoine P, Harroussean H, Borteyrn JP. Les enfants de parents alcooliques: anomalies observees. A propos de 127 cas. Quest Med 1968;25:477-82.
3. Ulleland CN. The offspring of alcoholic mothers. Ann NY Acad Sci 1972;197:167-9.
4. Jones KL, Smith DW, Ulleland CN, Streissguth AP. Pattern of malformation in offspring of chronic alcoholic mothers. Lancet 1973;1:1267-71.
5. Jones KL, Smith DW. Recognition of the fetal alcohol syndrome in early infancy. Lancet 1973;2:999-1001.
6. Scheiner AP, Donovan CM, Burtoshesky LE. Fetal alcohol syndrome in child whose parents had stopped drinking. Lancet 1979;1:1077-8.
7. Scheiner AP. Fetal alcohol syndrome in a child whose parents had stopped drinking. Lancet 1979;2:858.
8. Smith DW, Graham JM Jr. Fetal alcohol syndrome in child whose parents had stopped drinking. Lancet 1979;2:527.
9. FDA Drug Bulletin, Fetal Alcohol Syndrome, vol. 7. National Institute on Alcohol Abuse and Alcoholism, 1977:4.
10. Habbick BF, Casey R, Zaleski WA, Murphy F. Liver abnormalities in three patients with fetal alcohol syndrome. Lancet 1979;1:580-1.
11. Khan A, Bader JL, Hoy GR, Sinks LF. Hepatoblastoma in child with fetal alcohol syndrome. Lancet 1979;1:1403-4.
12. Harlap S, Shiono PH. Alcohol, smoking and incidence of spontaneous abortions in the first and second trimester. Lancet 1980;2:173-6.
13. Kline J, Shrout P, Stein Z, Susser M, Warburton D. Drinking during pregnancy and spontaneous abortion. Lancet 1980;2:176-80.
14. Sandor GGS, Smith DF, MacLeod PM. Cardiac malformations in the fetal alcohol syndrome. J Pediatr 1981;98:771-3.
15. Hanson JW, Jones KL, Smith DW. Fetal alcohol syndrome experience with 41 patients. JAMA 1976;235:1458-60.
16. Goetzman BW, Kagan J, Blankenship WJ. Expansion of the fetal alcohol syndrome. Clin Res 1975;23:100A.
17. DeBeukelaer MM, Randall CL, Stroud DR. Renal anomalies in the fetal alcohol syndrome. J Pediatr 1977;91:759-60.
18. Qazi Q, Masakawa A, Milman D, McGann B, Chua A, Haller J. Renal anomalies in fetal alcohol syndrome. Pediatrics 1979;63:886-9.
19. Steeg CN, Woolf P. Cardiovascular malformations in the fetal alcohol syndrome. Am Heart J 1979;98:636-7.
20. Anonymous. Update: drugs in breast milk. Med Lett Drugs Ther 1979;21:21.
21. Kesaniemi YA. Ethanol and acetaldehyde in the milk and peripheral blood of lactating women after ethanol administration. J Obstet Gynaecol Br Commonw 1974;81:84-6.
22. Wilson JT, Brown RD, Cherek DR, et al. Drug excretion in human breast milk. Principles, pharmacokinetics and projected consequences. Clin Pharmacol 1980;5:1-66.
23. Hoh TK. Severe hypoprothrombinaemic bleeding in the breast-fed young infants. Singapore Med J 1969;10:43-9.

24. Binkiewicz A, Robinson MJ, Senior B. Pseudo-Cushing syndrome caused by alcohol in breast milk. J Pediatr 1978;93:965.
25. Cobo E. Effect of different doses of ethanol on the milk-ejecting reflex in lactating women. Am J Obstet Gynecol 1973;115:817–21.

Name: **ETHCHLORVYNOL**

Class: **Hypnotic**   Risk Factor: **D**

Fetal Risk Summary

No reports linking the use of ethchlorvynol with congenital defects have been located. The Collaborative Perinatal Project reported 68 patients with 1st trimester exposure to non-barbiturate sedatives, 12 of which had been exposed to ethchlorvynol (1). For the group as a whole, a slight increase in the expected frequency of malformations was found. Specific data for the ethchlorvynol-exposed infants was not given. Animal data indicates that rapid equilibrium occurs between maternal and fetal blood with maximum fetal blood levels measured within 2 hours of maternal ingestion (2). The authors concluded that following maternal ingestion of a toxic or lethal dose, delivery should be accomplished before equilibrium occurs. Neonatal withdrawal symptoms consisting of mild hypotonia, poor suck, absent rooting, poor grasp and delayed onset jitteriness have been reported (3). The mother had been taking 500 mg daily during the 3rd trimester.

Breast Feeding Summary

No data available.

References

1. Heinonen OP, Slone D, Shapiro S. *Birth Defects and Drugs in Pregnancy.* Littleton: Publishing Sciences Group, 1977:336–7.
2. Hume AS, Williams JM, Douglas BH. Disposition of ethchlorvynol in maternal blood, fetal blood, amniotic fluid, and chorionic fluid. J Reprod Med 1971;6:54–6.
3. Personal communication. Rumack BH, Walravens PA. Department of Pediatrics, University of Colorado Medical Center, 1981.

Name: **ETHINYL ESTRADIOL**

Class: **Estrogenic Hormone**   Risk Factor: **D**

Fetal Risk Summary

Ethinyl estradiol is used frequently in combination with progestins for oral contraception (see Oral Contraceptives). The Collaborative Perinatal Project monitored 89 mother-child pairs who were exposed to ethinyl estradiol during the 1st trimester (1). An increased risk for malformations was found, although identification of the malformations was not provided. Estrogenic agents as a group were monitored in 614 mother-child pairs. An increase in the expected frequency of cardiovascular defects, eye and ear anomalies, and Down's syndrome was reported (2). In a smaller study, 12 mothers were exposed to ethinyl estradiol during the 1st trimester (3). No fetal abnormalities were observed. Ethinyl estradiol has also been used as a contraceptive when given with 72 hours of unprotected midcycle coitus (4). Use of estrogenic hormones during pregnancy is not recommended.

Breast Feeding Summary

Estrogens are frequently used for suppression of post–partum lactation (5, 6). Very small amounts are excreted in milk (6). Doses of 100 to 150 μg of ethinyl estradiol for 5 to 7 days are employed (5). Ethinyl estradiol when used in oral contraceptives has been associated with decreased milk production and decreased composition of nitrogen and protein content in human milk (7). The magnitude of these changes is low. However, the changes in milk production and composition may be of nutritional importance in malnourished mothers. If breast feeding is desired, the lowest dose of oral contraceptives should be chosen. Monitoring of infant weight gain and the possible need for nutritional supplementation should be considered (see Oral Contraceptives).

References

1. Heinonen OP, Slone D, Shapiro S. *Birth Defects and Drugs in Pregnancy*. Littleton: Publishing Sciences Group, 1977:389,391.
2. *Ibid*, 395.
3. Hagler S, Schultz A, Hankin H, Kunstadler RH. Fetal effects of steroid therapy during pregnancy. Am J Dis Child 1963;106:586–90.
4. Dixon GW, Schlesselman JJ, Ory HW, Blye RP. Ethinyl estradiol and conjugated estrogens as postcoital contraceptives. JAMA 1980;244:1336–9.
5. Gilman AG, Goodman LS, Gilman A. *The Pharmacological Basis of Therapeutics*. New York: MacMillan, 1980:1431.
6. Klinger G, Claussen C, Schroder S. Excretion of ethinyloestradiol sulfonate in the human milk. Zentralbl Gynaekol 1981;103:91–5.
7. Lonnerdal B, Forsum E, Hambraeus L. Effect of oral contraceptives on composition and volume of breast milk. Am J Clin Nutr 1980;33:816–24.

Name: **ETHISTERONE**

Class: **Progestogenic Hormone**   Risk Factor: **D**

Fetal Risk Summary

The Food and Drug Administration mandated deletion of pregnancy-related indications for all progestins because of a possible association with congenital anomalies. No reports linking the use of ethisterone alone with congenital defects have been located. The Collaborative Perinatal Project monitored 866 mother-child pairs with 1st trimester exposure to progestational agents (including 2 with exposure to ethisterone) (1). An increase in the expected frequency of cardiovascular defects and hypospadias was observed for the progestational agents as a group, but not for ethisterone as a single agent (2). In a subsequent report from the Collaborative Study a single case of tricuspid atresia and ventricular septal defect was identified with 3rd trimester exposure ethisterone and ethinyl estradiol (3). Use of progestational agents during pregnancy is not recommended (see Oral Contraceptives).

Breast Feeding Summary

See Oral Contraceptives.

References

1. Heinonen OP, Slone D, Shapiro S. *Birth Defects and Drugs in Pregnancy.* Littleton: Publishing Sciences Group, 1977:389,91.
2. *Ibid*, 394.
3. Heinonen OP, Slone D, Monson RR, Hook EB, Shapiro S. Cardiovascular birth defects and antenatal exposure to female sex hormones. N Engl J Med 1977;296:67–70.

Name: **ETHOHEPTAZINE**

Class: **Analgesic**   Risk Factor: **C**

Fetal Risk Summary

The Collaborative Perinatal Project monitored 50,282 mother-child pairs, 60 of which had 1st trimester exposure to ethoheptazine (1). For use anytime during pregnancy, 300 exposures were recorded (2). Although the numbers were small, a possible relationship may exist between this drug and major or minor malformations. Further, a possible association with individual defects was observed (3). The statistical significance of these associations is unknown and independent confirmation is required.

Congenital dislocation of the hip (3 cases)
Umbilical hernia (3 cases)
Inguinal hernia (8 cases)

Breast Feeding Summary

No data available.

References

1. Heinonen OP, Slone D, Shapiro S. *Birth Defects and Drugs in Pregnancy.* Littleton: Publishing Sciences Group, 1977:287–95.
2. *Ibid*, 434.
3. *Ibid*, 485.

Name: **ETHOPROPAZINE**

Class: **Parasympatholytic (Anticholinergic)**   Risk Factor: **C**

Fetal Risk Summary

Ethopropazine is a phenothiazine compound with anticholinergic activity that is used in the treatment of parkinsonism (see also Atropine and Promethazine). No reports of its use in pregnancy have been located.

Breast Feeding Summary

No data available (see also Atropine and Promethazine).

Name: **ETHOSUXIMIDE**

Class: **Anticonvulsant**   Risk Factor: **C**

Fetal Risk Summary

Ethosuximide is a succinimide anticonvulsant used in the treatment of petit mal epilepsy. The use of ethosuximide during pregnancy has been reported in 163 pregnancies (1-11). Due to the lack of specific information on the observed malformations, multiple drug therapies and differences in study methodology, conclusions linking the use of ethosuximide with congenital defects are difficult. Spontaneous hemorrhage in the neonate following *in utero* exposure to ethosuximide has been reported (see also Phenytoin and Phenobarbital) (6). Abnormalities identified with ethosuximide use in 10 pregnancies include:

Patent ductus arteriosus (8 cases)

Cleft lip and/or palate (7 cases)

Mongoloid facies, short neck, altered palmar crease and an accessory nipple (1 case)

Hydrocephalus (1 case)

Ethosuximide has a much lower teratogenic potential than the oxazolidinedione class of anticonvulsants (see also Trimethadione and Paramethadione) (11,12). The succinimide anticonvulsants should be considered the anticonvulsants of choice for the treatment of petit mal epilepsy during the 1st trimester.

Breast Feeding Summary

Ethosuximide freely enters the breast milk in concentrations similar to the maternal serum (13-15). Two reports measured similar milk:plasma ratios of 1.0 and 0.78 (13,14). No adverse effects on the nursing infant have been reported.

References

1. Speidel BD, Meadow SR. Maternal epilepsy and abnormalities of the fetus and newborn. Lancet 1972;2:839-43.
2. Fedrick J. Epilepsy and pregnancy: A report from the Oxford Record Linkage Study. Br Med J 1973;2:442-8.
3. Lowe CR. Congenital malformations among infants born to epileptic women. Lancet 1973;1:9-10.
4. Starreveld-Zimmerman AAE, van der Kolk WJ, Meinardi H, Elshve J. Are anticonvulsants teratogenic? Lancet 1973;2:48-9.
5. Kuenssberg EV, Knox JDE. Teratogenic effect of anticonvulsants. Lancet 1973;2:198.
6. Speidel BD, Meadow SR. Epilepsy, anticonvulsants and congenital malformations. Drugs

1974;8:354-65.
. Janz D. The teratogenic risk of antiepileptic drugs. Epilepsia 1975;16:159-69.
. Nakane Y, Okuma T, Takahashi R, et al. Multi-institutional study on the teratogenicity and fetal toxicity of antiepileptic drugs: a report of a collaborative study group in Japan. Epilepsia 1980;21:663-80.
. Heinonen OP, Slone D, Shapiro S. Birth Defects and Drugs in Pregnancy. Littleton: Publishing Sciences Group, 1977:358-9.
. Dansky L, Andermann E, Andermann F. Major congenital malformations on the offspring of epileptic patients: genetic and environment risk factors. In Epilepsy, Pregnancy and the Child. Proceedings of a workshop held in Berlin, September 1980. New York: Raven Press (in press), 1981.
. Fabro S, Brown NA. Teratogenic potential of anticonvulsants. N Engl J Med 1979;300:1280-1.
. The National Institute of Health. Anticonvulsants found to have teratogenic potential. JAMA 1981;241:36.
. Koup JR, Rose JQ, Cohen ME. Ethosuximide pharmacokinetics in pregnant patient and her newborn. Epilepsia 1978;19:535.
. Kaneko S, Sato T, Suzuki K. The levels of anticonvulsants in breast milk. Br J Clin Pharmacol 1979;7:624-6.
. Horning MG, Stillwell WG, Nowlin J, Lertratanangkoon K, Stillwill RN, Hill RM. Identification and quantification of drugs and drug metabolites in human breast milk using GC-MS-COM methods. Mod Prob Paediatr 1975;15:73-9.

---

ame: **ETHOTOIN**

lass: **Anticonvulsant**   Risk Factor: **D**

etal Risk Summary

thotoin is a low-potency hydantoin anticonvulsant (1). The fetal hydantoin yndrome has been associated with the use of the more potent phenytoin (see henytoin). Only 6 reports describing the use of ethotoin during the 1st imester have been located (2–4). Congenital malformations observed in two f these cases included cleft lip/palate and patent ductus arteriosus (3,4). No ause and effect relationship was established. Although the toxicity of ethotoin ppears to be lower than the more potent phenytoin, the occurrence of ongenital defects in two fetuses exposed to ethantoin suggests that a tera-genic potential may exist.

reast Feeding Summary

o data available.

eferences
. Schmidt RP, Wilder BJ. Epilepsy. In Contemporary Neurology Services, vol. 2. FA Davis Co. Philadelphia 1968:154.
. Heinonen OP, Slone D, Shapiro S. Birth Defects and Drugs in Pregnancy. Littleton: Publishing Sciences Group, 1977:358-9.
. Zablen M, Brand N. Cleft lip and palate with the anticonvulsant ethantoin. N Engl J Med 1978;298:285.
. Nakane Y, Okuma T, Takahashi R, et al. Multi-institutional study on the teratogenicity and fetal toxicity of antiepileptic drugs: a report of a collaborative study group in Japan. Epilepsia 1980;21:663-80.

Name: **ETHYL BISCOUMACETATE**

Class: **Anticoagulant**   Risk Factor: **D**

Fetal Risk Summary

See Coumarin Derivatives.

Breast Feeding Summary

See Coumarin Derivatives.

Name: **ETHYNODIOL**

Class: **Progestogenic Hormone**   Risk Factor: **D**

Fetal Risk Summary

Ethynodiol is used primarily in oral contraceptive products (see Oral Contraceptives).

Breast Feeding Summary

See Oral Contraceptives.

Name: **EVAN'S BLUE**

Class: **Dye**   Risk Factor: **C**

Fetal Risk Summary

No reports linking the use of Evan's blue with congenital defects have been located. The dye is teratogenic in some animal species (1). Evan's blue has been injected intra-amniotically for diagnosis of ruptured membranes without apparent effect on the fetus (2). When given within 48 hours of delivery, the newborn will be temporarily stained.

Breast Feeding Summary

No data available.

References

1. Wilson JG. Teratogenic activity of several azo dyes chemically related to trypan blue. Anat Rec 1955;123:313–34.
2. Atley RD, Sutherst JR. Premature rupture of the fetal membranes confirmed by intraamniotic injection of dye (Evans blue T-1824). Am J Obstet Gynecol 1970;108:993–4.

Name: **FENFLURAMINE**

Class: **Central Stimulant/Anorectant**   Risk Factor: **C**

Fetal Risk Summary

No data available (see Diethylpropion, Dextroamphetamine).

Breast Feeding Summary

No data available.

Name: **FENOPROFEN**

Class: **Nonsteroidal Anti-inflammatory**   Risk Factor: **B***

Fetal Risk Summary

No reports linking the use of fenoprofen with congenital defects have been located. The drug was used during labor in one study (1). No data was given except that the drug could not be detected in cord blood or amniotic fluid. If the drug did reach the fetus, fenoprofen, a prostaglandin synthetase inhibitor, could theoretically cause constriction of the ductus arteriosus *in utero* (2). Persistent pulmonary hypertension of the newborn should also be considered (2). Drugs in this class have been shown to inhibit labor and prolong pregnancy (3). The manufacturer recommends the drug not be used during pregnancy (4).

[* Risk Factor D if used in 3rd trimester or near delivery.]

Breast Feeding Summary

Fenoprofen passes into breast milk in very small quantities. The milk:plasma ratio in nursing mothers given 600 mg every 6 hours for 4 days was approximately 0.017 (1). The clinical significance of this amount is unknown.

References

1. Rubin A, Chernish SM, Crabtree R, et al. A profile of the physiological disposition and gastrointestinal effects of fenoprofen in man. Curr Med Res Opin 1974;2:529–44.
2. Levin DL. Effects of inhibition of prostaglandin synthesis on fetal development, oxygenation, and the fetal circulation. Semin Perinatol 1980;4:35–44.
3. Fuchs F. Prevention of prematurity. Am J Obstet Gynecol 1976;126:809–20.
4. Product information. Nalfon. Dista Products Company, 1982.

Name: **FENOTEROL**

Class: **Sympathomimetic (Adrenergic)**   Risk Factor: **B**

Fetal Risk Summary

No reports linking the use of fenoterol with congenital defects have been located. Fenoterol, a β-sympathomimetic, has been used to prevent premature labor (1, 2). The effects in the mother, fetus and newborn are similar to the parent compound (see Metaproterenol).

Fenoterol was administered to 11 patients 30 minutes prior to cesarean section under general anesthesia at an infusion rate of 3 μg per minute (3). No adverse effects were seen in the mother, fetus or newborn after this short exposure.

Breast Feeding Summary

No data available.

References

1. Lipshitz J, Baillie P, Davey DA. A comparison of the uterine beta-2-adrenoreceptor selectivity of fenoterol, hexoprenaline, ritodrine and salbutamol. S Afr Med J 1976;50:1969–72.
2. Lipshitz J. The uterine and cardiovascular effects of oral fenoterol hydrochloride. Br J Obstet Gynaecol 1977;84:737–9.
3. Jouppila R, Kauppila A, Tuimala R, Pakarinen A, Mailanen. Maternal, fetal and neonatal effects of beta-adrenergic stimulation in connection with cesarean section. Acta Obstet Gynecol Scand 1980;59:489–93.

Name: **FENTANYL**

Class: **Narcotic Analgesic**   Risk Factor: **B***

Fetal Risk Summary

No reports linking the use of fentanyl with congenital defects have been located. Use of the drug during labor should be expected to produce neonatal respiratory depression to the same degree as other narcotic analgesics. Respiratory depression has been observed in one infant whose mother received epidural fentanyl during labor (1). Fentanyl given during general anesthesia may produce loss of fetal heart rate variability without causing fetal hypoxia (2).

[* Risk Factor D if used for prolonged periods or in high doses at term.]

Breast Feeding Summary

No data available.

References

1. Carrie LES, O'Sullivan GM, Seegobin R. Epidural fentanyl in labour. Anaesthesia 1981;36:965–9.
2. Johnson ES, Colley PS. Effects of nitrous oxide and fentanyl anesthesia on fetal heart-rate variability intra- and postoperatively. Anesthesiology 1980;52:429–30.

Name: **FLUCYTOSINE**

Class: **Antifungal**   Risk Factor: **C**

Fetal Risk Summary

Flucytosine is embryotoxic and teratogenic in some species of animals, but its use in human pregnancy has not been studied. Following oral administration, about 4% of the drug is metabolized to 5-fluorouracil, an antineoplastic agent (1). Fluorouracil is suspected of producing congenital defects in humans (see Fluorouracil). Two case reports of pregnant patients treated in the 2nd trimester with flucytosine have been located (2, 3). No defects were observed in either of the newborns.

Breast Feeding Summary

No data available.

References

1. Diasio RB, Lakings DE, Bennett JE. Evidence for conversion of 5-fluorocytosine to 5-fluorouracil in humans: possible factor in 5-fluorocytosine clinical toxicity. Antimicrob Agents Chemother 1978;14:903–8.
2. Philpot CR, Lo D. Cryptococcal meningitis in pregnancy. Med J Aust 1972;2:1005–7.
3. Schonebeck J, Segerbrand E. Candida albicans septicaemia during first half of pregnancy successfully treated with 5-fluorocytosine. Br Med J 1973;4:337–8.

Name: **FLUNITRAZEPAM**

Class: **Hypnotic**   Risk Factor: **C**

Fetal Risk Summary

Flunitrazepam is a benzodiazepine (see also Diazepam). No reports linking the use of flunitrazepam with congenital defects have been located, but other drugs in this group have been suspected of causing fetal malformations (see also Diazepam or Chlordiazepoxide). In contrast to other benzodiazepines, flunitrazepam crosses the placenta slowly (1, 2). About 12 hours after a 1-mg oral dose, cord:maternal blood ratios in early and late pregnancy were about 0.5 and 0.22, respectively. Amniotic fluid:maternal serum ratios were in the

0.02 to 0.07 range in both cases. Accumulation in the fetus may occur after repeated doses (1).

Breast Feeding Summary

Flunitrazepam is excreted into breast milk. Following a single 2-mg oral dose in 5 patients, mean milk:plasma ratios at 11, 15, 27 and 39 hours were 0.61, 0.68, 0.9 and 0.75, respectively (1, 2). The effect of these levels on the nursing infant are unknown but they are probably insignificant.

References

1. Kanto J, Aaltonen L, Kangas L, Erkkola R, Pitkanen Y. Placental transfer and breast milk levels of flunitrazepam. Curr Ther Res 1979;26:539–46.
2. Kanto JH. Use of benzodiazepines during pregnancy, labour and lactation, with special reference to pharmacokinetic considerations. Drugs 1982;23:354–80.

Name: **FLUOROURACIL**

Class: **Antineoplastic**   Risk Factor: **D**

Fetal Risk Summary

Experience with fluorouracil during pregnancy is limited. Following systemic therapy, two reports have described possible teratogenic or toxic effects in the newborn (1, 2). There are no reports of fetal effects after topical use of the drug. Data from one review indicated that 40% of the infants exposed to anticancer drugs were of low birth weight (3). Long term studies of growth and mental development in offspring exposed to fluorouracil and other antineoplastic drugs during the 2nd trimester, the period of neuroblast multiplication, have not been conducted (4).

Amenorrhea has been observed in women treated with fluorouracil for breast cancer but this was probably due to concurrent administration of melphalan (see also Melphalan) (5, 6).

Author (ref)	No. Pts.	Indication	Gestational Age	Dose	Other Drugs	Fetal Effects	Comment
Stephens (1)	1	CA Large bowel	1st trimester	600 mg IV*	Tetracycline Radiation	Radial aplasia Absent thumbs and 3 fingers Hypoplasia of lungs, aorta, thymus, bile duct Aplasia of esophagus, duodenum and ureters	Patient was 41 years old. A therapeutic abortion was elected. Genetic or chromosomal abnormalities cannot be ruled out.
Stadler (2)	1	CA breast	3rd trimester	500 mg IV	Not stated	Cyanosis Jerking extremities	Symptoms persisted 24 hours.

* IV, intravenously

Breast Feeding Summary

No data available.

References

1. Stephens JD, Golbus MS, Miller TR, Wilber RR, Epstein CJ. Multiple congenital anomalies in a fetus exposed to 5-fluorouracil during the first trimester. Am J Obstet Gynecol 1980;137:747–9.
2. Stadler HE, Knowles J. Fluorouracil in pregnancy: effect on the neonate. JAMA 1971;217:214–5.
3. Nicholson HO. Cytotoxic drugs in pregnancy: review of reported cases. J Obstet Gynaecol Br Commonw 1968;75:307–12.
4. Dobbing J. Pregnancy and leukaemia. Lancet 1977;1:1155.
5. Fisher B, Sherman B, Rockette H, Redmond C, Margolese K, Fisher ER. L-phenylalanine (L-PAM) in the management of premenopausal patients with primary breast cancer. Cancer 1979;44:847–57.
6. Schilsky RL, Lewis BJ, Sherins RJ, Young RC. Gonadal dysfunction in patients receiving chemotherapy for cancer. Ann Intern Med 1980;93:109–14.

Name: **FLUPENTHIXOL**

Class: **Tranquilizer**   Risk Factor: **C**

Fetal Risk Summary

See Chlorpromazine.

Breast Feeding Summary

See Chlorpromazine.

Name: **FLUPHENAZINE**

Class: **Tranquilizer**   Risk Factor: **C**

Fetal Risk Summary

Fluphenazine is a piperazine phenothiazine in the same group as prochlorperazine. Phenothiazines readily cross the placenta (1). Extrapyramidal symptoms in the newborn have been attributed to *in utero* exposure to fluphenazine (see also Chlorpromazine) (2). An infant with multiple anomalies was born to a mother treated with fluphenazine enanthate injections throughout pregnancy (see table below) (3). Other reports have indicated that the phenothiazines are relatively safe during pregnancy (see also Prochlorperazine).

Author (ref)	No. Pts.	Indication	Gestational Age	Dose	Other Drugs	Fetal Effects	Comment
Donaldson (3)	1	Schizophrenia	Through-out	25 mg intra-muscularly 11 doses	Debendox Iron Folic acid Acetami-nophen Amytal	Ocular hypertelorism with telecanthus Cleft lip/palate Imperforate anus Hypospadias of peno-scro-tal type Jerky, roving eye move-ments Episodic rapid nystagmoid movements Rectourethral fistula Poor ossification of frontal skull bone	Debendox only other drug taken in 1st trimester

Breast Feeding Summary

No data available.

References

1. Moya F, Thorndike V. Passage of drugs across the placenta. Am J Obstet Gynecol 1962;84:1778–98.
2. Cleary MF. Fluphenazine decanoate during pregnancy. Am J Psychiatry 1977;134:815–6.
3. Donaldson GL, Bury RG. Multiple congenital abnormalities in a newborn boy associated with maternal use of fluphenazine enanthate and other drugs during pregnancy. Acta Paediatr Scand 1982;71:335–8.

Name: **FURAZOLIDONE**

Class: **Anti-infective**   Risk Factor: **C**

Fetal Risk Summary

No reports linking the use of furazolidone with congenital defects have been located. The Collaborative Perinatal Project monitored 50,282 mother-child pairs, 132 of which had 1st trimester exposure to furazolidone (1). No association with malformations was found. Theoretically, furazolidone could produce hemolytic anemia in a glucose-6-phosphate-dehydrogenase-deficient newborn if given at term. Placental passage of the drug has not been reported.

Breast Feeding Summary

No data available.

References

1. Heinonen OP, Slone D, Shapiro S. *Birth Defects and Drugs in Pregnancy*. Littleton: Publishing Sciences Group, 1977:299–302.

Name: FUROSEMIDE

Class: **Diuretic**   Risk Factor: **C**

Fetal Risk Summary

Furosemide is a potent diuretic. Cardiovascular disorders such as pulmonary edema, severe hypertension or congestive heart failure are probably the only valid indications for this drug in pregnancy. Furosemide crosses the placenta (1). Following oral doses of 25 to 40 mg, peak concentrations in cord serum of 330 ng/ml were recorded at 9 hours. Maternal and cord levels were equal at 8 hours. Increased fetal urine production after maternal furosemide therapy has been observed (2, 3). Newborns exposed to furosemide shortly before birth were found to diurese more than controls (4). Urinary sodium and potassium in the treated newborns were significantly greater than in the non-exposed controls.

Furosemide is rarely given during the 1st trimester. After the 1st trimester, furosemide has been used for edema, hypertension and toxemia of pregnancy without causing fetal or newborn adverse effects (5–27). Many investigators now consider diuretics contraindicated in pregnancy, except for patients with cardiovascular disorders, since they do not prevent or alter the course of toxemia and they may decrease placental perfusion (28–31).

Administration of the drug during pregnancy does not significantly alter amniotic fluid volume (26). Serum uric acid levels, which are increased in toxemia, are further elevated by furosemide (32). No association was found in a 1973 study between furosemide and low platelet counts in the neonate (33). Unlike the thiazide diuretics, neonatal thrombocytopenia has not been reported for furosemide.

Breast Feeding Summary

Furosemide is excreted into breast milk (34). While no reports of adverse effects in nursing infants have been found, the manufacturer recommends against breast feeding if furosemide must be given to the mother (34). Thiazide diuretics have been used to suppress lactation (see Chlorothiazide).

References

1. Beermann B, Groschinsky-Grind M, Fahraeus L, Lindstroem B. Placental transfer of furosemide. Clin Pharmacol Ther 1978;24:560–2.
2. Wladimiroff JW. Effect of frusemide on fetal urine production. Br J Obstet Gynaecol 1975;82:221–4.
3. Stein WW, Halberstadt E, Gerner R, Roemer E. Affect of furosemide on fetal kidney function. Arch Gynekol 1977;224:114–5.
4. Pecorari D, Ragni N, Autera C. Administration of furosemide to women during confinement, and its action on newborn infants. Acta Biomed (Italy) 1969;40:2–11.
5. Pulle C. Diuretic therapy in monosymptomatic edema of pregnancy. Minerva Med 1965;56:1622–3.
6. DeCecco L. Furosemide in the treatment of edema in pregnancy. Minerva Med 1965;56:1586–91.

7. Bocci A, Pupita F, Revelli E, Bartoli E, Molaschi M, Massobrio A. The water-salt metabolism in obstetrics and gynecology. Minerva Ginecol 1965;17:103–10.

8. Sideri L. Furosemide in the treatment of oedema in gynaecology and obstetrics. Clin Ter 1966;39:339–46.

9. Wu CC, Lee TT, Kao SC. Evaluation of new diuretic (Furosemide) on pregnant women. A pilot study. J Obstet Gynecol Republ China 1966;5:318–20.

10. Loch EG. Treatment of gestosis with diuretics. Med Klin 1966;61:1512–5.

11. Buchheit M, Nicolai. Influence of furosemide (Lasix) on gestational edemas. Med Klin 1966;61:1515–8.

12. Tanaka T. Studies on the clinical effect of Lasix in edema of pregnancy and toxemia of pregnancy. Sanka To Fujinka 1966;41:914–20.

13. Merger R, Cohen J, Sadut R. Study of the therapeutic effects of furosemide in obstetrics. Rev Fr Gynecol 1967;62:259–65.

14. Nascimento R, Fernandes R, Cunha A. Furosemide as an accessory in the therapy of the toxemia of pregnancy. Hospital (Portugal) 1967;71:137–40.

15. Finnerty FA Jr. Advantages and disadvantages of furosemide in the edematous states of pregnancy. Am J Obstet Gynecol 1969;105:1022–7.

16. Das Gupta S. Frusemide in blood transfusion for severe anemia in pregnancy. J Obstet Gynaecol India 1970;20:521–5.

17. Kawathekar P, Anusuya SR, Sriniwas P, Lagali S. Diazepam (Calmpose) in eclampsia: a preliminary report of 16 cases. Curr Ther Res 1973;15:845–55.

18. Pianetti F. Our results in the treatment of parturient patients with oedema during the five years 1966–1970. Atti Accad Med Lomb 1973;27:137–40.

19. Azcarte Sanchez S, Quesada Rocha T, Rosas Arced J. Evaluation of a plan of treatment in eclampsia (first report). Ginecol Obstet Mex 1973;34:171–86.

20. Bravo Sandoval J. Management of pre-eclampsia-eclampsia in the third gyneco-obstetrical hospital. Cir Cirjjands 1973;41:487–94.

21. Franck H, Gruhl M. Therapeutic experience with nortensin in the treament of toxemia of pregnancy. Munch Med Wochenschr 1974;116:521–4.

22. Cornu P, Laffay J, Ertel M, Lemiere J. Resuscitation in eclampsia. Rev Prat 1975;25:809–30.

23. Finnerty FA Jr. Management of hypertension in toxemia of pregnancy. Hosp Med 1975;11:52–65.

24. Saldana-Garcia RH. Eclampsia: maternal and fetal mortality. Comparative study of 80 cases. In: VIII World Congress of Gynecology and Obstetrics. Int Cong Ser 1976;396:58–9.

25. Palot M, Jakob L, Decaux J, Brundis JP, Quereux C, Wahl P. Arterial hypertensions of labor and the postpartum period. Rev Fr Gynecol Obstet 1979;74:173–6.

26. Votta RA, Parada OH, Windgrad RH, Alvarez OH, Tomassinni TL, Patori AA. Furosemide action on the creatinine concentration of amniotic fluid. Am J Obstet Gynecol 1975;123:621–4.

27. Clark AD, Sevitt LH, Hawkins DF. Use of furosemide in severe toxaemia of pregnancy. Lancet 1972;1:35–6.

28. Pitkin RM, Kaminetzky HA, Newton M, Pritchard JA. Maternal nutrition: a selective review of clinical topics. Obstet Gynecol 1972;40:773–85.

29. Lindheimer MD, Katz AI. Sodium and diuretics in pregnancy. N Engl J Med 1973;288:891–4.

30. Christianson R, Page EW. Diuretic drugs and pregnancy. Obstet Gynecol 1976;48:647–52.

31. Gant NF, Madden JD, Shteri PK, MacDonald PC. The metabolic clearance rate of dehydro-isoandrosterone sulfate. IV. Acute effects of induced hypertension, hypotension, and natriuresis in normal and hypertensive pregnancies. Am J Obstet Gynecol 1976;124:143–8.

32. Carswell W, Semple PF. The effect of furosemide on uric acid levels in maternal blood, fetal blood and amniotic fluid. J Obstet Gynaecol Br Commonw 1974;81:472–4.

33. Jerkner K, Kutti J, Victorin L. Platelet counts in mothers and their newborn infants with respect to antepartum administration of oral diuretics. Acta Med Scand 1973;194:473–5.

34. Product information. Lasix. Hoechst-Roussel Pharmaceuticals, 1980.

Name: **GENTAMICIN**

Class: **Antibiotic**   Risk Factor: **C**

Fetal Risk Summary

Gentamicin is an aminoglycoside antibiotic. The drug rapidly crosses the placenta into the fetal circulation and amniotic fluid (1–8). Following 40- to 80-mg intramuscular (IM) doses given to patients in labor, peak cord serum levels averaging 34 to 44% of maternal levels were obtained at 1 to 2 hours (1, 4, 8). No toxicity attributable to gentamicin was seen in any of the newborns. Patients undergoing 1st and 2nd trimester abortions were given 1 mg/kg IM (5). Gentamicin could not be detected in their cord serum before 2 hours. Amniotic fluid levels were undetectable at this dosage up to 9 hours post-injection. Doubling the dose to 2 mg/kg allowed detectable levels in the fluid in 1 of 2 samples 5 hours post-injection.

Intra-amniotic instillations of gentamicin were given to 11 patients with premature rupture of the membranes (9). Ten patients received 25 mg every 12 hours and one received 25 mg every 8 hours, for a total of 1 to 19 doses per patient. Maternal gentamicin serum levels ranged from 0.063 to 6 μg/ml (all but 1 were less than 0.6 μg/ml and that one was believed to be due to error). Cord serum levels varied from 0.063 to 2 μg/ml (all but 2 were less than 0.6 μg/ml). No harmful effects were seen in the newborns after prolonged exposure to high local concentrations of gentamicin.

No reports linking the use of gentamicin to congenital defects have been located. Ototoxicity, which is known to occur after gentamicin therapy, has not been reported as an effect of *in utero* exposure. However, eighth cranial nerve toxicity in the fetus is well known following exposure to other aminoglycosides (see Kanamycin and Streptomycin) and may potentially occur with gentamicin.

Breast Feeding Summary

Data on the excretion of gentamicin into breast milk is lacking. In one case report, a nursing infant developed two grossly bloody stools while his mother was receiving gentamicin and clindamycin (10). The condition cleared rapidly when breast feeding was discontinued. Clindamycin is known to be excreted into breast milk as are other aminoglycosides (see Amikacin, Kanamycin, Streptomycin and Tobramycin).

References
 1. Percetto G, Baratta A, Menozzi M. Observations on the use of gentamicin in gynecology and obstetrics. Minerva Ginecol 1969;21:1–10.

2. von Kobyletzki D. Experimental studies on the transplacental passage of gentamicin. Paper presented at Fifth International Congress on Chemotherapy, Vienna, 1967.
3. von Koblyetzki D, Wahlig H, Gebhardt F. Pharmacokinetics of gentamicin during delivery. Antimicrob Anticancer Chemother—Proceedings of the Sixth International Congress on Chemotherapy, Tokyo, 1969;1:650–2.
4. Yoshioka H, Monma T, Matsuda S. Placental transfer of gentamicin. J Pediatr 1972;80:121–3.
5. Garcia S, Ballard C, Martin C, Ivler D, Mathies A, Bernard B. Perinatal pharmacology of gentamicin. (Abstract). Clin Res 1972;20:252.
6. Daubenfeld O, Modde H, Hirsch H. Transfer of gentamicin to the foetus and the amniotic fluid during a steady state in the mother. Arch Gynecol 1974;217:233–40.
7. Kauffman R, Morris J, Azarnoff D. Placental transfer and fetal urinary excetion of gentamicin during constant rate maternal infusion. Pediatr Res 1975;9:104–7.
8. Weistein A, Gibbs R, Gallagher M. Placental transfer of clindamycin and gentamicin in term pregnancy. Am J Obstet Gynecol 1976;124:688–91.
9. Freeman D, Matsen J, Arnold N. Amniotic fluid and maternal and cord serum levels of gentamicin after intra-amniotic instillation in patients with premature rupture of the membranes. Am J Obstet Gynecol 1972;113:1138–41.
10. Mann CF. Clindamycin and breast-feeding. Pediatrics 1980;66:1030–1.

Name: **GENTIAN VIOLET**

Class: **Disinfectant/Anthelmintic**   Risk Factor: **C**

Fetal Risk Summary

The Collaborative Perinatal Project monitored 50,282 mother-child pairs, 40 of which had 1st trimester exposure to gentian violet (1). Evidence was found to suggest a relationship to malformations based on defects in 4 patients. Independent confirmation is required to determine the actual risk.

Breast Feeding Summary

No data available.

Reference

1. Heinonen OP, Slone D, Shapiro S. *Birth Defects and Drugs in Pregnancy.* Littleton:Publishing Sciences Group 1977:302.

Name: **GITALIN**

Class: **Cardiac Glycoside**   Risk Factor: **B**

Fetal Risk Summary

See Digitalis.

Breast Feeding Summary

See Digitalis.

Name: **GLYCERIN**

Class: **Diuretic** Risk Factor: **C**

Fetal Risk Summary

No data available.

Breast Feeding Summary

No data available.

Name: **GLYCOPYRROLATE**

Class: **Parasympatholytic (Anticholinergic)** Risk Factor: **C**

Fetal Risk Summary

Glycopyrrolate is an anticholinergic agent. In a large prospective study, 2,323 patients were exposed to this class of drugs during the 1st trimester, only 4 of whom took glycopyrrolate (1). A possible association was found between the total group and minor malformations. Glycopyrrolate has been used prior to cesarean section to decrease gastric secretions (2–4). Maternal heart rate, but not blood pressure, was increased. Uterine activity increased as expected for normal labor (3). Fetal heart rate and variability were not changed significantly confirming the limited placental transfer of this quaternary ammonium compound. No effects in the newborns were observed.

Breast Feeding Summary

No data available (see also Atropine).

References

1. Heinonen OP, Slone D, Shapiro S. *Birth Defects and Drugs in Pregnancy.* Littleton: Publishing Sciences Group, 1977:346–53.
2. Diaz DM, Diaz SF, Marx GF. Cardiovascular effects of glycopyrrolate and belladonna derivatives in obstetric patients. Bull NY Acad Med 1980;56:245–8.
3. Abboud TK, Read J, Miller F, Chen T, Valle R, Henriksen EH. Use of glycopyrrolate in the parturient: effect on the maternal and fetal heart and uterine activity. Obstet Gynecol 1981;57:224–7.
4. Roper RE, Salem MG. Effects of glycopyrrolate and atropine combined with antacid on gastric acidity. Br J Anaesth 1981;53:1277–80.

Name: **GRISEOFULVIN**

Class: **Antifungal**   Risk Factor: **C**

Fetal Risk Summary

Griseofulvin is embryotoxic and teratogenic in some species of animals, but its use in human pregnancy has not been studied. Because of the animal toxicity, at least one publication believes it should not be given during pregnancy (1). Placental transfer of griseofulvin has been demonstrated at term (2).

Breast Feeding Summary

No data available.

References

1. Anonymous. Griseofulvin: a new formulation and some old concerns. Med Lett Drugs Ther 1976;18:17.
2. Rubin A, Dvornik D. Placental transfer of griseofulvin. Am J Obstet Gynecol 1965;92:882–3.

Name: **GUAIFENESIN**

Class: **Expectorant**   Risk Factor: **C**

Fetal Risk Summary

The Collaborative Perinatal Project monitored 197 mother-child pairs with 1st trimester exposure to guaifenesin (1). An increase in the expected frequency of inguinal hernias was found. For use anytime during pregnancy, 1,336 exposures were recorded (2). In this latter case, no evidence for an association with malformations was found.

Breast Feeding Summary

No data available.

References

1. Heinonen OP, Slone D, Shapiro S. *Birth Defects and Drugs in Pregnancy*. Littleton: Publishing Sciences Group, 1977:478.
2. *Ibid*, 442.

Name: **HALOPERIDOL**

Class: **Tranquilizer**   Risk Factor: **C**

Fetal Risk Summary

Two reports describing limb reduction malformations after 1st trimester use of haloperidol have been located (1, 2). In one of these cases, high doses (15 mg/day) were used (2). Other investigations have not found these defects in their patients (3–6). In 98 of 100 patients treated with haloperidol for hyperemesis gravidarum in the 1st trimester, no effects were produced on birth weight, duration of pregnancy, sex ratio, fetal or neonatal mortality, and no malformations were found in abortuses, stillborns or liveborns (3). Two of the patients were lost to followup. In 31 infants with severe reduction deformities born over a 4-year period, none of the mothers remembered taking haloperidol (4). Haloperidol has been used for the control of chorea gravidarum and manic-depressive illness during the 2nd and 3rd trimesters (7, 8). During labor, the drug has been administered to the mother without causing neonatal depression or other effects in the newborn (5).

Author (ref)	No. Pts.	Indica-tion	Gestational Age	Dose	Other Drugs	Fetal Effects	Comment
Dieulangard (1)	1	Antie-metic	1st tri-mester	1.5 mg/day	"Other drugs"	Ectrophocomelia	—
Kopelman (2)	1	Agita-tion	1st tri-mester	15 mg/day	Methyl phenidate Phenytoin Tetracycline Decongestant Surgery (general anesthesia)	Multiple upper and lower limb defects Aortic valve defect Death at 2 hours due to sub-dural hemorrhage	Doubtful rela-tionship to haloperidol

Breast Feeding Summary

Haloperidol is excreted into breast milk. In one patient receiving an average of 29.2 mg per day, a milk level of 5 ng/ml was detected (9). When the dose was decreased to 12 mg, a level of 2 ng/ml was measured. In a second patient taking 10 mg daily, milk levels up to 23.5 ng/ml were found (10). A milk:plasma ratio of 0.6 to 0.7 was calculated. No adverse effects were noted in the nursing infant.

References

1. Dieulangard P, Coignet J, Vidal JC. Sur un cas d'ectro-phocomelie peut-etre d'origine medicamenteuse. Bull Fed Gynecol Obstet 1966;18:85–7.
2. Kopelman AE, McCullar FW, Heggeness L. Limb malformations following maternal use of haloperidol. JAMA 1975;231:62–4.
3. Van Waes A, Van de Velde E. Safety evaluation of haloperidol in the treatment of hyperemesis gravidarum. J Clin Pharmacol 1969;9:224–7.
4. Hanson JW, Oakley GP. Haloperidol and limb deformity. JAMA 1975;231:26.
5. Ayd FJ Jr. Haloperidol: fifteen years of clinical experience. Dis Nerv Syst 1972;33:459–69.
6. Magnier P. On hyperemesis gravidarum; a therapeutical study of R 1625. Gynecol Prat 1964;15:17–23.
7. Donaldson JO. Control of chorea gravidarum with haloperidol. Obstet Gynecol 1982;59:381–2.
8. Nurnberg HG. Treatment of mania in the last six months of pregnancy. Hosp Community Psychiatry 1980;31:122–6.
9. Stewart RB, Karas B, Springer PK. Haloperidol excretion in human milk. Am J Psychiatry 1980;137:849–50.
10. Whalley LJ, Blain PG, Prime JK. Haloperidol secreted in breast milk. Br Med J 1981;282:1746–7.

Name: **HEPARIN**

Class: **Anticoagulant** Risk Factor: **D**

Fetal Risk Summary

No reports linking the use of heparin during gestation with congenital defects have been located. Other problems, at times lethal to the fetus or neonate, may be related to heparin or to the severe maternal disease necessitating anticoagulant therapy. Hall and co-workers reviewed the use of heparin and other anticoagulants during pregnancy (167 references) (see also Coumarin Derivatives) (1). They concluded from the published cases in which heparin was used without other anticoagulants that significant risks existed for the mother and fetus and that heparin was not a clearly superior form of antico-agulation during pregnancy. Nageotte and others analyzed the same data to arrive at a different conclusion (2).

	Hall	Nageotte
Total number of cases	135	119
Term liveborn—no complications	86	86
Premature—survived without complications	19	19
Liveborn—complications (not specified)	1	1
Premature—expired		
heparin therapy appropriate*	10	5
heparin therapy not appropriate*	—	4[a]
severe maternal disease making successful outcome of pregnancy unlikely	—	1[b]

Spontaneous abortions		
unknown cause	2	1
maternal death due to pulmonary embolism	—	1
Stillbirths		
heparin therapy appropriate*	17	8
heparin therapy not appropriate*	—	7[c]
heparin and coumadin used	—	2

* Appropriateness as determined by current standards
[a] Hypertension of pregnancy (4)
[b] Tricuspid atresia (1)
[c] Hypertension of pregnancy (6); proliferative glomerulonephritis (1)

By eliminating the 15 cases in which maternal disease or other drugs were the most likely cause of the fetal problem, Nageotte's analysis results in a 13% (15/119) unfavorable outcome *vs* Hall's 22% (30/135). This new value appears to be significantly better than the 31% (133/426) abnormal outcome reported for coumarin derivatives (see Coumarin Derivatives). Further, in contrast to coumarin derivatives where a definitive drug-induced pattern of malformations has been observed (fetal warfarin syndrome), heparin has not been related to congenital defects nor does it cross the placenta (3–5). Consequently, the mechanism of heparin's adverse effect on the fetus, if it exists, must be indirect. Hall theorized that fetal effects may be due to calcium (or other cation) chelation resulting in the deficiency of that ion(s) in the fetus (1). A more likely explanation, in light of Nageotte's report, is severe maternal disease that could be relatively independent of heparin. In summary, heparin appears to have major advantages over oral anticoagulants as treatment of choice during pregnancy.

Breast Feeding Summary

Heparin is not excreted into breast milk due to its high molecular weight (15,000) (6).

References

1. Hall JG, Pauli RM, Wilson KM. Maternal and fetal sequelae of anticoagulation during pregnancy. Am J Med 1980;68:122–40.
2. Nageotte MP, Freeman RK, Garite TJ, Block RA. Anticoagulation in pregnancy. Am J Obstet Gynecol 1981;141:472.
3. Flessa HC, Kapstrom AB, Glueck HI, Will JJ, Miller MA, Brinker B. Placental transport of heparin. Am J Obstet Gynecol 1965;93:570–3.
4. Russo R, Bortolotti U, Schivazappa L, Girolami A. Warfarin treatment during pregnancy: a clinical note. Haemostasis 1979;8:96–8.
5. Moe N. Anticoagulant-therapy in the prevention of placental infarction and perinatal death. Obstet Gynecol 1982;59:481–3.
6. O'Reilly RA. Anticoagulant, antithrombotic, and thrombolytic drugs. In Gilman AG, Goodman LS, Gilman A, eds. The Pharmacological Basis of Therapeutics, ed. 6. New York: MacMillan, 1980:1350.

Name: **HEROIN**

Class: **Narcotic Analgesic**   Risk Factor: **B***

Fetal Risk Summary

In the United States, heroin exposure during pregnancy is confined to illicit use as opposed to other countries, such as Great Britain, where the drug is commercially available. The documented fetal toxicity of heroin derives from the illicit use and resulting maternal-fetal addiction. In the form available to the addict, heroin is adulterated with various substances such as lactose, glucose, mannitol, starch, quinine, amphetamines, strychnine, procaine or lidocaine or contaminated with bacteria, viruses or fungi (1, 2). Maternal use of other drugs, abuse and non-abuse, is likely. It is, therefore, difficult to separate entirely the effects of heroin on the fetus from the possible effects of other chemical agents, multiple diseases with addiction, and life style.

Heroin rapidly crosses the placenta, entering fetal tissues within one hour of administration. Withdrawal of the drug from the mother causes the fetus to undergo simultaneous withdrawal. Intrauterine death may occur from meconium aspiration (3, 4).

Assessment of fetal maturity and status is often difficult due to uncertain dates and an accelerated appearance of mature lecithin/sphingomyelin ratios (5).

Until recently, the incidence of congenital anomalies was not thought to be increased (6-8). Current data, however, suggests that a significant increase in major anomalies can occur (9). Abnormalities reported with heroin addiction are shown in the table below (6-13). A discernible pattern of defects is not evident.

Characteristics of the infant delivered from a heroin-addicted mother may be (14):

> Accelerated liver maturity with a lower incidence of jaundice (8, 15)
>
> Lower incidence of hyaline membrane disease after 32 weeks gestation (5, 16)
>
> Normal Apgar scores (6)

(*Note:* The findings of Ostrea are in disagreement with the above statements) (9).

> Low birth weight; up to 50% weigh less than 2500 g
>
> Small size for gestational age
>
> Narcotic withdrawal in about 85% (58-91%); symptoms apparent usually within the first 48 hours with some delaying up to 6 days; incidence is directly related to daily dose and length of maternal addiction; hyperactivity, respiratory distress, fever, diarrhea, mucus secretion, sweating, convulsions, yawning and face scratching (7, 8)
>
> Meconium staining of amniotic fluid
>
> Elevated serum magnesium levels when withdrawal signs are present (up to twice normal)
>
> Increased perinatal mortality; rates up to 37% in some series (13)

Random chromosome damage was significantly higher when Apgar scores were 6 or less (12, 17). However, only one case has appeared relating chromosome abnormalities to congenital anomalies (12). The lower incidence of hyaline membrane disease may be due to elevated prolactin blood levels in fetuses of addicted members (18).

Long term effects on growth and behavior have been reported (19). As compared to controls, children age 3 to 6 years delivered from addicted mothers were found to have lower weights, lower heights and impaired behavior, perceptual and organizational abilities.

	No. Pts.	Indication	Gestational Age	Dose	Other Drugs	Fetal Effects	Comment
	40	Maternal addiction	Through-out	Various	Other abuse drugs likely	3 inguinal hernias	—
	382	Maternal addiction	Through-out	Various	Barbiturates Tranquilizers Other abuse drugs likely	1 tracheoesophaged fistula, imperforate anus, hypospadias, congenital fused kidney 1 congenital heart lesion 1 arthrogryposis multiplex 1 incontinenti pigmenti 7 inguinal hernias	—
	830	Maternal addiction	Through-out	Various	Methadone Barbiturates Amphetamines Benzodiazepines Other abuse drugs likely	2 hydrocephalus 2 interrupted aortic arch 4 patent ductus arteriosus 1 ventricular septal defect 1 malrotation of intestines 2 posterior urethral valves 1 multicystic kidney 3 hypospadias 1 cleft lip 2 inguinal hernias 4 metatarsus adductus 8 polydactylism 1 genu recurvatum 2 skin tags 1 clinodactyly 2 hemangiomas	Incidence of defects significantly higher than control group (400 pts). Conclusions differ from previous reports in that authors found higher rates of jaundice, respiratory distress syndrome, low Apgar scores than in controls. 37 infants were found to have defects.
er	22	Maternal addiction	Through-out	Various	Other abuse drugs likely	1 positive phenylketonuria, imperforate anus, rectovaginal fistula, cataracts 1 paraphimosis 1 inguinal hernia	—
	18	Maternal addiction	Through-out	Various	Other abuse drugs likely	1 mongol, talipes equinovarus, bilateral polycystic kidneys 1 umbilical hernia, divergent strabismus	—
	1	Maternal addiction	1st trimester	Not known	Cocaine Other abuse drugs likely	Chromosome aneuploidy 45, X, bilaterally absent fifth toes features consistent with Turner's syndrome phenotype	Only report of chromosome defect related to a congenital anomaly after heroin use
	82	Maternal addiction	Through-out	Various	Other abuse drugs likely	1 cardiac malformation 1 tracheoesophageal fistula 1 clubfeet 1 diaphragmatic hernia	

* Risk Factor D if used for prolonged periods or in high doses at term.]

Breast Feeding Summary

Heroin crosses into breast milk in sufficient quantities to cause addiction in the infant (20). A milk:plasma ratio has not been reported. Previous investigators have considered nursing as one method for treating the addicted newborn (21).

References

1. Anonymous. Diagnosis and management of reactions to drug abuse. Med Lett Drugs Ther 1980;22:74.
2. Thomas L. Notes of a biology-watcher. N Engl J Med 1972;286:531–3.
3. Chappel JN. Treatment of morphine-type dependence. JAMA 1972;221:1516.
4. Rementeria JL, Nunag NN. Narcotic withdrawal in pregnancy: stillbirth incidence with a case report. Am J Obstet Gynecol 1973;116:1152–6.
5. Gluck L, Kulovich MV. Lecithin/sphingomyelin ratios in amniotic fluid in normal and abnormal pregnancy. Am J Obstet Gynecol 1973;115:539–46.
6. Reddy AM, Harper RG, Stern G. Observations on heroin and methadone withdrawal in the newborn. Pediatrics 1971;48:353–8.
7. Stone ML, Salerno LJ, Green M, Zelson C. Narcotic addiction in pregnancy. Am J Obstet Gynecol 1971;109:716–23.
8. Zelson C, Rubio E, Wasserman E. Neonatal narcotic addiction: 10 year observation. Pediatrics 1971;48:178–89.
9. Ostrea EM, Chavez CJ. Perinatal problems (excluding neonatal withdrawal) in maternal drug addiction: a study of 830 cases. J Pediatr 1979;94:292–5.
10. Perlmutter JF. Drug addiction in pregnant women. Am J Obstet Gynecol 1967;99:569–72.
11. Krause SO, Murray PM, Holmes JB, Burch RE. Heroin addiction among pregnant women and their newborn babies. Am J Obstet Gynecol 1958;75:754–8.
12. Kushnick T, Robinson M, Tsao C. 45, X chromosome abnormality in the offspring of a narcotic addict. Am J Dis Child 1972;124:772–3.
13. Naeye RL, Blanc W, Leblanc W, Khatamee MA. Fetal complications of maternal heroin addiction: abnormal growth, infections and episodes of stress. J Pediatr 1973;83:1055–61.
14. Perlmutter JF. Heroin addiction and pregnancy. Obstet Gynecol Surv 1974;29:439–46.
15. Nathenson G, Cohen MI, Liff IF, McNamara H. The effect of maternal heroin addiction on neonatal jaundice. J Pediatr 1972;81:899–903.
16. Glass L, Rajegowda BK, Evans HE. Absence of respiratory distress syndrome in premature infants of heroin-addicted mothers. Lancet 1971;2:685–6.
17. Amarose AP, Norusis MJ. Cytogenetics of methadone-managed and heroin-addicted pregnant women and their newborn infants. Am J Obstet Gynecol 1976;124:635–40.
18. Parekh A, Mukherjee TK, Jhaveri R, Rosenfeld W, Glass L. Intrauterine exposure to narcotics and cord blood prolactin concentrations. Obstet Gynecol 1981;57:447–9.
19. Wilson GS, McCreary R, Kean J, Baxter JC. The development of preschool children of heroin-addicted mothers: a controlled study. Pediatrics 1979;63:135–41.
20. Lichlenstein PM. Infant drug addiction. NY Med J 1915;102:905. As reported by Cobrinik RW, et al, in Pediatrics 1959;24:288–304.
21. Cobrinik RW, Hood RT Jr, Chusid E. The effect of maternal narcotic addiction on the newborn infant. Pediatrics 1959;24:288–304.

Name: **HETACILLIN**

Class: **Antibiotic**   Risk Factor: **B**

Fetal Risk Summary

Hetacillin, a penicillin antibiotic, breaks down in aqueous solution to ampicillin and acetone (see Ampicillin).

Breast Feeding Summary

See Ampicillin.

Name: **HEXAMETHONIUM**

Class: **Antihypertensive**   Risk Factor: **C**

Fetal Risk Summary

No reports linking the use of hexamethonium with congenital defects have been located. Hexamethonium crosses the placenta and accumulates in the amniotic fluid. The drug has been used in the treatment of pre-eclampsia and essential hypertension. Its use in these conditions is no longer recommended. Three cases of paralytic ileus and one case of delayed passage of meconium have been reported (1, 2).

Breast Feeding Summary

No data available.

References

1. Morris N. Hexamethonium in the treatment of pre-eclampsia and essential hypertension during pregnancy. Lancet 1953;1:322–4.
2. Hallum JL, Hatchuel WLF. Congenital paralytic ileus in a premature baby as a complication of hexamethonium bromide therapy for toxemia of pregnancy. Arch Dis Child 1954;29:354–6.

Name: **HEXOCYCLIUM**

Class: **Parasympatholytic (Anticholinergic)**   Risk Factor: **C**

Fetal Risk Summary

Hexocyclium is an anticholinergic agent. No reports of its use in pregnancy have been located (see also Atropine).

Breast Feeding Summary

No data available (see also Atropine).

Name: **HOMATROPINE**

Class: **Parasympatholytic (Anticholinergic)**   Risk Factor: **C**

Fetal Risk Summary

Homatropine is an anticholinergic agent. The Collaborative Perinatal Project monitored 50,282 mother-child pairs, 26 of which used homatropine in the 1st trimester (1). For use anytime during pregnancy, 86 exposures were recorded (2). Only for anytime use was a possible association with congenital defects discovered. In addition, when the group of parasympatholytics were taken as a whole (2,323 exposures), a possible association with minor malformations was found (1).

Breast Feeding Summary

See Atropine.

References

1. Heinonen OP, Slone D, Shapiro S. *Birth Defects and Drugs in Pregnancy.* Littleton: Publishing Sciences Group, 1977:346–53.
2. *Ibid,* 439.

Name: **HORMONAL PREGNANCY TEST TABLETS**

Class: **Estrogenic/Progestogenic Hormones**   Risk Factor: **D**

Fetal Risk Summary

See Oral Contraceptives.

Breast Feeding Summary

See Oral Contraceptives.

Name: **HYDRALAZINE**

Class: **Antihypertensive**   Risk Factor: **B**

Fetal Risk Summary

No reports linking the use of hydralazine with congenital defects have been located. Neonatal thrombocytopenia and bleeding secondary to maternal ingested hydralazine has been reported in three infants (1). In each case, the mother had consumed the drug daily throughout the 3rd trimester. The condition returned to normal within a few weeks. The Collaborative Perinatal Project monitored 50,282 mother-child pairs, 8 of which had 1st trimester exposure to hydralazine (2). For use anytime during pregnancy, 136 cases were recorded (3). No defects were observed with 1st trimester use although there were 8 infants born with defects who were exposed in the 2nd or 3rd trimesters. This incidence (5.8%) is greater than the expected frequency of occurrence; however, no major category or individual malformations were identified. Patients with pre-eclampsia are at risk for having a marked increase in fetal mortality (4–7). Use of hydralazine in 194 pre-eclamptic or eclamptic women was not associated with adverse fetal effects (4–7). Fatal maternal ypotension has been reported in one patient after combined therapy with ydralazine and diazoxide (8).

reast Feeding Summary

o reports of hydralazine's excretion into breast milk have been located. A redicted milk:plasma ratio of 1.1 to 1.45 has been calculated from the pK_a alue (9).

eferences

1. Widerlov E, Karlman I. Storsater J. Hydralazine-induced neonatal thrombocytopenia. N Engl J Med 1980;303:1235.
2. Heinonen OP, Slone D, Shapiro S. *Birth Defects and Drugs in Pregnancy.* Littleton: Publishing Sciences Group, 1977:372.
3. *Ibid*, 441.
4. Bott-Kanner G, Schweitzer A, Schoenfeld A, Joel-Cohen J, Rosenfeld JB. Treatment with propranolol and hydralazine throughout pregnancy in a hypertensive patient. Isr J Med Sci 1978;14:466–8.
5. Pritchard JA, Pritchard SA. Standardized treatment of 154 consecutive cases of eclampsia. Am J Obstet Gynecol 1975;123:543–52.
6. Chapman ER, Strozier WE, Magee RA. The clinical use of Apresoline in the toxemias of pregnancy. Am J Obstet Gynecol 1954;68:1109–17.
7. Johnson GT, Thompson RB. A clinical trial of intravenous Apresoline in the management of toxemia of late pregnancy. J Obstet Gynecol 1958;65:360–6.
8. Henrich WL, Cronin R, Miller PD, Anderson RJ. Hypotensive sequelae of diazoxide and hydralazine therapy. JAMA 1977;237:264–5.
9. Daily JW. Anticoagulant and cardiovascular drugs. In Wilson JT, ed. *Drugs in Breast Milk.* Australia: ADIS Press, 1981:61–4.

Name: **HYDROCHLOROTHIAZIDE**

Class: **Diuretic**   Risk Factor: **D**

etal Risk Summary

See Chlorothiazide.

Breast Feeding Summary

See Chlorothiazide.

Name: **HYDROCODONE**

Class: **Narcotic Analgesic/Antitussive**   Risk Factor: **B***

Fetal Risk Summary

No reports linking the use of hydrocodone with congenital defects have been located. Due to its narcotic properties, withdrawal could theoretically occur in infants exposed *in utero* to prolonged maternal ingestion of hydrocodone.
* Risk Factor D if used for prolonged periods or if high doses given at term.]

Breast Feeding Summary

No data available.

Name: **HYDROFLUMETHIAZIDE**

Class: **Diuretic**   Risk Factor: **D**

Fetal Risk Summary

See Chlorothiazide.

Breast Feeding Summary

See Chlorothiazide.

Name: **HYDROMORPHONE**

Class: **Narcotic Analgesic**   Risk Factor: **B***

Fetal Risk Summary

No reports linking the use of hydromorphone with congenital defects have been located. Withdrawal could occur in infants exposed *in utero* to prolonged maternal ingestion of hydromorphone. Use of the drug in pregnancy is primarily confined to labor. Respiratory depression in the neonate similar to that produced by meperidine or morphine should be expected (1).

[* Risk Factor D if used for prolonged periods or if high doses given at term.]

Breast Feeding Summary

No data available.

Reference

1. Bonica J. *Principles and Practice of Obstetric Analgesia and Anesthesia.* Philadelphia: FA Davis, 1967:251.

Name: **HYDROXYPROGESTERONE**

Class: **Progestogenic Hormone**   Risk Factor: **D**

Fetal Risk Summary

The Food and Drug Administration mandated deletion of pregnancy-related indications from all progestins because of a possible association with congenital anomalies. Ambiguous genitalia of both male and female fetuses have been reported with hydroxyprogesterone (see Norethindrone, Norethynodrel) (1–3). The Collaborative Perinatal Project monitored 866 mother-child pairs with 1st trimester exposure to progestational agents (including 162 with exposure to hydroxyprogesterone) (4). An increase in the expected frequency of cardiovascular defects and hypospadias was observed for both estrogens and progestogens (3). Because of overlap and the rigor of multivariate analysis, there was insufficient data to support an increase in risk for hydroxyprogesterone. Dillion reported 6 infants with malformations exposed to hydroxyprogesterone during various stages of gestation (7, 8). The congenital defects included spina bifida, anencephalus, hydrocephalus, Fallot's tetralogy, common truncus arteriosus, cataract and ventricular septal defect. Complete absence of both thumbs and dislocated head of the right radius in a child has been associated with hydroxyprogesterone (9). Use of diazepam in early pregnancy and the lack of similar reports makes an association doubtful. Developmental changes in the psychosexual performance of boys has been attributed to *in utero* exposure to hydroxyprogesterone (10). The mothers received an estrogen/progestogen regimen for their diabetes. Hormone-exposed males demonstrated a trend to have less heterosexual experience and fewer masculine interests than controls. The use of high dose hydroxprogesterone during the 2nd and 3rd trimesters has been advocated for the prevention of premature labor (10, 11). However, the use of this steroid was ineffective for this indication in twin pregnancies (12). Fetal adverse effects were not observed.

Breast Feeding Summary

No data available.

References

1. Dayan E, Rosa FW. Fetal ambiguous genitalia associated with sex hormone use early in pregnancy. ADR Highlights 1981:1–14. Food and Drug Administration, Division of Drug Experience.
2. Wilkins L. Masculinization of female fetus due to use of orally given progestins. JAMA 1960;172;1028–32.
3. Wilkins L, Jones HW, Holman GH, Stempfel RS Jr. Masculinization of the female fetus associated with administration of oral and intramuscular progestins during gestation: nonadrenal female pseudohermaphrodism. J Clin Endocrin Metab 1958;68:559–85
4. Heinonen OP, Slone D, Shapiro S. *Birth Defects and Drugs in Pregnancy.* Littleton: Publishing Sciences Group, 1977:389,391.
5. *Ibid*, 394.
6. Heinonen OP, Slone D, Monson RR, Hook EB, Shapiro S. Cardiovascular birth defects and antenatal exposure to female sex hormones. N Engl J Med 1977;296:67–70.
7. Dillion S. Congenital malformations and hormones in pregnancy. Br Med J 1976;2:1446.
8. Dillon S. Progestogen therapy in early pregnancy and associated congenital defects. Practioner 1970;205:80–4.
9. Yalom ID, Green R, Fisk N. Prenatal exposure to female hormones. Effect on psychosexual development in boys. Arch Gen Psychiatry 1973;28:554–61.
10. Johnson JWC, Austin KL, Jones GS, Davis GH, King TM. Efficacy of 17-hydroxyprogesterone caproate in the prevention of premature labor. N Engl J Med 1975;293:675–80.
11. Johnson JWC, Lee PA, Zachary AS, Calhoun S, Migeon CJ. High-risk prematurity-progestin treatment and steroid studies. Obstet Gynecol 1979;54:412–18.
12. Hartikainen-Sorri AL, Kauppila A, Tuimala R. Inefficacy of 17-hydroxyprogesterone caproate in the prevention of prematurity in twin pregnancy. Obstet Gynecol 1980;56:692–5.

Name: **HYDROXYZINE**

Class: **Tranquilizer**   Risk Factor: **C**

Fetal Risk Summary

Hydroxyzine belongs to the same class of compounds as buclizine, cyclizine and meclizine. Although an animal teratogen in high doses, human teratogenicity has not been proven. In 100 patients treated in the 1st trimester with oral hydroxyzine (50 mg daily) for nausea and vomiting, no significant difference from non-treated controls was found in fetal wastage or anomalies (1). The Collaborative Perinatal Project monitored 50,282 mother-child pairs, 50 of which had 1st trimester exposure to hydroxyzine (2). For use anytime during pregnancy, 187 exposures were recorded (3). Based on 5 malformed children, a possible relationship was found between 1st trimester use and congenital defects, but the numbers were too small to determine statistical significance. The manufacturer considers the drug contraindicated in early pregnancy (4). During labor, hydroxyzine has been shown to be safe and effective for the relief of anxiety (5). No effect on the progress of labor or on neonatal Apgar scores was observed.

Breast Feeding Summary

No data available.

References

1. Erez S, Schifrin BS, Dirim O. Double-blind evaluation of hydroxyzine as an antiemetic in pregnancy. J Reprod Med 1971;7:57–9.
2. Heinonen OP, Slone D, Shapiro S. Birth Defects and Drugs in Pregnancy. Littleton: Publishing Sciences Group, 1977:335–7,341.
3. Ibid, 438.
4. Product information. Vistaril. Pfizer Laboratories, 1981.
5. Zsigmond EK, Patterson RL. Double-blind evaluation of hydroxyzine hydrochloride in obstetric anesthesia. Anesth Analg (Cleve) 1967;46:275.

Name: **L-HYOSCYAMINE**

Class: **Parasympatholytic (Anticholinergic)**   Risk Factor: **C**

Fetal Risk Summary

L-Hyoscyamine is an anticholinergic agent. No reports of its use in pregnancy have been located (see also Belladonna or Atropine).

Breast Feeding Summary

See Atropine.

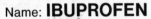

Name: **IBUPROFEN**

Class: **Nonsteroidal Anti-inflammatory**   Risk Factor: **B***

Fetal Risk Summary

No published reports linking the use of ibuprofen with congenital defects have been located. The manufacturer has nearly a dozen reports of ibuprofen use during pregnancy, all but one resulting in normal term infants (1). The one malformation involved an anencephalic infant exposed during the 1st trimester to ibuprofen and Bendectin (doxylamine succinate and pyridoxine hydrochloride). No cause and effect relationship could be established.

Theoretically, ibuprofen, a prostaglandin synthetase inhibitor, could cause constriction of the ductus arteriosus *in utero* (2). Persistent pulmonary hypertension of the newborn should also be considered (2). Drugs in this class have been shown to inhibit labor and prolong pregnancy (3). The manufacturer recommends that the drug not be used during pregnancy (4).

[*Risk Factor D if used in 3rd trimester.]

Breast Feeding Summary

Ibuprofen apparently does not enter human milk in significant quantities. In 12 patients taking 400 mg every 6 hours for 24 hours, an assay capable of detecting 1 μg/ml failed to demonstrate ibuprofen in the milk (5). In another case report, a woman was treated with 400 mg twice daily for 3 weeks (6). Milk levels shortly before and up to 8 hours after drug administration were all less than 0.5 μg/ml.

References

1. Personal communication. MM Westland, The Upjohn Company, 1981.
2. Levin DL. Effects of inhibition of prostaglandin synthesis on fetal development, oxygenation, and the fetal circulation. Semin Perinatol 1980;4:35–44.
3. Fuchs F. Prevention of prematurity. Am J Obstet Gynecol 1976;126:809–20.
4. Product information. Motrin. The Upjohn Company, 1982.
5. Townsend RJ, Benedetti T, Erickson S, Gillespie WR, Albert KS. A study to evaluate the passage of ibuprofen into breast milk (Abstract). Drug Intell Clin Pharm 1982;16:482–3.
6. Weibert RT, Townsend RJ, Kaiser DG, Naylor AJ. Lack of ibuprofen secretion into human milk. Clin Pharm 1982;1:457–8.

Name: **IDOXURIDINE**

Class: **Antiviral**   Risk Factor: **C**

Fetal Risk Summary

Idoxuridine has not been studied in human pregnancy. The drug is teratogenic in some species of animals after injection and ophthalmic use (1, 2).

Breast Feeding Summary

No data available.

References

1. Nishimura H, Tanimura T. *Clinical Aspects of the Teratogenicity of Drugs.* Amsterdam: Excerpta Medica, 1976: 148, 258–9.
2. Itoi M, Gefter JW, Kaneko N, Ishii Y, Ramer RM, Gasset AR. Teratogenicities of ophthalmic drugs. I. Antiviral ophthalmic drugs. Arch Ophthalmol 1975;93:46–51.

Name: **IMIPRAMINE**

Class: **Antidepressant**   Risk Factor: **D**

Fetal Risk Summary

Imipramine has been shown to cross the placenta in the rat (1). Data for placental transfer in humans has not been located. Bilateral amelia was reported in one child whose mother had injested imipramine during pregnancy (2). Analysis of 546,505 births, 161 with 1st trimester exposure to imipramine, were unable to confirm an association with limb reduction defects (3–15). Reported malformations other than limb reduction include (7, 10, 11):

    Defective abdominal muscles (1 case)
    Diaphragmatic hernia (2 cases)
    Exencephaly, cleft palate, adrenal hypoplasia (1 case)
    Cleft palate (2 cases)
    Renal cystic degeneration (1 case)

These reports indicate that imipramine is not a major cause of congenital limb deformities.

Neonatal withdrawal symptoms have been reported with the use of imipramine during pregnancy. The symptoms observed were colic, cyanosis and irritability during the 1st week of life (16, 17). Urinary retention in the neonate has been associated with maternal use of nortriptyline (chemically related to imipramine) (18).

Breast Feeding Summary

Imipramine and its metabolite, desipramine, enter breast milk in low concentrations (19, 20). A milk:plasma ratio of 1 has been suggested (19). Assuming a therapeutic serum level of 200 ng/ml, a 5-kg infant consuming 1000 ml of

breast milk would ingest a daily dose of about 0.2 mg. The significance of this
amount is not known.

Author (ref)	No. Pts.	Dose	Concentrations (µg/ml) Serum	Concentrations (µg/ml) Milk	M:P Ratio	Effect on Infant
Sovner (19)	1	Not stated	0.021	0.004–0.029	0.2–1.4	Not stated

References

1. Douglas BH, Hume AS. Placental transfer of imipramine: a basic, lipid-soluble drug. Am J Obstet Gynecol 1967;99:573–7.
2. McBride WG. Limb deformities associated with iminodibenzyl hydrochloride. Med J Aust 1972; 1:492.
3. Heinonen OP, Slone D, Shapiro S. Birth Defects and Drugs in Pregnancy. Littleton: Publishing Sciences Group, 1977:336–7.
4. Crombie DL, Pinsent R, Fleming D. Imipramine in pregnancy. Br Med J 1972; 1:745.
5. Sim M. Imipramine and pregnancy. Br Med J 1972; 2:45.
6. Scanlon FJ. Use of antidepressant drugs during the first trimester. Med J Aust 1969;2:1077.
7. Kuenssberg EV, Knox JDE. Imipramine in pregnancy. Br Med J 1972;2:29.
8. Rachelefsky GS, Flynt JW, Eggin AJ, Wilson MG. Possible teratogenicity of tricyclic antidepressants. Lancet 1972; 1:838.
9. Banister P, Dafoe C, Smith ESO, Miller J. Possible teratogenicity of tricyclic antidepressants. Lancet 1972; 1:838–9.
10. Barson AJ. Malformed infant. Br Med J 1972; 2:45.
11. Idanpaan-Heikkila J, Saxen L. Possible teratogenicity of imipramine/chloropyramine. Lancet 1973;2:282–3.
12. Jacobs D. Imipramine (Tofranil). S Afr Med J 1972;46:1023.
13. Australian Drug Evaluation Committee. Tricyclic antidepressant and limb reduction deformities. Med J Aust 1973;1:766–9.
14. Morrow AW. Imipramine and congenital abnormalities. N Z Med J 1972;75:228–9.
15. Wilson JG. Present status of drugs as teratogens in man. Teratology 1973;7:3–15.
16. Hill RM. Will this drug harm the unborn infant? South Med J 1977;67:1476–80.
17. Eggermont E. Withdrawal symptoms in neonate associated with maternal imipramine therapy. Lancet 1973;2:680.
18. Shearer WT, Schreiner RL, Marshall RE. Urinary retention in a neonate secondary to maternal ingestion of nortriptyline. J Pediatr 1972;81:570–2.
19. Sovner R, Orsulak PJ. Excretion of imipramine and desipramine in human breast milk. Am J Psychiatry 1979;136:451–2.
20. Erickson SH, Smith GH, Heidrich F. Tricyclics and breast feeding. Am J Psychiatry 1979;136:1483.

Name: **INDIGO CARMINE**

Class: **Dye**   Risk Factor: **B**

Fetal Risk Summary

Indigo carmine is used as a diagnostic dye and for food coloring. No reports linking its use with congenital defects have been located. Intra-amniotic injection has been accomplished without apparent effect on the fetus (1). Due to its known toxicities after intravenous administration, however, one author cautioned that the dye should not be considered totally safe (2).

Breast Feeding Summary

No data available.

References

1. Elias S, Gerbie AB, Simpson JL, Nadler HL, Sabbagha RE, Shkolnik A. Genetic amniocentesis in twin gestations. Am J Obstet Gynecol 1980;138:169–74.
2. Fribourg S. Safety of intraamniotic injection of indigo carmine. Am J Obstet Gynecol 1981;140:350–1.

Name: **INDOMETHACIN**

Class: **Nonsteroidal Anti-inflammatory Analgesic**   Risk Factor: **D**

Fetal Risk Summary

Phocomelia and agenesis of the penis have been attributed to *in utero* exposure to indomethacin (1). The drug has been used for the prevention of premature labor based on its action as a prostaglandin synthetase inhibitor (2–14). This use may cause *in utero* constriction of the ductus arteriosus resulting in persistent pulmonary hypertension (PPHN) in the newborn (2–9). Severe oligohydramnion, meconium staining and hemorrhage have been reported in 3 infants (11). The manufacturer recommends that the drug not be used during pregnancy (15).

hor (f)	No. Pts.	Indication	Gestational Age	Dose	Other Drugs	Fetal Effects	Comment
sta	1	—	—	—	—	Phocomelia Agenesis of Penis	
man	50	Premature labor	<27–36 weeks	Total 200–1100 mg	Not stated	Surviving: 38 mature, 7 premature. Deaths in 5 premature: 1 stillborn, 4 neonatal	No "ill effects" noted in surviving infants
ester	7	Premature labor	1 33 weeks, 1 27–34 weeks, 5 not stated	Total: 1 550 mg (4 days), 1 2500–2800 mg (53 days), 5 not stated	1 alcohol infusion; ampicillin, kanamycin, thiopental, and nitrous oxide; 1 Maalox, intravenous antibiotics, oxytocin, mepivacaine, morphine, secobarbital; 5 not stated	2 PPHN, 5 asymptomatic	
tz	3	Premature labor	1 34 weeks, 1 33 weeks, 1 32 weeks	Total: 1 550 mg (4 days), 1 2500–2800 mg (53 days), 5 not stated	Not stated	1 died after 3 hours of life; meconium stained, gastric hemorrhage. 1 stillborn; meconium stained, severe oligohydramnion, intraperitoneal hemorrhage. 1 stillborn; meconium stained, severe oligohydramnion	Ductus arteriosus internal diameters were 2.0, 2.0 and 2.5 mm respectively; normal in term babies is 4.4 mm
	10	Premature labor	Average at birth: 38.5 weeks (35–41 weeks)	100 mg rectal then 25 mg p.o. every 6 hr	Not stated	5 PPHN, 2 died on 1st day, no hyaline membrane disease found	
	1	Premature labor	36 weeks	25 mg/day for 3 days	Not stated	Died at 55 hours of age; patent ductus arteriosus; increase in pulmonary arterial muscle due to increased smooth muscle; hypoxemia	
elli	29	Premature labor	29–36 weeks	100 mg/day for 5 days, repeated as needed	Ritodrine	5 PPHN, 1 hyaline membrane disease, died from intraventricular hemorrhage	

Breast Feeding Summary

Indomethacin is excreted in human breast milk, but a milk:plasma ratio has not been reported. It is known that milk levels are similar to maternal plasma (16). One case report of possible indomethacin-induced convulsions in a breast-fed infant has appeared, although the causal link between the two events has been questioned (16, 17). The mother was taking 200 mg per day (3 mg/kg/day). The manufacturer recommends that the drug not be used when breast feeding (15).

References

1. Di Battista C, Landizi L, Tamborino G. Focomelia ed agenesia del pene in neonato. Minerva Pediatr 1975;27:675. As cited in Dukes MNG, ed. Side Effects of Drugs Annual 1. Amsterdam: Excerpta Medica, 1977:89.
2. Levin DL. Effects of inhibition of prostaglandin synthesis on fetal development, oxygenation, and the fetal circulation. Semin Perinatol 1980;4:35–44.
3. Zuckerman H, Reiss U, Rubinstein I. Inhibition of human premature labor by indomethacin. Obstet Gynecol 1974;44:787–92.
4. Reiss U, Atad J, Rubinstein I, Zuckerman H. The effect of indomethacin in labour at term. Int J Gynaecol Obstet 1976;14:369–74.
5. Manchester D, Margolis HS, Sheldon RE. Possible association between maternal indomethacin therapy and primary pulmonary hypertension of the newborn. Am J Obstet Gynecol 1976;126:467–9.
6. Csaba IF, Sulyok E, Ertl T. Relationship of maternal treatment with indomethacin to persistence of fetal circulation syndrome. J Pediatr 1978;92:484.
7. Levin DL, Fixler DE, Morriss FC, Tyson J. Morphologic analysis of the pulmonary vascular bed in infants exposed in utero to prostaglandin synthetase inhibitors. J Pediatr 1978;92:478–83.
8. Grella P, Zanor P. Premature labor and indomethacin. Prostaglandins 1978;16:1007–17.
9. Rubaltelli FF, Chiozza ML, Zanardo V, Cantarutti F. Effect on neonate of maternal treatment with indomethacin. J Pediatr 1979;94:161.
10. Wiqvist N, Lundstrom V, Green K. Premature labor and indomethacin. Prostaglandins 1975;10:515–26.
11. Itskovitz J, Abramovici H, Brandes JM. Oligohydramnion, meconium and perinatal death concurrent with indomethacin treatment in human pregnancy. J Reprod Med 1980;24:137–40.
12. Gamissans O, Canas E, Cararach V, Ribas J, Puerto B, Edo A: A study of indomethacin combined with ritodrine in threatened preterm labor. Eur J Obstet Reprod Biol 1978;8:123–8.
13. Tinga DJ, Aranoudse JG. Post-partum pulmonary oedema associated with preventive therapy for premature labor. Lancet 1979;1:1026.
14. Souka AR, Osman N, Sibaie F, Einen MA. Therapeutic value of indomethacin in threatened abortion. Prostaglandins 1980;19:457–60.
15. Product information. In Physicians' Desk Reference, vol. 34. Oradell, N.J.: Medical Economics Company, 1980.
16. Eeg-Olofsson O, Malmros I, Elwin CE, Steen B. Convulsions in a breast-fed infant after maternal indomethacin. Lancet 1978;2:215.
17. Fairhead FW. Convulsions in a breast-fed infant after maternal indomethacin. Lancet 1978;2:576.

Name: **INSULIN**

Class: **Antidiabetic**   Risk Factor: **B**

Fetal Risk Summary

Insulin, a natural occurring hormone, is the drug of choice for the control of diabetes mellitus in pregnancy. Infants of diabetic mothers are at risk for an increased incidence of congenital anomalies, up to 2 to 4 times that of normal controls (1–4). The rate of malformations seems to be related to the severity of the maternal disease. The exact mechanisms causing this increase are unknown. Human insulin does not cross the placenta, at least when administered in the 2nd trimester (5). Studies prior to this time have not been conducted. This distinction is of interest since most major malformations observed in infants of diabetic mothers were induced sometime prior to the 7th week of gestation (1). Several mechanisms have been offered as a cause of the malformations, including exogenous insulin itself and insulin-induced hypoglycemia. However, a recent study using hemoglobin A_{1c}, a normal minor hemoglobin whose levels are indicative of diabetic control, found a significantly higher percentage of major congenital anomalies in the offspring of mothers with elevated levels of this hemoglobin (3). The authors concluded that poorly controlled diabetes (i.e., hyperglycemia) was associated with an increased risk of defects. Congenital malformations are now the most common cause of perinatal death in infants of diabetic mothers (1, 2). Not only is the frequency of major defects increased, but also the frequency of multiple malformations (affecting more than one organ system) (1). Malformations observed in infants of diabetic mothers usually involve one or more of five systems (1):

Most common
> skeletal: vertebrae and limbs
> cardiovascular: transposition of great vessels; ventricular septal defects; coarctation of the aorta
> central nervous system: neural tube defects

Less common
> genitourinary: varied
> gastrointestinal: tracheoesophageal fistula; bowel atresias; imperforate anus; narrowed colon

Infants of diabetic mothers may have significant perinatal morbidity, even when the mothers have been under close diabetic control (6). Perinatal morbidity in one series affected 65% (169/260) of the infants and included hypoglycemia, hyperbilirubinemia, hypocalcemia and polycythemia (6).

Breast Feeding Summary

Insulin is a naturally occurring constituent of the blood. It does not pass into breast milk.

References

1. Dignan PSJ. Teratogenic risk and counseling in diabetes. Clin Obstet Gynecol 1981;24:149–59.
2. Friend JR. Diabetes. Clin Obstet Gynaecol 1981;8:353–82.
3. Miller E, Hare JW, Cloherty JP, et al. Elevated maternal hemoglobin A_{1c} in early pregnancy and major congenital anomalies in infants in diabetic mothers. N Engl J Med 1981;304:1331–4.
4. Soler NG, Walsh CH, Malins JM. Congenital malformations in infants of diabetic mothers. Q J Med 1976;45:303–13.
5. Adam PAJ, Teramo K, Raiha N, Gitlin D, Schwartz R. Human fetal insulin metabolism early in gestation. Diabetes 1969;18:409–16.
6. Gabbe SG, Mestman JH, Freeman RK, et al. Management and outcome of pregnancy in diabetes mellitus, classes B to R. Am J Obstet Gynecol 1977;129:723–32.

Name: **IPRINDOLE**
Class: **Antidepressant**   Risk Factor: **D**

Fetal Risk Summary

No data available (see Imipramine).

Breast Feeding Summary

No data available (see Imipramine).

Name: **IPRONIAZID**
Class: **Antidepressant**   Risk Factor: **C**

Fetal Risk Summary

No data available (see Phenelzine).

Breast Feeding Summary

No data available (see Phenelzine).

Name: **ISOCARBOXAZID**
Class: **Antidepressant**   Risk Factor: **C**

Fetal Risk Summary

Isocarboxazid is a monoamine oxidase inhibitor. The Collaborative Perinatal Project monitored 21 mother-child pairs exposed to these drugs during the 1st trimester, 1 which was exposed to isocarboxazid (1). An increased risk of malformations was found. Details of the single case with exposure to isocarboxazid were not given.

Breast Feeding Summary

No data available.

Reference

1. Heinonen OP, Slone D, Shapiro S. *Birth Defects and Drugs in Pregnancy*. Littleton: Publishing Sciences Group, 1977:336–7.

Name: **ISOETHARINE**

Class: **Sympathomimetic (Adrenergic)**   Risk Factor: **C**

Fetal Risk Summary

No reports linking the use of isoetharine with congenital defects have been located. Isoetharine-like drugs are teratogenic in some animal species, but human teratogenicity has not been suspected (1, 2). Recent data may require a reappraisal of this opinion. The Collaborative Perinatal Project monitored 50,282 mother-child pairs, 3,082 of which had 1st trimester exposure to sympathomimetic drugs (3). For use anytime during pregnancy, 9,719 exposures were recorded (4). An association in the 1st trimester was found between the sympathomimetic class of drugs as a whole and minor malformations (not life-threatening or major cosmetic defects), inguinal hernia, and clubfoot (3). Sympathomimetics are often administered in combination with other drugs to alleviate the symptoms of upper respiratory infections. Thus, the fetal effects of sympathomimetics, other drugs and viruses cannot be totally separated. However, indiscriminate use of this class of drugs, especially in the 1st trimester, is not without risk.

Breast Feeding Summary

No data available.

References

1. Nishimura H, Tanimura T. *Clinical Aspects of the Teratogenicity of Drugs.* Amsterdam: Excerpta Medica, 1976:231.
2. Shepard TH. *Catalog of Teratogenic Agents*, ed. 3. Baltimore: Johns Hopkins University Press, 1980:134–5.
3. Heinonen OP, Slone D, Shapiro S. *Birth Defects and Drugs in Pregnancy.* Littleton: Publishing Sciences Group, 1977:345–56.
4. *Ibid*, 439.

Name: **ISOFLUROPHATE**

Class: **Parasympathomimetic (Cholinergic)**   Risk Factor: **C**

Fetal Risk Summary

Isoflurophate is used in the eye. No reports of its use in pregnancy have been located. As a quaternary ammonium compound, it is ionized at physiologic pH and transplacental passage in significant amounts would not be expected (see also Neostigmine).

Breast Feeding Summary

No data available.

Name: **ISONIAZID**

Class: **Antituberculosis Agent**   Risk Factor: **C**

Fetal Risk Summary

Available reports discussing fetal effects of isoniazid during pregnancy reflect multiple drug therapies. These reports have identified retarded psychomotor activity, myoclonia, myelomeningocele with spina bifida and talipes, and hypospadias as possible effects related to isoniazid therapy during pregnancy (1, 2). The Collaborative Perinatal Project also monitored a small series of 85 patients who received isoniazid during the 1st trimester (3). They reported 10 malformations, an incidence almost twice the expected rate. The above observations have not been confirmed by other studies (4–8). Retrospective analysis of over 4,900 pregnancies in which isoniazid was administered demonstrated rates of malformations similar to control populations (0.7% to 2.3%). A case report of a malignant mesothelioma in a 9-year-old child who was exposed to isoniazid *in utero* has appeared (9). The authors suggest a possible carcinogenic effect because of the rarity of malignant mesotheliomas during the 1st decade and supportive animal data. Hammond reported an earlier study which followed 660 children up to 16 years of age (10). No carcinogenic effects were observed in this study. The bulk of clinical experience apparently supports the use of isoniazid during gestation for the treatment and prophylaxis of tuberculosis.

Author (ref)	No. Pts.	Indication	Gestational Age	Dose	Other Drugs	Fetal Effects	Comment
Weinstein (1)	4	Tuberculosis	1st trimester	Not stated	Not stated	4 Retarded psychomotor activity 3 Psychic retardation 2 Convulsions 1 Myoclonia 2 Abnormal EEG	—
Lowe (2)	71	Tuberculosis	1st trimester	Not stated	p-aminosalicylic acid	1 Myelomeningocele with spina bifida and talipes 1 Hypospadias	Incidence of defects higher in untreated tuberculosis

Breast Feeding Summary

No reports of isoniazid-induced effects in the nursling have been located. A milk:plasma ratio of 1.0 has been reported (11). Timing of single-dose isoniazid regimens may limit the total amount of drug available to the infant. Patients who choose to breast feed should be counselled that experimental studies have suggested carcinogenic effects.

Author (ref)	No. Pts.	Dose	Concentrations (μg/ml)		M:P Ratio	Effect on Infant
			Serum	Milk		
Ricci (12)	1	5 mg/kg	—	6 (3 hr)	—	—
	1	10 mg/kg	—	12	—	—

References

1. Weinstein L, Dalton AC. Host determinants of response to antimicrobial agents. N Engl J Med 1968;279:524–31.
2. Lowe CR. Congenital defects among children born to women under supervision or treatment for pulmonary tuberculosis. Br J Prev Soc Med 1964;18:14–6.
3. Heinonen OP, Slone D, Shapiro S. Birth Defects and Drugs in Pregnancy. Littleton: Publishing Sciences Group, 1977:299, 313.
4. Marynowski A, Sianozecka E. Comparison of the incidence of congenital malformations in neonates from healthy mothers and from patients treated because of tuberculosis. Ginekol Pol 1972;43:713.
5. Jentgens H. Antituberkulose chimotherapie und schwangerschaft sabbruch. Prax Klin Pneumol 1973;27:479.
6. Ludford J, Doster B, Woolpert SF. Effect of isoniazid on reproduction. Am Rev Resp Dis 1973;108:1170–4.
7. Scheinhorn DJ, Angelillo VA. Antituberculosis therapy in pregnancy; risks to the fetus. West J Med 1977;127:195–8.
8. Good JT, Iseman MD, Davidson PT, Lakshminarayan S, Sahn SA. Tuberculosis in association with pregnancy. Am J Obstet Gynecol 1981;140:492–8.
9. Tuman KJ, Chilcote RR, Gerkow RI, Moohr JW. Mesothelioma in child with prenatal exposure to isoniazid. Lancet 1980;2:362.
10. Hammond DC, Silidoff IJ, Robitzek EH. Isoniazid therapy in relation to later occurrence of cancer in adults and in infants. Br Med J 1967;2:792–5.
11. Vorherr H. Drugs excretion in breast milk. Postgrad Med 1974;56:97–104.
12. Ricci G, Copaitich T. Modalta di eliminazione dili'isoniazide somministrata per via orale attraverso il latte di donna. Rass Clin Ter 1954–5;209:53–4.

Name: **ISOPROPAMIDE**

Class: **Parasympatholytic**   Risk Factor: **C**

Fetal Risk Summary

Isopropamide is an anticholinergic quaternary ammonium iodide. The Collaborative Perinatal Project monitored 50,282 mother-child pairs, 180 of which used isopropamide in the 1st trimester (1). For use anytime during pregnancy, 1,071 exposures were recorded (2). In neither case was evidence found for an association with malformations. However, when the group of parasympatholytics were taken as a whole (2,323 exposures), a possible association with minor malformations was found (1).

Breast Feeding Summary

No data available (see also Atropine).

References

1. Heinonen OP, Slone D, Shapiro S. *Birth Defects and Drugs in Pregnancy.* Littleton: Publishing Sciences Group, 1977:346–53.
2. *Ibid,* 439.

Name: **ISOPROTERENOL**

Class: **Sympathomimetic (Adrenergic)**   Risk Factor: **C**

Fetal Risk Summary

No reports linking the use of isoproterenol with congenital defects have been located. Isoproterenol is teratogenic in some animal species, but human teratogenicity has not been suspected (1, 2). Recent data may require a reappraisal of this opinion. The Collaborative Perinatal Project monitored 50,282 mother-child pairs, 31 of which had 1st trimester exposure to isoproterenol (3). No evidence was found to suggest a relationship between large categories of major or minor malformations or to individual defects. However, an association in the 1st trimester was found between the sympathomimetic class of drugs as a whole and minor malformations (not life-threatening or major cosmetic defects), inguinal hernia and clubfoot (4). Sympathomimetics are often administered in combination with other drugs to alleviate the symptoms of upper respiratory infections. Thus, the fetal effects of sympathomimetics, other drugs, and viruses cannot be totally separated. However, indiscriminate use of this class of drugs, especially in the 1st trimester, is not without risk.

Breast Feeding Summary

No data available.

References

1. Nishimura H, Tanimura T. *Clinical Aspects of the Teratogenicity of Drugs.* Amsterdam: Excerpta Medica, 1976;231–2.
2. Shepard TH. *Catalog of Teratogenic Agents*, ed. 3. Baltimore: Johns Hopkins University Press, 1980;191.
3. Heinonen OP, Slone D, Shapiro S. *Birth Defects and Drugs in Pregnancy.* Littleton: Publishing Sciences Group, 1977:346–7.
4. *Ibid*, 345–56.

Name: **ISOSORBIDE**

Class: **Diuretic** Risk Factor: **C**

Fetal Risk Summary

No data available.

Breast Feeding Summary

No data available.

Name: **ISOSORBIDE DINITRATE**

Class: **Vasodilator** Risk Factor: **C**

Fetal Risk Summary

See Nitroglycerin or Amyl Nitrite.

Breast Feeding Summary

No data available.

Name: **ISOXSUPRINE**

Class: **Sympathomimetic (Adrenergic)** Risk Factor: **C**

Fetal Risk Summary

No reports linking the use of isoxsuprine with congenital defects have been located. Isoxsuprine, a β-sympathomimetic, is indicated for vasodilation, but it has been used to prevent premature labor (1–6). Uterine inhibitory effects usually require high intravenous doses which increase the risk for serious adverse effects (7, 8). Maternal heart rate increases and blood pressure decreases are usually mild at lower doses (2, 4, 6). A decrease in the incidence of neonatal respiratory distress syndrome has been observed (9). However, in one study, neonatal respiratory depression was increased if cord serum levels exceeded 10 ng/ml (10). The depression was always associated with hypotension, so the mechanism of the defect may have been related to pulmonary hypoperfusion. Neonatal toxicity is generally rare if cord levels of isoxsuprine are less than 2 ng/ml (corresponding to a drug-free interval of more than 5 hours) but levels greater than 10 ng/ml (drug-free interval of 2 hours of less) were associated with severe neonatal problems (10). These problems include hypocalcemia, hypoglycemia, ileus, hypotension and death (10–12). Hypotension and neonatal death occurred primarily in infants of 26 to 31 weeks gestation, especially if cord levels exceeded 10 ng/ml, and in infants whose mothers developed hypotension or tachycardia during isoxsuprine infusion (10, 11). Neonatal ileus, up to 33% in some series, was not related to cord isoxsuprine concentrations, but hypotension and hypocalcemia were directly related, reaching 89% and 100%, respectively, when cord levels exceeded 10 ng/ml (10, 12). Fetal tachycardia is a common side effect. As compared to controls, no increase in late or variable decelerations was seen (10). In contrast to the above, infusion of isoxsuprine 30 minutes prior to cesarean section under general anesthesia was not observed to produce adverse effects in the mother, fetus or newborn (13). Cord concentrations were not measured. Long term evaluation of infants exposed to β-mimetics *in utero* has been reported, but not specifically for isoxsuprine (14). No harmful effects in the infants resulting from this exposure were observed.

Breast Feeding Summary

No data available.

References

1. Bishop EH, Woutersz TB. Isoxsuprine, a myometrial relaxant. A preliminary report. Obstet Gynecol 1961;17:442–6.
2. Hendricks CH, Cibils LA, Pose SV, Eskes TKAB. The pharmacological control of excessive uterine activity with isoxsuprine. Am J Obstet Gynecol 1961;82:1064–78.
3. Bishop EH, Woutersz TB. Arrest of premature labor. JAMA 1961;178:812–4.
4. Stander RW, Barden TP, Thompson JF, Pugh WR, Werts CE. Fetal cardiac effects of maternal isoxsuprine infusion. Am J Obstet Gynecol 1964;89:792–800.
5. Hendricks CH. The use of isoxsuprine for the arrest of premature labor. Clin Obstet Gynecol 1964;7:687–94.
6. Allen HH, Short H, Fraleigh DM. The use of isoxsuprine in the management of premature labor. Appl Ther 1965;7:544–7.
7. Anonymous. Drugs acting on the uterus. Br Med J 1964;1:1234–6.
8. Briscoe CC. Failure of oral isoxsuprine to prevent prematurity. Am J Obstet Gynecol 1966;95:885–6.
9. Kero P, Hirvonen T, Valimaki I. Perinatal isoxsuprine and respiratory distress syndrome. Lancet 1973;2:198.
10. Brazy JE, Little V, Grimm J, Pupkin M. Risk:benefit considerations for the use of isoxsuprine in the treatment of premature labor. Obstet Gynecol 1981;58:297–303.
11. Brazy JE, Pupkin MJ. Effects of maternal isoxsuprine administration on preterm infants. J Pediatr 1979;94:444–8.
12. Brazy JE, Little V, Grimm J. Isoxsuprine in the perinatal period. II. Relationships between

neonatal symptoms, drug exposure, and drug concentration at the time of birth. J Pediatr 1981;98:146–51.

13. Jouppila R, Kauppila A, Tuimala R, Pakarinen A, Moilanen K. Maternal, fetal and neonatal effects of beta-adrenergic stimulation in connection with cesarean section. Acta Obstet Gynecol Scand 1980;59:489–93.

14. Freysz H, Willard D, Lehr A, Messer J. Boog G. A long term evaluation of infants who received a beta-mimetic drug while in utero. J Perinat Med 1977;5:94–9.

15. Heinonen OP, Slone D, Shapiro S. *Birth Defects and Drugs in Pregnancy.* Littleton: Publishing Sciences Group, 1977:345–56.

16. *Ibid*, 439.

Name: **KANAMYCIN**

Class: **Antibiotic**   Risk Factor: **D**

Fetal Risk Summary

Kanamycin is an aminoglycoside antibiotic. At term, the drug is detectable in cord serum 15 minutes after a 500-mg intramuscular (IM) maternal dose (1). Mean cord serum levels at 3 to 6 hours were 6 µg/ml. Amniotic fluid levels were undetectable during the first hours, then rose during the next 6 hours to a mean value of 5.5 µg/ml. No effects on the infants were mentioned.

Eighth cranial nerve damage has been reported following *in utero* exposure to kanamycin (2, 3). In a retrospective survey of 391 mothers who had received kanamycin, 50 mg/kg, for prolonged periods during pregnancy, 9 children were found to have hearing loss (2.3% incidence) (2). Complete hearing loss in a mother and her infant was reported after the mother had been treated during pregnancy with kanamycin, 1 g IM per day for 4.5 days (3). Ethacrynic acid, an ototoxic diuretic, was also given to the mother during pregnancy.

Except for ototoxicity, no reports of congenital defects due to kanamycin have been located. Embryos were examined from 5 patients who aborted during the 11th to 12th week of pregnancy and who had been treated with kanamycin during the 6th and 8th week (2). No abnormalities in the embryos were found.

Breast Feeding Summary

Kanamycin is excreted in breast milk. Milk:plasma ratios of 0.05 to 0.40 have been reported (4). A 1-g IM dose produced peak milk levels of 18.4 µg/ml (5). No effects were reported in the nursing infants. Since oral absorption of kanamycin is poor, ototoxicity would not be expected. However, three potential problems exist for the nursing infant: modification of bowel flora, direct effects on the infant and interference with the interpretation of culture results if a fever work-up is required.

References

1. Good R, Johnson G. The placental transfer of kanamycin during late pregnancy. Obstet Gynecol 1971;38:60–2.
2. Nishimura H, Tanimura T. *Clinical Aspects of the Teratogenicity of Drugs.* Amsterdam: Excerpta Medica, 1976:131.
3. Jones HC. Intrauterine ototoxicity. A case report and review of literature. J Natl Med Assoc 1973;65:201–3.

4. Wilson JT. Milk/plasma ratios and contraindicated drugs. In Wilson JT, ed. *Drugs in Breast Milk*. Australia: ADIS Press, 1981:79.
5. O'Brien T. Excretion of drugs in human milk. Am J Hosp Pharm 1974;31:844–54.

Name: **LACTULOSE**

Class: **Laxative/Ammonia Detoxicant**   Risk Factor: **C**

Fetal Risk Summary

No data available.

Breast Feeding Summary

No data available.

Name: **LAETRILE**

Class: **Unclassified/Antineoplastic**   Risk Factor: **C**

Fetal Risk Summary

Laetrile is a non-approved agent used for the treatment of cancer. There are no studies of laetrile in pregnancy. A concern for possible gestational cyanide poisoning has been reported (1). Due to an increased amount of β-glycosidase present in the intestinal flora, the oral route would theoretically be more toxic than the parenteral route in liberation of hydrogen cyanide, which is present in various sources of laetrile (1). Long term follow-up has been recommended as neurological evidence of chronic cyanide exposure may not be recognizable in the infant.

Breast Feeding Summary

No data available.

Reference

1. Peterson RG, Ruman BH. Laetrile and pregnancy. Clin Toxicol 1979;15:181–4.

Name: **LANATOSIDE C**

Class: **Cardiac Glycoside**   Risk Factor: **B**

Fetal Risk Summary

See Digitalis.

Breast Feeding Summary

See Digitalis.

Name: **LEVALLORPHAN**

Class: **Narcotic Antagonist**   Risk Factor: **D**

Fetal Risk Summary

Levallorphan is a narcotic antagonist that is used to reverse respiratory depression from narcotic overdose. It has been used in combination with alphaprodine or meperidine during labor to reduce neonatal depression (1–6). Although some benefits were initially claimed, caution in the use of levallorphan during labor has been advised for the following reasons (7):

1. A statistically significant reduction in neonatal depression has not been demonstrated;
2. The antagonist also reduces analgesia; and
3. The antagonist may increase neonatal depression if an improper narcotic-narcotic antagonist ratio is used.

   As indicated above, levallorphan may cause respiratory depression in the absence of narcotics or if a critical ratio is exceeded (7). Because of these considerations, the use of levallorphan either alone or in combination therapy in pregnancy should be discouraged. If a narcotic antagonist is indicated, other agents that do not cause respiratory depression, such as naloxone, are preferred.

Breast Feeding Summary

No data available.

References

1. Backner DD, Foldes FF, Gordon EH. The combined use of alphaprodine (Nisentil) hydrochloride and levallorphan tartrate for analgesia in obstetrics. Am J Obstet Gynecol 1957;74:271–82.
2. Roberts H, Kuck MAC. Use of alphaprodine and levallorphan during labour. Can Med Assoc J 1960;83:1088–93.
3. Roberts H, Kane KM, Percival N, Snow P, Please NW. Effects of some analgesic drugs used in childbirth. Lancet 1957;1:128–32.
4. Bullough J. Use of premixed pethidine and antagonists in obstetrical analgesia with special reference to cases in which levallorphan was used. Br Med J 1959;2:859–62.

5. Posner AC. Combined pethidine and antagonists in obstetrics. Br Med J 1960;1:124–5.
6. Bullough J. Combined pethidine and antagonists in obstetrics. Br Med J 1960;1:125.
7. Bonica JJ. *Principles and Practice of Obstetric Analgesia and Anesthesia.* Philadelphia: FA Davis, 1967;254–9.

Name: **LEVARTERENOL**

Class: **Sympathomimetic (Adrenergic)**   Risk Factor: **D**

Fetal Risk Summary

Levarterenol is a sympathomimetic used in emergency situations to treat hypotension. Because of the nature of its indication, experience in pregnancy is limited. Levarterenol readily crosses the placenta (1). Uterine vessels are normally maximally dilated, and they have only α-adrenergic receptors (2). Use of the α- and β-adrenergic stimulant, levarterenol, could cause constriction of these vessels and reduce uterine blood flow, thereby producing fetal hypoxia (bradycardia). Levarterenol may also interact with oxytocics or ergot derivatives to produce severe persistent maternal hypertension (2). Rupture of a cerebral vessel is possible. If a pressor agent is indicated, other drugs such as ephedrine should be considered.

Breast Feeding Summary

No data available.

References

1. Morgan CD, Sandler M, Panigel M. Placental transfer of catecholamines in vitro and in vivo. Am J Obstet Gynecol 1972;112:1068–75.
2. Smith NT, Corbascio AN. The use and misuse of pressor agents. Anesthesiology 1970;33:58–101.

Name: **LEVORPHANOL**

Class: **Narcotic Analgesic**   Risk Factor: **B***

Fetal Risk Summary

No reports linking the use of levorphanol with congenital defects have been located. Use of the drug during labor should be expected to produce neonatal depression to the same degree as other narcotic analgesics (1).

[* Risk Factor D if used for prolonged periods or in high doses at term.]

Breast Feeding Summary

No data available.

Reference

1. Bonica JJ. *Principles and Practice of Obstetric Analgesia and Anesthesia.* Philadelphia: FA Davis, 1967:251.

Name: **LINCOMYCIN**

Class: **Antibiotic**   Risk Factor: **B**

Fetal Risk Summary

No reports linking the use of lincomycin with congenital defects have been located. The antibiotic crosses the placenta, achieving cord serum levels about 25% of the maternal serum (1, 2). Multiple intramuscular injections of 600 mg did not result in accumulation in the amniotic fluid (2). No effects on the newborn were observed.

The progeny of 302 patients treated at various stages of pregnancy with oral lincomycin, 2 g per day for 7 days, were evaluated at various intervals up to 7 years after birth (3). As compared to a control group, no increase in malformations or delayed developmental defects were observed.

Breast Feeding Summary

Lincomycin is excreted into breast milk. Six hours following oral dosing of 500 mg every 6 hours for 3 days, serum and milk levels in 9 patients averaged 1.37 and 1.28 μg/ml respectively, a milk:plasma ratio of 0.9 (1). Much lower milk:plasma ratios of 0.13 to 0.17 have also been reported (4). Although no adverse effects have been reported, three potential problems exist for the nursing infant: modification of bowel flora, direct effects on the infant and interference with the interpretation of culture results if a fever work-up is required.

References

1. Medina A, Fiske N, Hjelt-Harvey I, Brown CD, Prigot A. Absorption, diffusion, and excretion of a new antibiotic, lincomycin. Antimicrob Agents Chemother 1963;189–96.
2. Duignan NM, Andrews J, Williams JD. Pharmacological studies with lincomycin in late pregnancy. Br Med J 1973;3:75–8.
3. Mickal A, Panzer JD. The safety of lincomycin in pregnancy. Am J Obstet Gynecol 1975;121:1071–4.
4. Wilson JT. Milk/plasma ratios and contraindicated drugs. In Wilson JT, ed. *Drugs in Breast Milk.* Australia: ADIS Press, 1981:78–9.

Name: LITHIUM

Class: **Tranquilizer**   Risk Factor: **D**

Fetal Risk Summary

The use of lithium during the 1st trimester may be related to an increased incidence of congenital defects, particularly of the cardiovascular system. The drug freely crosses the placenta, equilibrating between maternal and cord serum (1–5). Amniotic fluid concentrations exceed cord serum levels (2). Frequent reports have described the fetal effects of lithium, the majority from data accumulated by the Lithium Baby Register (1, 6–12). The Register, founded in Denmark in 1968 and later expanded internationally, collects data on known cases of 1st trimester exposure to lithium. By 1977, the Register included 183 infants, 20 (11%) with major congenital anomalies (12). Of the 20 malformed infants, 15 involved cardiovascular defects, including 5 with the rare Ebstein's anomaly. Others have also noted the increased incidence of Ebstein's anomaly in lithium-exposed babies (13). Two new case reports bring the total number of infants with cardiovascular defects to 17, or 77% (17/22) of the known malformed children (14, 15). Details on 16 of these infants are shown below.

In 60 of the children born without malformations, follow-up comparisons with non-exposed siblings did not show an increased frequency of physical or mental anomalies (16).

Author (ref)	Case No.	Defect
Weinstein (11)	1	Coarctation of aorta
	2	High intraventricular septal defect
	3	Stenosis of aqueduct with hydrocephalus, spina bifida with sacral meningomyelocele, bilateral talipes equinovarus with paralysis; atonic bladder, patulous rectal sphincter and rectal prolapse (see also reference 7)
	4	Unilateral microtia
	5	Mitral atresia, rudimentary left ventricle without inlet or outlet, aorta and pulmonary artery arising from right ventricle, patent ductus arteriosus, left superior vena cava
	6	Mitral atresia
	7	Ebstein's anomaly
	8	Single umbilical artery, bilateral hypoplasia of maxilla
	9	Ebstein's anomaly
	10	Atresia of tricuspid valve
	11	Ebstein's anomaly
	12	Patent ductus arteriosus, ventricular septal defect
	13	Ebstein's anomaly
Rane (14)	14	Dextrocardia and situs solitus, patent ductus arteriosus, juxtaductal aortic coarctation
Weinstein (12)	15	Ebstein's anomaly
Arnon (15)	16	Massive tricuspid regurgitation, atrial flutter, congestive heart failure

Lithium toxicity in the newborn has been reported frequently:
  Cyanosis (2, 14, 17–20)
  Hypotonia (2, 10, 17–23)
  Bradycardia (14, 18, 22, 24)
  Thyroid depression with goiter (2, 10, 23)
  Electrocardiogram abnormalities (T wave inversion) (18, 24)
  Cardiomegaly (19)
  Gastrointestinal bleeding (24)
  Diabetes insipidus (2)

Most of these toxic effects are self-limiting, returning to normal in 1 to 2 weeks. This corresponds with the renal elimination of lithium from the infant. The serum half-life of lithium in newborns is prolonged, averaging 68 to 96 hours, as compared to the adult value of 10 to 20 hours (3, 14). The one reported case of nephrogenic diabetes insipidus persisted for 2 months (2).

In the mother, renal lithium clearance rises during pregnancy, returning to pre-pregnancy levels shortly after delivery (25). In 4 patients, the mean clearance before delivery was 29 ml/minute, declining to 15 ml/minute 6 to 7 weeks after delivery, a statistically significant difference ($P < 0.01$). This data emphasizes the need to closely monitor lithium levels before and after pregnancy.

In summary, lithium should be avoided, if possible, during pregnancy, especially in the 1st trimester. Use of the drug near term may produce severe toxicity in the newborn, which is usually reversible.

Breast Feeding Summary

Lithium is excreted into breast milk (5, 18, 26, 27). Milk levels average 40% of the maternal serum concentration (18, 27). Infant serum and milk levels are approximately equal. Although no toxic effects in the nursing infant have been reported, long term effects from this exposure have not been studied.

Author (ref)	No. Pts.	Dose	Concentrations Serum	Milk	M:P Ratio	Effect on Infant
Tunnessen (18)	1	600–1200 mg/day	1.5 mEq/l	0.6 mEq/l	0.4	Infant serum = 0.6 mEq/l
Fries (26)	1	900 mg/day	—	0.3 mEq/l	—	Infant serum = 0.3 mEq/l
Schou (27)	8	Not stated	0.78 mmol/l	0.35 mmol/l	0.4	Infant serum = 0.28 mmol/l

References

1. Weinstein MR, Goldfield M. Lithium carbonate treatment during pregnancy: report of a case. Dis Nerv Syst 1969;30:828–32.
2. Mizrahi EM, Hobbs JF, Goldsmith DI. Nephrogenic diabetes insipidus in transplacental lithium intoxication. J Pediatr 1979;94:493–5.
3. Mackay AVP, Loose R, Glen AIM. Labour on lithium. Br Med J 1976;1:878.
4. Schou M, Amdisen A. Lithium and placenta. Am J Obstet Gynecol 1975;122:541.
5. Sykes PA, Quarrie J, Alexander FW. Lithium carbonate and breast-feeding. Br Med J 1976;2:1299.

6. Schou M, Amdisen A. Lithium in pregnancy. Lancet 1970;1:1391.
7. Aoki FY, Ruedy J. Severe lithium intoxication: management without dialysis and report of a possible teratogenic effect of lithium. Can Med Assoc J 1971;105:847-8.
8. Goldfield M, Weinstein MR. Lithium in pregnancy: a review with recommendations. Am J Psychiatry 1971;127:888-93.
9. Goldfield MD, Weinstein MR. Lithium carbonate in obstetrics: guidelines for clinical use. Am J Obstet Gynecol 1973;116:15-22.
10. Schou M, Goldfield MD, Weinstein MR, Villeneuve A. Lithium and pregnancy. I. Report from the register of lithium babies. Br Med J 1973;2:135-6.
11. Weinstein MR, Goldfield MD. Cardiovascular malformations with lithium use during pregnancy. Am J Psychiatry 1975;132:529-31.
12. Weinstein MR. Recent advances in clinical psychopharmacology. I. Lithium carbonate. Hosp Form 1977;12:759-62.
13. Nora JJ, Nora AH, Toews WH. Lithium, Ebstein's anomaly, and other congenital heart defects. Lancet 1974;2:594-5.
14. Rane A, Tomson G, Bjarke B. Effects of maternal lithium therapy in a newborn infant. J Pediatr 1978;93:296-7.
15. Arnon RG, Marin-Garcia J, Peeden JN. Tricuspid valve regurgitation and lithium carbonate toxicity in a newborn infant. Am J Dis Child 1981;135:941-3.
16. Schou M. What happened later to the lithium babies? A follow-up study of children born without malformations. Acta Psychiatr Scand 1976;54:193-7.
17. Woody JN, London WL, Wilbanks GD Jr. Lithium toxicity in a newborn. Pediatrics 1971;47:94-6.
18. Tunnessen WW Jr, Hertz CG. Toxic effects of lithium in newborn infants: a commentary. J Pediatr 1972;81:804-7.
19. Piton M, Barthe ML, Laloum D, Davy J, Poilpre E, Venezia R. Acute lithium intoxication. Report of two cases: mother and her newborn. Therapie 1973;28:1123-44.
20. Wilbanks GD, Bressler B, Peete CH Jr, Cherny WB, London WL. Toxic effects of lithium carbonate in a mother and newborn infant. JAMA 1970;213:865-7.
21. Silverman JA, Winters RW, Strande C. Lithium carbonate therapy during pregnancy: apparent lack of effect upon the fetus. Am J Obstet Gynecol 1971;109:934-6.
22. Strothers JK, Wilson DW, Royston N. Lithium toxicity in the newborn. Br Med J 1973;3:233-4.
23. Karlsson K, Lindstedt G, Lundberg PA, Selstam U. Transplacental lithium poisoning: reversible inhibition of fetal thyroid. Lancet 1975;1:1295.
24. Stevens D, Burman D, Midwinter A. Transplacental lithium poisoning. Lancet 1974;2:595.
25. Schou M, Amdisen A, Steenstrup OR. Lithium and pregnancy. II. Hazards to women given lithium during pregnancy and delivery. Br Med J 1973;2:137-8.
26. Fries H. Lithium in pregnancy. Lancet 1970;1:1233.
27. Schou M, Amdisen A. Lithium and pregnancy. III. Lithium ingestion by children breast-fed by women on lithium treatment. Br Med J 1973;2:138.

Name: **LOPERAMIDE**

Class: **Antidiarrheal**   Risk Factor: **C**

Fetal Risk Summary

No reports linking the use of loperamide with congenital defects have been located. Animal studies did not indicate a teratogenic effect (1).

Breast Feeding Summary

Data relating to the excretion of loperamide into breast milk is lacking. One source recommends that the drug should not be used in the lactating mother (2).

References

1. Product information. Imodium. Ortho Pharmaceutical Corporation, 1982.
2. Stewart JJ. Gastrointestinal drugs. In Wilson JT, ed. *Drugs in Breast Milk.* Australia: ADIS Press, 1981:71.

Name: **LORAZEPAM**

Class: **Sedative**   Risk Factor: **C**

Fetal Risk Summary

Lorazepam is a benzodiazepine. No reports linking the use of lorazepam with congenital defects have been located. Other drugs in this group have been suspected of causing fetal malformations (see also Diazepam or Chlordiazepoxide). Lorazepam crosses the placenta, achieving cord levels similar to maternal serum concentrations (1–4). Placental transfer is slower than diazepam, but high intravenous doses may produce the "floppy infant" syndrome (2).

Breast Feeding Summary

Lorazepam is excreted into breast milk in low concentrations (5). No effects in the nursing infant have been reported.

References

1. de Groot G, Maes RAA, Defoort P, Thiery M. Placental transfer of lorazepam. IRCS Med Science 1975;3:290.
2. McBride RJ, Dundee JW, Moore J, Toner W, Howard PJ. A study of the plasma concentrations of lorazepam in mother and neonate. Br J Anaesth 1979;51:971–8.
3. Kanto J, Aaltonen L, Liukko P, Maenpaa K. Transfer of lorazepam and its conjugate across the human placenta. Acta Pharmacol Toxicol (Copenh) 1980;47:130–4.
4. Kanto JH. Use of benzodiazepines during pregnancy, labour and lactation, with particular reference to pharmacokinetic considerations. Drugs 1982;23:354–80.
5. Whitelaw AGL, Cummings AJ, McFadyen IR. Effect of maternal lorazepam on the neonate. Br Med J 1981;282:1106–8.

Name: **LOXAPINE**

Class: **Tranquilizer**   Risk Factor: **C**

Fetal Risk Summary

No data available.

Breast Feeding Summary

No data available.

Name: **LYNESTRENOL**

Class: **Progestogenic Hormone**   Risk Factor: **D**

Fetal Risk Summary

The Food and Drug Administration mandated deletion of pregnancy-related indications from all progestins because of a possible association with congenital anomalies. No reports linking the use of lynestrenol with congenital defects have been located (see Hydroxyprogesterone, Norethynodrel, Norethindrone, Medroxyprogesterone, Ethisterone). Ravn observed 16 women who had used lynestrenol for contraception and gave birth to normal infants following cessation of treatment (1). No conclusions can be made from this report. Use of progestogens during pregnancy are not recommended.

Breast Feeding Summary

See Oral Contraceptives.

Reference

1. Ravn J. Pregnancy and progeny after long-term contraceptive treatment with low-dose progestogens. Curr Med Res Opin 1975;2:616–9.

Name: **LYPRESSIN**

Class: **Pituitary Hormone, Synthetic**   Risk Factor: **B**

Fetal Risk Summary

Lypressin is a synthetic polypeptide structurally identical to the major active component of vasopressin. See Vasopressin.

Breast Feeding Summary

See Vasopressin.

Name: MAFENIDE
Class: **Anti-infective**   Risk Factor: **B***

Fetal Risk Summary

See Sulfonamides.

* Risk Factor D if administered near term.]

Breast Feeding Summary

See Sulfonamides.

Name: MAGNESIUM SALICYLATE
Class: **Analgesic/Antipyretic**   Risk Factor: **C***

Fetal Risk Summary

See Aspirin.

* Risk Factor D if used in the 3rd trimester.]

Breast Feeding Summary

See Aspirin.

Name: MAGNESIUM SULFATE
Class: **Anticonvulsant/Cathartic**   Risk Factor: **B**

Fetal Risk Summary

No reports linking the use of magnesium sulfate with congenital defects have been located. The Collaborative Perinatal Project monitored 50,282 mother-child pairs, 141 of which had exposure to magnesium sulfate during pregnancy (1). No evidence was found to suggest a relationship to congenital malformations. Magnesium sulfate is routinely used for the management of toxemia and premature labor. Hypocalcemia and hypermagnesia have been reported in the mother, but it is apparently not a problem for the newborn (2–5).

Breast Feeding Summary

Magnesium salts may be encountered by nursing mothers using over-the-counter laxatives. A study in which 50 mothers received an emulsion of magnesium and liquid petrolatum or mineral oil found no evidence of changes or frequency of stools in nursing infants (6). In 10 preeclamptic patients receiving magnesium sulfate, 1 g per hour intravenously during the first 24 hours after delivery, magnesium levels in breast milk were 64 μg/ml as compared to 48 μg/ml in non-treated controls (7). Twenty-four hours after stopping the drug, milk levels in treated and non-treated patients were 38 and 32 μg/ml, respectively. By 48 hours, the levels were identical in the two groups. Milk:plasma ratios were 1.9 and 2.1 in treated and nontreated patients, respectively.

References

1. Heinonen OP, Slone D, Shapiro S. *Birth Defects and Drugs in Pregnancy.* Littleton: Publishing Sciences Group, 1977:440.
2. Lipsitz PJ, English IC. Hypermagnesemia in the newborn infant. Pediatrics 1967;40:856–62.
3. Monif GRG, Savory J. Iatrogenic maternal hypocalcemia following magnesium sulfate therapy. JAMA 1972;219:1469–70.
4. Cruikshank DP, Pitkin RM, Reynolds WA, Williams GA, Hargis GK. Effects of magnesium sulfate treatment on perinatal calcium metabolism. I. Maternal and fetal responses. Am J Obstet Gynecol 1979;134:243–9.
5. Kyank VH, During R. Pro und kontra bei der behandlung der hypertensiven gestosen. Teil I. Praeklampsie und eklampsie. Zentrable Gynaekol 1978;100:1465–71.
6. Baldwin WF. Clinical study of senna administration to nursing mothers: assessment of effects on infant bowel habits. Can Med Assoc J 1963;89:566–8.
7. Cruikshank DP, Varner MW, Pitkin RM. Breast milk magnesium and calcium concentrations following magnesium sulfate treatment. Am J Obstet Gynecol 1982;143:685–8.

Name: **MANDELIC ACID**

Class: **Urinary Germicide**   Risk Factor: **C**

Fetal Risk Summary

Mandelic acid is available as a single agent and in combination with methenamine (see also Methenamine). The Collaborative Perinatal Project reported 30 1st trimester exposures for this drug (1). For use anytime in pregnancy, 224 exposures were recorded (2). Only in the latter group was a possible association with malformations found. The statistical significance of this association is not known. Independent confirmation is required.

Breast Feeding Summary

Mandelic acid is excreted into breast milk. In 6 mothers given 12 g per day, milk levels averaged 550 μg/ml (3). The drug was found in the urine of all infants. It was estimated than an infant would receive an average dose of 86 mg/kg/day by this route. The significance of this amount is not known.

References

. Heinonen OP, Slone D, Shapiro S. *Birth Defects and Drugs in Pregnancy.* Littleton: Publishing
   Sciences Group, 1977:299, 302.
. *Ibid*, 435.
. Berger H. Excretion of mandelic acid in breast milk. Am J Dis Child 1941;61:256–61.

Name: **MANNITOL**

Class: Diuretic Risk Factor: **C**

Fetal Risk Summary

Mannitol is an osmotic diuretic. No reports of its use in pregnancy following intravenous administration have been located. Mannitol, given by intra-amniotic injection, has been used for the induction of abortion (1).

Breast Feeding Summary

No data available.

Reference

. Craft IL, Mus BD. Hypertonic solutions to induce abortions. Br Med J 1971;2:49.

Name **MAPROTILINE**

Class: Antidepressant Risk Factor: B_M

Fetal Risk Summary

No reports linking the use of maprotiline with congenital defects have been located. Animal studies have failed to demonstrate teratogenicity, carcinogenicity, mutagenicity or impairment of fertility (1).

Breast Feeding Summary

Maprotiline is excreted into breast milk (2). Milk:plasma ratios of 1.5 and 1.3 have been reported following a 100-mg single dose and 150 mg in divided doses for 120 hours. Multiple dosing resulted in milk concentrations of unchanged maprotiline of 0.2 μg/ml. Although this amount is low, the significance to the nursing infant is not known.

References

1. Product information. Ludiomil. CIBA Pharmaceutical Co. Summit, New Jersey, 1981.
2. Reiss W. The relevance of blood level determinations during the evaluation of maprotiline in
   man. In *Research and Clinical Investigation in Depression.* Cambridge Medical Publications,
   1980:19–38.

Name: **MAZINDOL**

Class: **Central Stimulant/Anorectant**   Risk Factor: C

Fetal Risk Summary

No data available.

Breast Feeding Summary

No data available.

Name: **MEBANAZINE**

Class: **Antidepressant**   Risk Factor: C

Fetal Risk Summary

No data available (see Phenelzine).

Breast Feeding Summary

No data available (see Phenelzine).

Name: **MECHLORETHAMINE**

Class: **Antineoplastic**   Risk Factor: D

Fetal Risk Summary

Mechlorethamine is an alkylating antineoplastic agent. The drug has been used in pregnancy, usually in combination with other antineoplastic drugs. Most reports have not shown an adverse effect in the fetus even when mechlorethamine was given during the 1st trimester (1–4). Two malformed infants have resulted following 1st trimester use of mechlorethamine (see table below) (5, 6). Data from one review indicated that 40% of the infants exposed to anticancer drugs were of low birth weight (3). Long term studies of growth and mental development in offspring exposed to mechlorethamine during the 2nd trimester, the period of neuroblast multiplication, have not been conducted (7).

Ovarian function has been evaluated in 27 women previously treated with mechlorethamine and other antineoplastic drugs (8). Excluding 3 patients who received pelvic radiation, 13 (54%) maintained regular cyclic menses and overall, 13 normal children were born after therapy. Other successful pregnancies have been reported following combination chemotherapy with mech-

rethamine (9–11). Ovarian failure is apparently often gradual in onset and is
ɪe-related (8). Mechlorethamine therapy in males has been observed to
ɪoduce testicular germinal cell depletion and azoospermia (11–13).

ɪthor ɪef)	No. Pts.	Indica- tion	Gestactional Age	Dose	Other Drugs	Fetal Effects	Comments
ɪrett 5)	1	Hodgkin's	1st tri- mester	Not stated	Procarbazine Vinblastine	Spontaneous abortion at 24 weeks gestation Oligodactyly of both feet with webbing of 3rd and 4th toes 4 metatarsals on left, 3 on right Bowing of right tibia Cerebral hemorrhage	
ɪnnuti 6)	1	Hodgkin's	1st tri- mester	200 mg/ day	Procarbazine Vincristine	Elective abortion Malformed kidneys—mark- edly reduced size and malposition	

ɪreast Feeding Summary

ɪo data available.

ɪferences

1. Hennessy JP, Rottino A. Hodgkin's disease in pregnancy with a report of twelve cases. Am J Obstet Gynecol 1952;63:756–64.
2. Riva HL, Andreson PS, O'Grady JW. Pregnancy and Hodgkin's disease: a report of eight cases. Am J Obstet Gynecol 1953;66:866–70.
3. Nicholson HO. Cytotoxic drugs in pregnancy: review of reported cases. J Obstet Gynaecol Br Commonw 1968;75:307–12.
4. Jones RT, Weinerman ER. MOPP (nitrogen mustard, vincristine, procarbazine, and predni- sone) given during pregnancy. Obstet Gynecol 1979;54:477–8.
5. Garrett MJ. Teratogenic effects of combination chemotherapy. Ann Intern Med 1974;80:667.
6. Mennuti MT, Shepard TH, Mellman WJ. Fetal renal malformation following treatment of Hodgkin's disease during pregnancy. Obstet Gynecol 1975;46:194–6.
7. Dobbing J. Pregnancy and leukaemia. Lancet 1977;1:1155.
8. Schilsky RL, Sherins RJ, Hubbard SM, Wesley MN, Young RC, DeVita VT Jr. Long-term follow-up of ovarian function in women treated with MOPP chemotherapy for Hodgkin's disease. Am J Med 1981;71:552–6.
9. Ross GT. Congenital anomalies among children born of mothers receiving chemotherapy for gestational trophoblastic neoplasms. Cancer 1976;37:1043–7.
10. Johnson SA, Goldman JM, Hawkins DF. Pregnancy after chemotherapy for Hodgkin's disease. Lancet 1979;2:93.
11. Schilsky RL, Lewis BJ, Sherins RJ, Young RC. Gonadal dysfunction in patients receiving chemotherapy for cancer. Ann Intern Med 1980;93:109–14.
12. Sherins RJ, Olweny CLM, Ziegler JL. Gynecomastia and gonadal dysfunction in adolescent boys treated with combination chemotherapy for Hodgkin's disease. N Engl J Med 1978;299:12–6.
13. Sherins RJ, DeVita VT Jr. Effect of drug treatment for lymphoma on male reproductive capacity: studies of men in remission after therapy. Ann Intern Med 1973;79:216–20.

Name: **MECLIZINE**

Class: **Antihistamine/Antiemetic**   Risk factor: **B**

Fetal Risk Summary

Meclizine is a piperazine antihistamine which is frequently used as an anti-emetic (see also Buclizine and Cyclizine). The drug is teratogenic in animals but apparently not in humans. Since late 1962, the question of meclizine's effect on the fetus has been argued in numerous citations, the bulk of which are case reports and letters (1-27). Three studies involving large numbers of patients have concluded that meclizine is not a human teratogen (28-32).

The Collaborative Perinatal Project (CPP) monitored 50,282 mother-child pairs, 1,014 of which had exposure to meclizine in the 1st trimester (28). For use anytime during pregnancy, 1,463 exposures were recorded (29). In neither case was evidence found to suggest a relationship to large categories of major or minor malformations. Several possible associations with individual malformations were found, but the statistical significance of these are unknown (28-30). Independent confirmation is required to determine the actual risk.

Respiratory defects (7 cases)

Eye and ear defects (7 cases)

Inguinal hernia (18 cases)

Hypoplasia cordis (3 cases)

Hypoplastic left heart syndrome (3 cases)

The FDA's OTC Laxative Panel, acting on the data from the CPP study, concluded that meclizine was not teratogenic (33).

A second large prospective study covering 613 1st-trimester exposures supported these negative findings (31). No harmful effects were found in the exposed offspring as compared to the total sample.

Finally, in a 1971 report, significantly fewer infants with malformations were exposed to antiemetics in the 1st trimester as compared to controls (32). Meclizine was the third most commonly used antiemetic.

Breast Feeding Summary

No data available.

References

1. Watson GI. Meclozine ("Ancoloxin") and foetal abnormalities. Br Med J 1962;2:1446.
2. Smithells RW. "Ancloxin" and foetal abnormalities. Br Med J 1962;2:1539.
3. Diggorg PLC, Tomkinson JS. Meclozine and foetal abnormalities. Lancet 1962;2:1222.
4. Carter MP, Wilson FW. "Ancoloxin" and foetal abnormalities. Br Med J 1962;2:1609.
5. Macleod M, *Ibid*.
6. Lask S, *Ibid*.
7. Leck IM, *Ibid*., 1610.
8. McBride WG. Drugs and foetal abnormalities. Br Med J 1962;2:1681.
9. Fagg CG, *Ibid*.
10. Barwell TE, *Ibid*.
11. Woodall J. *Ibid*, 1682.
12. McBride WG. Drugs and congenital abnormalities. Lancet 1962;2:1332.
13. Lenz W. *Ibid*.

14. David A. Goodspeed AH. "Ancoloxin" and foetal abnormalities. Br Med J 1963;1:121.
15. Gallagher C, *Ibid*, 121–2.
16. Watson GI, *Ibid*, 122.
17. Mellin GW, Katzenstein M. Meclozine and foetal abnormalities. Lancet 1963;1:222–3.
18. Salzmann KD. "Ancloxin" and foetal abnormalities. Br Med J 1963;1:471.
19. Burry AF. Meclozine and foetal abnormalities. Br Med J 1963;1:1476.
20. Smithells RW, Chinn ER. Meclozine and feotal abnormalities. Br Med J 1963;1:1678.
21. O'Leary JL, O'Leary JA. Nonthalidomine ectromelia. Report of a case. Obstet Gynecol 1964;23:17–20.
22. Smithells RW, Chinn ER. Meclozine and foetal malformations: a prospective study. Br Med J 1964;1:217–8.
23. Pettersson F. Meclozine and congenital malformations. Lancet 1964;1:675.
24. Yerushalmy J, Milkovich L. Evaluation of the teratogenic effect of meclizine in man. Am J Obstet Gynecol 1965;93:553–62.
25. Sadusk JF Jr, Palmisano PA. Teratogenic effect of meclizine, cyclizine, and chlorcyclizine. JAMA 1965;194:987–9.
26. Lenz W. Malformations caused by drugs in pregnancy. Am J Dis Child 1966;112:99–106.
27. Lenz W. How can the teratogenic action of a factor be established in man? S Med J 1971;64 (Supplement No. 1):41–7.
28. Heinonen OP, Slone D, Shapiro S, *Birth Defects and Drugs in Pregnancy*. Littleton: Publishing Sciences Group, 1977:328.
29. *Ibid*, 437.
30. *Ibid*, 475.
31. Milkovich L, Van den Berg BJ. An evaluation of the teratogenicity of certain antinauseant drugs. Am J Obstet Gynecol 1976;125:244–8.
32. Nelson MM, Forfar JO. Associations between drugs administered during pregnancy and congenital abnormalities of the fetus. Br Med J 1971;1:523–7.
33. Anonymous. Pink Sheets. Meclizine, cyclizine not teratogenic. FDC Reports 1974; 2.

Name: **MECLOFENAMATE**

Class: **Nonsteroidal Anti-inflammatory**   Risk Factor: **B***

Fetal Risk Summary

No reports linking the use of meclofenamate with congenital defects have been located. Theoretically, meclofenamate, a prostaglandin synthetase inhibitor, could cause constriction of the ductus arteriosus *in utero* (1). Persistent pulmonary hypertension of the newborn should also be considered (2). Drugs in this class have been shown to inhibit labor and prolong pregnancy (2). The manufacturer recommends that the drug not be used during pregnancy (3).

[* Risk Factor D if used in 3rd trimester.]

Breast Feeding Summary

No data available. The manufacturer recommends that the drug not be used when breast feeding (3).

References

1. Levin DL. Effects of inhibition of prostaglandin synthesis on fetal development, oxygenation, and the fetal circulation. Semin Perinatol 1980;4:35–44.
2. Fuchs F. Prevention of prematurity. Am J Obstet Gynecol 1976;126:809–20.
3. Product information. Meclomen. Parke-Davis, 1982.

Name: **MEDROXYPROGESTERONE**

Class: **Progestogenic Hormone**   Risk Factor: **D**

Fetal Risk Summary

The Food and Drug Administration mandated deletion of pregnancy-related indications from all progestins because of a possible association with congenital anomalies. Fourteen cases of ambiguous genitalia of the fetus have been reported to the FDA, although the literature is more supportive of the 19-nortestosterone derivatives (see Norethindrone, Norethynodrel) (1). The Collaborative Perinatal Project monitored 866 mother-child pairs with 1st trimester exposure to progestational agents (including 130 with exposure to medroxyprogesterone) (2). An increase in the expected frequency of cardiovascular defects and hypospadias was observed for the progestational agents as a group (3). The cardiovascular defects included a ventricular septal defect and tricuspid atresia (4). Use of synthetic or naturally occurring progestational agents during pregnancy is not recommended.

Breast Feeding Summary

Medroxyprogesterone has not been shown to adversely affect lactation (5, 6). Milk production and duration of lactation may be increased if given in the puerperium. If breast feeding is desired, medroxyprogesterone may be used safely.

References

1. Dayan E, Rosa FW. Fetal ambiguous genitalia associated with sex hormones use early in pregnancy. Food and Drug Administration, Division of Drug Experience. ADR Highlights 1981:1–14.
2. Heinonen OP, Slone D, Shapiro S. *Birth Defects and Drugs in Pregnancy.* Littleton: Publishing Sciences Group, 1977:389.
3. *Ibid,* 394.
4. Heinonen OP, Slone D, Monson RR, Hook EB, Shapiro S. Cardiovascular birth defects and antenatal exposure to female sex hormones. N Engl J Med 1977;296:67–70.
5. Guiloff E, Ibarra-Polo A, Zanartu J, Toscanini C, Mischler TW, Gomez-Rogers C. Effect of contraception on lactation. Am J Obstet Gynecol 1974;118:42–5.
6. Karim M, Ammar R, El Mahgoub S, El Ganzoury B, Fikri F, Abdou Z. Injected progesterone and lactation. Br Med J 1971;1:200–3.

Name: **MELPHALAN**

Class: **Antineoplastic**   Risk Factor: **D**

Fetal Risk Summary

No reports linking the use of melphalan with congenital defects have been located. Melphalan is mutagenic as well as carcinogenic (1–8). These effects have not been described in infants following *in utero* exposure. Data from one review indicated that 40% of the infants exposed to anticancer drugs were of low birth weight (9). Long term studies of growth and mental development in offspring exposed to melphalan and other antineoplastic drugs during the 2nd trimester, the period of neuroblast multiplication, have not been conducted (10).

Melphalan has caused suppression of ovarian function resulting in amenorrhea (10–13). These effects should be considered prior to administering the drug to patients in their reproductive years. Although there are no supportive data to suggest a teratogenic effect, melphalan is structurally similar to other alkylating agents which have produced defects (see Chlorambucil, Mechlorethamine, Cyclophosphamide).

Breast Feeding Summary

No data available.

References

1. Sharpe HB. Observations on the effect of therapy with nitrogen mustard or a derivative on chromosomes of human peripheral blood lymphocytes. Cell Tissue Kinet 1971;4:501–4.
2. Kyle RA, Pierre RV, Bayrd ED. Multiple myeloma and acute myelomonocytic leukemia. N Engl J Med 1970;283:1121–5.
3. Kyle RA. Primary amyloidosis in acute leukemia associated with melphalan. Blood 1974;44:333–7.
4. Burton IE, Abbott CR, Roberts BE, Antonis AH. Acute leukemia after four years of melphalan treatment for melanoma. Br Med J 1976;1:20.
5. Peterson HS. Erythroleukemia in a melphalan treated patient with primary macroglobulinaemia. Scand J Haematol 1973;10:5–11.
6. Stavem P, Harboe M. Acute erythroleukaemia in a patient treated with melphalan for the cold agglutinin syndrome. Scand J Haematol 1971;8:375–9.
7. Einhorn N. Acute leukemia after chemotherapy (Melphalan). Cancer 1978;41:444–7.
8. Reimer RR, Hover R, Fraumen JF, Young RC. Acute leukemia after alkylating agent therapy of ovarian cancer. N Engl J Med 1977;297:177–81.
9. Nicholson HO. Cytotoxic drugs in pregnancy: review of reported cases. J Obstet Gynaecol Br Commonw 1968;75:307–12.
10. Dobbing J. Pregnancy and leukaemia. Lancet 1977;1:11–15.
11. Rose DP, David PE. Ovarian function in patients receiving adjuvant chemotherapy for breast cancer. Lancet 1977;1:1174–6.
12. Ahmann DL. Repeated adjuvant chemotherapy with phenylalanine mustard or 5-fluorouracil, cyclophosphamide and prednisone with or without radiation. Lancet 1978;1:893–6.
13. Schilsky RL, Lewis BJ, Sherins RJ, Young RC. Gonadal dysfunction in patients receiving chemotherapy for cancer. Ann Intern Med 1980;93:109–14.

Name: **MEPENZOLATE**

Class: **Parasympatholytic (Anticholinergic)**   Risk Factor: **C**

Fetal Risk Summary

Mepenzolate is an anticholinergic quaternary ammonium bromide. In a large prospective study, 2,323 patients were exposed to this class of drugs during the 1st trimester, 1 of whom took mepenzolate (1). A possible association was found between the total group and minor malformations.

Breast Feeding Summary

No data available (see also Atropine).

Reference

1. Heinonen OP, Slone D, Shapiro S. *Birth Defects and Drugs in Pregnancy*. Littleton: Publishing Sciences Group, 1977:346–53.

Name: **MEPERIDINE**

Class: **Narcotic Analgesic**   Risk Factor: **B***

Fetal Risk Summary

Fetal problems have not been reported from the therapeutic use of meperidine in pregnancy except when it has been given during labor. Like all narcotics, maternal and neonatal addiction are possible from inappropriate use. Neonatal depression, at times fatal, has historically been the primary concern following obstetrical meperidine analgesia. Controversy has now risen over the potential long-term adverse effects resulting from this use.

Meperidine's placental transfer is very rapid, appearing in cord blood within 2 minutes following intravenous administration (1). It is detectable in amniotic fluid 30 minutes after intramuscular (IM) injection (2). Cord blood concentrations average 70 to 77% (range 45 to 106%) of maternal plasma levels (3, 4). The drug has been detected in the saliva of newborns for 48 hours following maternal administration during labor (5). Concentrations in pharyngeal aspirates were higher than either arterial or venous cord blood.

Respiratory depression in the newborn following use of the drug in labor is time- and dose-dependent. The incidence of depression increases markedly if delivery occurs 60 minutes or longer after injection, reaching a peak around 2 to 3 hours (6, 7). Whether this depression is due to metabolites of meperidine (e.g., normeperidine) or the drug itself is currently not known (2, 8–10). However, recent work by Belfrage suggests these effects are related to unmetabolized meperidine and not to normeperidine (7).

Impaired behavioral response and EEG changes persisting for several days have been observed (11, 12). These persistent effects may be partially explained by the slow elimination of meperidine and normeperidine by the neonate over several days (13, 14). Belsey related depressed attention and social responsiveness during the first 6 weeks of life to high cord blood levels of meperidine (15). An earlier study reported long term follow-up of 70 healthy neonates born to mothers who had received meperidine within 2 hours of birth (16, 17). Psychological and physical parameters at age 5 years were similar in both exposed and control groups. Academic progress and behavior during the 3rd and 4th year in school were also similar.

The Collaborative Perinatal Project monitored 50,282 mother-child pairs, 268 of which had 1st trimester exposure to meperidine (18). For use anytime during pregnancy, 1,100 exposures were recorded (19). No evidence was found to suggest a relationship to large categories of major or minor malformations. A possible association between the use of meperidine in the 1st trimester and inguinal hernia was found based on 6 cases (20). The statistical significance of this association is unknown and independent confirmation is required.

[* Risk Factor D if used for prolonged periods or in high doses at term.]

Breast Feeding Summary

Meperidine is excreted into breast milk (21, 22). In a group of mothers who had received meperidine during labor, the breast-fed infants had higher saliva levels of the drug for up to 48 hours after birth than a similar group that was bottle-fed (5). In nine nursing mothers, a single 50-mg IM dose produced peak levels of 0.13 μg/ml at 2 hours (22). After 24 hours, the concentrations decreased to 0.02 μg/ml. Average milk:plasma ratios for the nine patients were greater than 1.0. No adverse effects in nursing infants were reported in any of the above studies.

References

1. Crawford JS, Rudofsky S. The placental transmission of pethidine. Br J Anaesth 1965;37:929–33.
2. Szeto HH, Zervoudakis IA, Cederquist LL, Inturrise CE. Amniotic fluid transfer of meperidine from maternal plasma in early pregnancy. Obstet Gynecol 1978;52:59–62.
3. Apgar V, Burns JJ, Brodie BB, Papper EM. The transmission of meperidine across the human placenta. Am J Obstet Gynecol 1952;64:1368–70.
4. Shnider SM, Way EL, Lord MJ. Rate of appearance and disappearance of meperidine in fetal blood after administration of narcotic to the mother. Anesthesiology 1966;27:227–8.
5. Freeborn SF, Calvert RT, Black P, MacFarlane T, D'Souza SW. Saliva and blood pethidine concentrations in the mother and the newborn baby. Br J Obstet Gynaecol 1980;87:966–9.
6. Morrison JC, Wiser WL, Rosser SI, et al. Metabolites of meperidine related to fetal depression. Am J Obstet Gynecol 1973;115:1132–7.
7. Belfrage P, Boreus LO, Hartvig P, Irestedt L, Raabe N. Neonatal depression after obstetrical analgesia with pethidine. The role of the injection-delivery time interval and the plasma concentrations of pethidine and norpethidine. Acta Obstet Gynecol Scand 1981;60:43–9.
8. Morrison JC, Whybrew WD, Rosser SI, Bucovaz ET, Wiser WL, Fish SA. Metabolites of meperidine in the fetal and maternal serum. Am J Obstet Gynecol 1976;126:97–1002.
9. Clark RB, Lattin DL. Metabolites of meperidine in serum. Am J Obstet Gynecol 1978;130:113–5.
0. Morrison JC. Reply to Drs. Clark and Lattin. Am J Obstet Gynecol 1978;130:115–7.

11. Borgstedt AD, Rosen MG. Medication during labor correlated with behavior and EEG of the newborn. Am J Dis Child 1968;115:21–4.
12. Hodgkinson R, Bhatt M, Wang CN. Double-blind comparison of the neurobehaviour of neonates following the administration of different doses of meperidine to the mother. Can Anaesth Soc J 1978;25:405–11.
13. Cooper LV, Stephen GW, Aggett PJA. Elimination of pethidine and bupivacaine in the newborn. Arch Dis Child 1977;52:638–41.
14. Kuhnert BR, Kuhnert PM, Prochaska AL, Sokol RJ. Meperidine disposition in mother, neonate and nonpregnant females. Clin Pharmacol Ther 1980;27:486–91.
15. Belsey EM, Rosenblatt DB, Lieberman BA, et al. The influence of maternal analgesia on neonatal behaviour. I. Pethidine. Br J Obstet Gynaecol 1981;88:398–406.
16. Buck C, Gregg R, Stavraky K, Subrahmaniam K, Brown J. The effect of single prenatal and natal complications upon the development of children of mature birthweight. Pediatrics 1969;43:942–55.
17. Buck C. Drugs in pregnancy. Can Med Assoc J 1975;112:1285.
18. Heinonen O, Slone D, Shapiro S. Birth Defects and Drugs in Pregnancy. Littleton: Publishing Sciences Group, 1977:287–95.
19. Ibid, 434.
20. Ibid, 471.
21. Vorherr H. Drug excretion in breast milk. Postgrad Med 1974;56:97–104. 1974.
22. Peiker G, Muller B, Ihn W, Noschel H. Excretion of pethidine in mother's milk. Zentralbl Gynaekol 1980;102:537–41.

Name: MEPHENTERMINE

Class: Sympathomimetic (Adrenergic)   **Risk Factor: C**

Fetal Risk Summary

Mephentermine is a sympathomimetic used in emergency situations to treat hypotension. Because of the nature of its indication, experience in pregnancy with mephentermine is limited. Mephentermine's primary action is an increase in cardiac output due to enhanced cardiac contraction and, to a lesser extent, from peripheral vasoconstriction (1, 2). Its effect on uterine blood flow should be minimal (2).

Breast Feeding Summary

No data available.

References

1. Product information. Wyamine sulfate. Wyeth Laboratories, 1972.
2. Smith NT, Corbascio AN. The use and misuse of pressor agents. Anesthesiology 1970;33:58–101.

Name: **MEPHENYTOIN**

Class: **Anticonvulsant**   Risk Factor: **C**

Fetal Risk Summary

Mephenytoin is a hydantoin anticonvulsant similar to phenytoin (see Phenytoin). The drug is infrequently prescribed because of the greater incidence of
serious side effects than with phenytoin (1). There have been reports of 12
infants with 1st trimester exposure to mephenytoin (2–5). No evidence of
adverse fetal effects were found.

Breast Feeding Summary

No data available.

References

1. Rall TW, Shleifer LS. Drugs effective in the treatment of the epilepsies. In Goodman AG,
   Goodman LS, Gilman A, eds. *The Pharmacological Basis of Therapeutics*, ed. 6. New York:
   Macmillan Publishing, 1980:456.
2. Fedrick J. Epilepsy and pregnancy: a report from the Oxford Linkage Study. Br Med J
   1973;2:442–8.
3. Heinonen O, Slone D, Shapiro S. *Birth Defects and Drugs in Pregnancy.* Littleton: Publishing
   Sciences Group, 1977:358–9.
4. Annegers JF, Elveback LR, Hauser WA, Kurland LT. Do anticonvulsants have a teratogenic
   effect? Arch Neurol 1974;31:364–73.
5. Speidel BD, Meadow SR. Maternal epilepsy and abnormalities of the fetus and newborn.
   Lancet 1972;2:839–43.

Name: **MEPHOBARBITAL**

Class: **Anticonvulsant/Sedative**   Risk Factor: **C**

Fetal Risk Summary

No reports linking the use of mephobarbital with congenital defects have been
located. The drug is demethylated by the liver to phenobarbital (see Phenobarbital). The Collaborative Perinatal Project monitored 50,282 mother-child
pairs, 8 of which had 1st trimester exposure to mephobarbital (1). No evidence
was found to suggest a relationship to large categories of major or minor
malformations or to individual defects. Hemorrhagic disease of the newborn
and barbiturate withdrawal are theoretically possible, although no reports have
appeared with the use of mephobarbital.

Breast Feeding Summary

See Phenobarbital.

Reference

1. Heinonen O, Slone D, Shapiro S. *Birth Defects and Drugs in Pregnancy.* Littleton: Publishing
   Sciences Group, 1977:336.

Name: **MEPROBAMATE**

Class: **Sedative**   Risk Factor: **D**

Fetal Risk Summary

Meprobamate use in pregnancy has been reported to be associated with an increased risk of congenital anomalies (1.9 to 12.1%) (1, 2). In 395 patients, Milkovich observed 8 defects (1):

Congenital heart disease (2 with multiple other defects) (5 cases)
Down's syndrome (1 case)
Deafness (partial) (1 case)
Deformed elbows and joints (1 case)

Other reports describing congenital heart defects after exposure to meprobamate have not been located. The Collaborative Perinatal Project monitored 50,282 mother-child pairs, 356 of which were exposed in the 1st trimester to meprobamate (3, 4). No association of meprobamate with large classes of malformations or to individual defects was found. Others have also failed to find a relationship between the use of meprobamate and congenital malformations (5). However, since few indications exist for this drug in the pregnant woman, it should be used with extreme caution, if at all, during pregnancy.

Breast Feeding Summary

Meprobamate is excreted into breast milk (6). Milk concentrations are 2 to 4 times that of maternal plasma (6, 7). The effect of this amount of drug on the nursing infant is not known.

References

1. Milkovich L, van den Berg BJ. Effects of prenatal meprobamate and chlordiazepoxide hydrochloride on human embryonic and fetal development. N Engl J Med 1974;291:1268–71.
2. Crombie DL, Pinsent RJ, Fleming DM, Rumeau-Rouguette C, Goujard J, Huel G. Fetal effects of tranquilizers in pregnancy. N Engl J Med 1975;293:198–9.
3. Heinonen OP, Slone D, Shapiro S. *Birth Defects and Drugs in Pregnancy.* Littleton: Publishing Sciences Group, 1977:336–7.
4. Hartz SC, Heinonen OP, Shapiro S, Siskind V, Slone D. Antenatal exposure to meprobamate and chlordiazepoxide in relation to malformations, mental development, and childhood mortality. N Engl J Med 1975;292:726–8.
5. Belafsky HA, Breslow S, Hirsch LM, Shangold JE, Stahl MB. Meprobamate during pregnancy. Obstet Gynecol 1969;34:378–86.
6. Product information. Equanil. Wyeth Laboratories, 1980.
7. Wilson JT, Brown RD, Cherek DR, et al. Drug excretion in human breast milk: principles pharmacokinetics and projected consequences. Clin Pharmacokinet 1980;5:1–66.

Name: **MERCAPTOPURINE**

Class: **Antineoplastic**   Risk Factor: **D**

Fetal Risk Summary

Mercaptopurine is an antimetabolite antineoplastic agent. Experience with mercaptopurine in pregnancy has been reviewed by Moloney (1964) and Nicholson (1968) (1, 2). A total of 62 exposed pregnancies have been described, including 29 in the 1st trimester (1–9). Excluding those pregnancies that ended in abortion or stillbirths, abnormalities were found in three infants:

Pancytopenia (infant exposed to six antineoplastic agents in 3rd trimester) (5)

Microangiopathic hemolytic anemia (8)

Multiple congenital anomalies: cleft palate, microphthalmia, hypoplasia of the ovaries and thyroid gland, corneal opacity, cytomegaly and intra-uterine growth retardation (also exposed to busulfan and radiation) (9).

Except for these 3 cases, no other abnormalities were noted in the exposed offspring. Data from one review indicated that 40% of the infants exposed to anticancer drugs were of low birth weight (2). This finding was not related to the timing of exposure. In addition, long term studies of growth and mental development in infants exposed to mercaptopurine during the 2nd trimester, the period of neuroblast multiplication, have not been conducted (10).

Severe oligospermia has been described in a 22-year-old male receiving sequential chemotherapy of cyclophosphamide, methotrexate and mercapto-purine for leukemia (11). After treatment was stopped, the sperm count returned to normal and the patient fathered a healthy female child. Others have also observed reversible testicular dysfunction (12). Ovarian function in females exposed to mercaptopurine does not seem to be adversely affected (13–17). However, long term analysis of human reproduction following mer-captopurine therapy has not been reported (18).

Breast Feeding Summary

No data available.

References

1. Moloney WC. Management of leukemia in pregnancy. Ann NY Acad Sci 1964;114:857–67.
2. Nicholson HO. Cytotoxic drugs in pregnancy: review of reported cases. J Obstet Gynaecol Br Commonw 1968;75:307–12.
3. Wegelius R. Successful pregnancy in acute leukaemia, Lancet 1975;2:1301.
4. Nicholson HO. Leukaemia and pregnancy: a report of five cases and discussion of manage-ment. J Obstet Gynaecol Br Commonw 1968;75:517–20.
5. Pizzuto J, Aviles A, Noriega L, Niz J, Morales M, Romero F. Treatment of acute leukemia during pregnancy: presentation of nine cases. Cancer Treat Rep 1980;64:679–83.
6. Burnier AM. Discussion. In Plows CW. Acute myelomonocytic leukemia in pregnancy: report of a case. Am J Obstet Gynecol 1982;143:41–3.
7. Dara P, Slater LM, Armentrout SA. Successful pregnancy during chemotherapy for acute leukemia. Cancer 1981;47:845–6.
8. McConnell JF, Bhoola R. A neonatal complication of maternal leukemia treated with 6-mercaptopurine. Postgrad Med J 1973;49:211–3.

9. Diamond J, Anderson MM, McCreadie SR. Transplacental transmission of busulfan (Myleran) in a mother with leukemia: production of fetal malformation and cytomegaly. Pediatrics 1960;25:85–90.
10. Dobbing J. Pregnancy and leukaemia. Lancet 1977;1:1155.
11. Hinkes E, Plotkin D. Reversible drug-induced sterility in a patient with acute leukemia. JAMA 1973;223:1490–1.
12. Lendon M, Palmer MK, Hann IM, Shalet SM, Jones PHM. Testicular histology after combination chemotherapy in childhood for acute lymphoblastic leukaemia. Lancet 1978;2:439–41.
13. Schilsky RL, Lewis BJ, Sherins RJ, Young RC. Gonadal dysfunction in patients receiving chemotherapy for cancer. Ann Intern Med 1980;93:109–14.
14. Gasser C. Long-term survival (cures) in childhood acute leukemia. Paediatrician 1980;9:344–57.
15. Bacon C, Kernahan J. Successful pregnancy in acute leukaemia. Lancet 1975;2:515.
16. Walden PAM, Bagshawe KD. Pregnancies after chemotherapy for gestational trophoblastic tumours. Lancet 1979;2:1241.
17. Sanz MH, Rafecas FJ. Successful pregnancy during chemotherapy for acute promyelocytic leukemia. N Engl J Med 1982;306:939.
18. Steckman ML. Treatment of Chohn's disease with 6-mercaptopurine: what effects on fertility? N Engl J Med 1980;303:817.

Name: **MESORIDAZINE**

Class: **Tranquilizer**   Risk Factor: **C**

Fetal Risk Summary

Mesoridazine is a piperidyl phenothiazine. Phenothiazines readily cross the placenta (1). No specific information on its use in pregnancy has been located. Although occasional reports have attempted to link various phenothiazine compounds with congenital malformations, the bulk of the evidence indicates that these drugs are safe for the mother and fetus (see Chlorpromazine).

Breast Feeding Summary

No data available.

Reference

1. Moya F, Thorndike V. Passage of drugs across the placenta. Am J Obstet Gynecol 1962;84:1778–98.

Name: **MESTRANOL**

Class: **Estrogenic Hormone**   Risk Factor: **D**

Fetal Risk Summary

Mestranol is the 3-methyl ester of ethinyl estradiol. Mestranol is used frequently in combination with progestins for oral contraception (see Oral Contraceptives). Congenital malformations attributed to the use of mestranol alone have not been located. The Collaborative Perinatal Project monitored 614 mother-child pairs with 1st trimester exposure to estrogenic agents (including 179 with exposure to mestranol) (1). An increase in the expected frequency of cardiovascular defects, eye and ear anomalies and Down's syndrome was found (2). An increased risk of malformations due to 1st trimester exposure to mestranol was not found (1). Use of estrogenic hormones during pregnancy is not recommended.

Breast Feeding Summary

Estrogens are frequently used for suppression of postpartum lactation (3). Doses of 100 to 150 μg of ethinyl estradiol (equivalent to 160 to 240 μg of mestranol) for 5 to 7 days are employed (3). Mestranol, when used in oral contraceptives with doses of 30 to 80 μg, has been associated with decreased milk production, infant weight gain and composition of nitrogen and protein content of human milk (4–6). The magnitude of these changes is low. However, the changes in milk production and composition may be of nutritional importance in malnourished mothers. If breast feeding is desired, the lowest dose of oral contraceptives should be chosen. Monitoring of infant weight gain and the possible need for nutritional supplementation should be considered (see Oral Contraceptives).

References

1. Heinonen OP, Slone D, Shapiro S. *Birth Defects and Drugs in Pregnancy.* Littleton: Publishing Sciences Group, 1977:389, 391.
2. *Ibid*, 395.
3. Gilman AG, Goodman LS, Gilman A. *The Pharmacological Basis of Therapeutics.* New York: MacMillan, 1980:1431.
4. Kora SJ. Effect of oral contraceptives on lactation. Fertil Steril 1969;20:419–23.
5. Miller GH, Hughs LR. Lactation and genital involution effects of a new low-dose oral contraceptive on breast-feeding mothers and their infants. Obstet Gynecol 1970;35:44–50.
6. Lonnerdal B, Forsum E, Hambraeus L. Effect of oral contraceptives on composition and volume of breast milk. Am J Clin Nutr 1980;33:816–24.

Name: **METAPROTERENOL**

Class: **Sympathomimetic (Adrenergic)**   Risk Factor: **B**

Fetal Risk Summary

No reports linking the use of metaproterenol with congenital defects have been located. Metaproterenol, a β-sympathomimetic, has been used to prevent premature labor (1–3). Its use for this purpose has been largely assumed by ritodrine, albuterol or terbutaline. Like all β-mimetics, metaproterenol causes maternal, and to a lesser degree, fetal tachycardia. Maternal hypotension, hyperglycemia and neonatal hypoglycemia should be expected (see also Ritodrine, Albuterol or Terbutaline). Long term evaluation of infants exposed to *in utero* β-mimetics has been reported, but not specifically for metaproterenol (4). No harmful effects in the infants were observed.

Breast Feeding Summary

No data available.

References

1. Baillie P, Meehan FP, Tyack AJ. Treatment of premature labour with orciprenaline. Br Med J 1970;4:154–5.
2. Tyack AJ, Baillier P, Meehan FP. In-vivo response of the human uterus to orciprenaline in early labour. Br Med J 1971;2:741–3.
3. Zilianti M, Aller J. Action of orciprenaline on uterine contractility during labor, maternal cardiovascular system, fetal heart rate, and acid-base balance. Am J Obstet Gynecol 1971;109:1073–9.
4. Freysz H, Willard D, Lehr A, Messer J, Boog G. A long term evaluation of infants who received a beta-mimetic drug while in utero. J Perinat Med 1977;5:94–9.

Name: **METARAMINOL**

Class: **Sympathomimetic (Adrenergic)**   Risk Factor: **D**

Fetal Risk Summary

Metaraminol is a sympathomimetic used in emergency situations to treat hypotension. Because of the nature of its indications, experience in pregnancy with metaraminol is limited. Uterine vessels are normally maximally dilated and they have only α-adrenergic receptors (1). Use of the predominantly α-adrenergic stimulant, metaraminol, could cause constriction of these vessels and reduce uterine blood flow, thereby producing fetal hypoxia (bradycardia). Metaraminol may also interact with oxytocics or ergot derivatives to produce severe persistent maternal hypertension (1). Rupture of a cerebral vessel is possible. If a pressor agent is indicated, other drugs such as ephedrine should be considered.

Breast Feeding Summary

No data available.

Reference

1. Smith NT, Corbascio AN. The use and misuse of pressor agents. Anesthesiology 1970;33:58–101.

Name: **METHACYCLINE**

Class: **Antibiotic**   Risk Factor: **D**

Fetal Risk Summary

See Tetracycline.

Breast Feeding Summary

See Tetracycline.

Name: **METHADONE**

Class: **Narcotic Analgesic**   Risk Factor: **B***

Fetal Risk Summary

Methadone use in pregnancy is almost exclusively related to the treatment of heroin addiction. No increase in congenital defects have been observed. However, since these patients normally consume a wide variety of drugs, it is not possible to completely separate the effects of methadone from the effects of other agents. Neonatal narcotic withdrawal and low birth weight seem to be the primary problems.

Withdrawal symptoms occur in approximately 60 to 90% of the infants (1–6). One study concluded that the intensity of withdrawal was increased if the daily maternal dosage exceeded 20 mg (5). When withdrawal symptoms do occur, they normally start within 48 hours after delivery, but a small percentage may be delayed up to 7 to 14 days (1). One report observed initial withdrawal symptoms appearing up to 28 days after birth, but the authors do not mention if mothers of these infants were breast feeding (6). Methadone concentrations in breast milk are reported to be sufficient to prevent withdrawal in addicted infants (See Breast Feeding Summary below). Some authors believe methadone withdrawal is more intense than that occurring with heroin (1). Less than one third of symptomatic infants require therapy (1–5). A lower incidence of hyaline membrane disease is seen in infants exposed *in utero* to chronic methadone and may be due to elevated blood levels of prolactin (7).

Infants of drug-addicted mothers are often small for gestational age. In some series, one third or more of the infants weigh less than 2500 g (1, 2, 4). The newborn of methadone addicts may have a higher birth weight than comparable offspring of heroin addicts for reasons that remain unclear (4).

Other problems occurring in the offspring of methadone addicts are increased mortality, sudden infant death syndrome (SIDS), jaundice and thrombocytosis. A relationship between methadone and SIDS may exist (4, 8, 9). In one study, a positive correlation was found between severity of neonatal withdrawal and the incidence of SIDS (9). Maternal withdrawal during pregnancy has been observed to produce a marked response of the fetal adrenal glands and sympathetic nervous system (10). An increased stillborn and neonatal mortality rate has also been reported (11). Both reports recommend against detoxification of the mother during gestation. Jaundice is comparatively infrequent in both heroin- and methadone-exposed newborns. However, a higher rate of severe hyperbilirubinemia in methadone infants than in a comparable group of heroin infants has been observed (1). Thrombocytosis developing in the second week of life, with some platelet counts exceeding $1,000,000/mm^3$ and persisting for over 16 weeks, has been reported (12). The condition was not related to withdrawal symptoms or neonatal treatment. Some of these infants also had increased circulating platelet aggregates.

Respiratory depression is not a significant problem, as Apgar scores are comparable to a non-addicted population (1–5). Long term effects on the behavior and gross motor development skills are not known.

Author (ref)	No. Pts.	Indication	Gestational Age	Dose	Other Drugs	Fetal Effects	Comment
Newman (4)	313 live births	Maternal addiction	Various	40 to >100 mg/ day	Heroin Other abuse drugs likely	SIDS—2 (0.6%)	Infant mortality rate similar to overall experience in New York City
Pierson (8)	14	Maternal addiction	Various	40–60 mg/day average	Heroin Other abuse drugs likely	SIDS—3 (12%)	Unable to establish correlation between SIDS and methadone
Chavez (9)	688	Maternal addiction	Various	Various	Heroin Other abuse drugs likely	SIDS-17 (2.5%)	Correlation is suggested between drug addiction and SIDS but unable to correlate to a single drug

[* Risk Factor D if used for prolonged periods or in high doses at term.]

Breast Feeding Summary

Methadone enters breast milk in concentrations approaching plasma levels and may prevent withdrawal symptoms in addicted infants. One study reported an average milk concentration in 10 patients of 0.27 μg/ml, representing an average milk:plasma ratio of 0.83 (13). The same investigators earlier reported levels ranging from 0.17 μg/ml to 5.6 μg/ml in the milk of mothers on methadone maintenance (2). At least one infant death has been attributed to methadone obtained through breast milk (14). However, a recent report claimed that methadone enters breast milk in very low quantities which are clinically insignificant (15).

Author (ref)	No. Pts.	Dose	Concentrations µg/ml		M:P Ratio	Effect on Infant
			Serum	Milk		
Blinick (2)	Not stated	80–140 mg/day	—	0.17–5.6	—	—
Blinick (13)	10	10–80 mg/day	—	0.27	0.83	—
Smialek (14)	1	Not stated	—	—	—	Baby died Blood level 0.4 µg/ml

References

1. Zelson C, Lee SJ, Casalino M. Neonatal narcotic addiction. N Engl J Med 1973;289:1216–20.
2. Blinick G, Jerez E, Wallach RC. Methadone maintenance, pregnancy and progeny. JAMA 1973;225:477–9.
3. Strauss ME, Andresko M, Stryker JC, Wardell JN, Dunkel LD. Methadone maintenance during pregnancy: pregnancy, birth and neonate characteristics. Am J Obstet Gynecol 1974;120:895–900.
4. Newman RG, Bashkow S, Calko D. Results of 313 consecutive live births of infants delivered to patients in the New York City methadone maintenance program. Am J Obstet Gynecol 1975;121:233–7.
5. Ostrea EM, Chavez CJ, Strauss ME. A study of factors that influence the severity of neonatal narcotic withdrawal. J Pediatr 1976;88:642–5.
6. Kandall SR, Gartner LM. Delayed presentation of neonatal methadone withdrawal. Pediatr Res 1973;7:320.
7. Parekh A, Mukherjee TK, Jhaveri R, Rosenfeld W, Glass L. Intrauterine exposure to narcotics and cord blood prolactin concentrations. Obstet Gynecol 1981;57:447–9.
8. Pierson PS, Howard P, Kleber HD. Sudden deaths in infants born to methadone-maintained addicts. JAMA 1972;220:1733–4.
9. Chavez CJ, Ostrea EM, Stryker JC, Smialek Z. Sudden infant death syndrome among infants of drug-dependent mothers. J Pediatr 1979;95:407–9.
10. Zuspan FP, Gumpel JA, Mejia-Zelaya A, Madden J, David R. Fetal stress from methadone withdrawal. Am J Obstet Gynecol 1975;122:43–6.
11. Rementeria JL, Nunag NN. Narcotic withdrawal in pregnancy: stillbirth incidence with a case report. Am J Obstet Gynecol 1973;116:1152–6.
12. Burstein Y, Giardina PJV, Rausen AR, Kandall SR, Siljestrom K, Peterson CM. Thrombocytosis and increased circulating platelet aggregates in newborn infants of polydrug users. J Pediatr 1979;94:895–9.
13. Blinick G, Inturrisi CE, Jerez E, Wallach RC. Methadone assays in pregnant women and progeny. Am J Obstet Gynecol 1975;121:617–21.
14. Smialek JE, Monforte JR, Aronow R, Spitz WU. Methadone deaths in children—a continuing problem. JAMA 1977;238:2516–7.
15. Anonymous. Methadone in breast milk. Med Lett Drugs Ther 1979;21:52.

Name: **METHANTHELINE**

Class: **Parasympatholytic (Anticholinergic)**   Risk Factor: **C**

Fetal Risk Summary

Methantheline is an anticholinergic quaternary ammonium bromide. In a large prospective study, 2,323 patients were exposed to this class of drugs during the 1st trimester, 2 of whom took methantheline (1). A possible association was found between the total group and minor malformations.

Breast Feeding Summary

No data available (see also Atropine).

Reference

1. Heinonen OP, Slone D, Shapiro S. *Birth Defects and Drugs in Pregnancy.* Littleton: Publishing Sciences Group, 1977:346–53.

Name: **METHAQUALONE**

Class: **Hypnotic**   Risk Factor: **D**

Fetal Risk Summary

No reports linking the use of methaqualone with congenital defects have been located. One manufacturer is not aware of any adverse effects following 1st trimester use (1). Methaqualone is often used as an illicit abuse drug. Separating fetal effects from adulterants or other drugs is not possible. Due to the abuse potential, methaqualone is not recommended during pregnancy.

Breast Feeding Summary

No data available.

Reference

1. Personal communication. Smith RR. William H. Rorer, Inc., 1972.

Name: **METHARBITAL**

Class: **Anticonvulsant/Sedative**   Risk Factor: **B**

Fetal Risk Summary

No reports linking the use of metharbital with congenital defects have been located. Metharbital is demethylated to barbital by the liver (see also Phenobarbital).

Breast Feeding Summary

Metharbital's metabolite, barbital, has been demonstrated in breast milk in trace amounts (1). No reports linking the use of metharbital with adverse effects in the nursing infant have been located.

Reference

1. Kwit NT, Hatcher RA. Excretion of drugs in milk. Am J Dis Child 1935;40:900–4.

Name: **METHENAMINE**

Class: **Urinary Germicide**   Risk Factor: **B**

Fetal Risk Summary

Methenamine, in either the mandelate or hippurate salt form, is used for chronic suppressive treatment of bacteriura. In two studies, the mandelate form was given to 120 patients and the hippurate to 70 patients (1, 2). No increase in congenital defects or other problems as compared to controls were observed. The Collaborative Perinatal Project reported 49 1st trimester exposures to methenamine (3). For use anytime in pregnancy, 299 exposures were recorded (4). Only in the latter group was a possible association with malformations found. The statistical significance of this is not known. Independent confirmation is required.

Methenamine interferes with the determination of urinary estrogen (5). Urinary estrogen was formerly used to assess the condition of the fetoplacental unit, depressed levels being associated with fetal distress. This assessment is now made by measuring unconjugated estriol, which is not affected by methenamine.

Breast Feeding Summary

Methenamine is excreted into breast milk. Peak levels occur at 1 hour (6). No adverse effects on the nursing infant have been reported.

References

1. Gordon SF. Asymptomatic bacteriura of pregnancy. Clin Med 1972;79:22–4.
2. Furness ET, McDonald PJ, Beasley NV. Urinary antiseptics in asymptomatic bacteriuria of pregnancy. N Z Med J 1975;81:417–9.
3. Heinonen OP, Slone D, Shapiro S. *Birth Defects and Drugs in Pregnancy.* Littleton: Publishing Sciences Group, 1977:299, 302.
4. *Ibid*, 435.
5. Kivinen S, Tuimala R. Decreased urinary oestriol concentrations in pregnant women during hexamine hippurate treatment. Br Med J 1977;2:682.
6. Sapeika N. The excretion of drugs in human milk—a review. J Obstet Gynaecol Br Emp 1947;54:426–31.

Name: **METHICILLIN**

Class: **Antibiotic**   Risk Factor: **B**

Fetal Risk Summary

Methicillin is a penicillin antibiotic (see also Penicillin G). The drug rapidly crosses the placenta into the fetal circulation and amniotic fluid (1, 2). Following a 500-mg intravenous dose over 10 to 15 minutes, peak levels of 13.0 and 10.5 μg/ml were measured in maternal and fetal serums, respectively, at 30 minutes (1). Equilibration occurred between the two serums within 1 hour. No effects were reported in the infants.

No reports linking the use of methicillin with congenital defects have been located. The Collaborative Perinatal Project monitored 50,282 mother-child pairs, 3,546 of which had 1st trimester exposure to penicillin derivatives (3). For use anytime during pregnancy, 7,171 exposures were recorded (4). In neither case was evidence found to suggest a relationship to large categories of major or minor malformations or to individual defects.

Breast Feeding Summary

No data available (see Penicillin G).

References

1. Depp R, Kind A, Kirby W, Johnson W. Transplacental passage of methicillin and dicloxacillin into the fetus and amniotic fluid. Am J Obstet Gynecol 1970;107:1054–7.
2. MacAulay M, Molloy W, Charles D. Placental transfer of methicillin. Am J Obstet Gynecol 1973;115:58–65.
3. Heinonen OP, Slone D, Shapiro S. *Birth Defects and Drugs in Pregnancy.* Littleton: Publishing Sciences Group, 1977:297–313.
4. *Ibid*, 435.

Name: **METHIXENE**

Class: **Parasympatholytic**   Risk Factor: **C**

Fetal Risk Summary

Methixene is an anticholinergic agent. No reports of its use in pregnancy have been located (see also Atropine).

Breast Feeding Summary

No data available (see also Atropine).

Name: **METHOTREXATE**

Class: **Antineoplastic**

Risk Factor: **D**

Fetal Risk Summary

Methotrexate is a folic acid antagonist. References describing the use of this antineoplastic agent in 15 pregnancies, 8 in the 1st trimester, have been located (1–7). Three of the eight 1st-trimester exposures resulted in malformed infants (2, 3, 6). Methotrexate-induced congenital defects are similar to those produced by another folic acid antagonist, aminopterin (see also Aminopterin) (6). Two such infants are described in the table below. Possible retention of methotrexate in maternal tissues prior to conception was suggested as the cause of desquamating fibrosing alveolitis in a newborn (8). Previous studies have shown that methotrexate may persist for prolonged periods in human tissues (9). The only other apparent adverse effect observed following methotrexate use in pregnancy was in a 1000-g male infant born with pancytopenia after exposure to 6 different antineoplastic agents in the 3rd trimester (4). However, data from one review indicated that 40% of the infants exposed to cytotoxic drugs were of low birth weight (1). This finding was not related to the timing of the exposure. Long term studies of growth and mental development in offspring exposed to antineoplastic agents during the 2nd trimester, the period of neuroblast multiplication, have not been conducted (10, 11).

Successful pregnancies have followed the use of methotrexate prior to conception (8, 12–16). Apparently, ovarian and testicular dysfunction are reversible (11, 17–19).

Author (ref)	No. Pts.	Indication	Gestational Age	Dose	Other Drugs	Fetal Effects	Comments
Milunsky (2)	1	Attempted abortion	1st trimester	12.5 mg, 5 doses	Not stated	Absence of lambdoid and coronal sutures Oxycephaly Absence of frontal bone Low set ears Hypertelorism Dextroposition of heart Absence of digits on feet Growth retardation Very wide posterior fontanel Hypoplastic mandible Multiple anomalous ribs	
Powell (3)	1	Psoriasis	1st trimester	5 mg/day (total dose 240 mg)	Not stated	Oxycephaly due to absent coronal sutures Larger anterior fontanel Depressed/wide nasal bridge Low set ears Long webbed fingers Wide set eyes	

Breast Feeding Summary

Methotrexate is excreted into breast milk in low concentrations (20). After a dose of 22.5 mg per day, milk concentrations of 6×10^{-9} M (0.26 μg/dl) have been measured (milk:plasma ratio 0.08). The significance of this small amount is not known. However, since the drug may accumulate in neonatal tissues, breast feeding is not recommended.

References

1. Nicholson HO. Cytotoxic drugs in pregnancy: review of reported cases. J Obstet Gynaecol Br Commonw 1968;75:307-12.
2. Milunsky A, Graef JW, Gaynor MF. Methotrexate-induced congenital malformations. J Pediatr 1968;72:790-5.
3. Powell HR, Ekert H. Methotrexate-induced congenital malformations. Med J Aust 1971;2:1076-7.
4. Pizzuto J, Aviles A, Noriega L, Niz J, Morales M, Romero F. Treatment of acute leukemia during pregnancy: presentation of nine cases. Cancer Treat Rep 1980;64:679-83.
5. Dara P, Slater LM, Armentrout SA. Successful pregnancy during chemotherapy for acute leukemia. Cancer 1981;47:845-6.
6. Warkany J. Teratogenicity of folic acid antagonists. Cancer Bull 1981;33:76-7.
7. Burnier AM. Discussion. In Plows CW. Acute myelomonocytic leukemia in pregnancy: report of a case. Am J Obstet Gynecol 1982;143:41-3.
8. Walden PAM, Bagshawe KD. Pregnancies after chemotherapy for gestational trophoblastic tumours. Lancet 1979;2:1241.
9. Charache S, Condit PT, Humphreys SR. Studies on the folic acid vitamins. IV. The persistance of amethopterin in mammalian tissues. Cancer 1960;13:236-40.
10. Dobbing J. Pregnancy and leukaemia. Lancet 1977;1:1155.
11. Schilsky RL, Lewis BJ, Sherins RJ, Young RC. Gonadal dysfunction in patients receiving chemotherapy for cancer. Ann Intern Med 1980;93:109-14.
12. Bacon C, Kernahan J. Successful pregnancy in acute leukaemia. Lancet 1975;2:515.
13. Wegelius R. Successful pregnancy in acute leukaemia. Lancet 1975;2:1301.
14. Ross GT. Congenital anomalies among children born of mothers receiving chemotherapy for gestational trophoblastic neoplasms. Cancer 1976;37:1043-7.
15. Gasser C. Long-term survival (cures) in childhood acute leukemia. Paediatrician 1980;9:344-57.
16. Sanz MA, Rafecas FJ. Successful pregnancy during chemotherapy for acute promyelocytic leukemia. N Engl J Med 1982;306:939.
17. Hinkes E, Plotkin D. Reversible drug-induced sterility in a patient with acute leukemia. JAMA 1973;223:1490-1.
18. Sherins RJ, DeVita VT Jr. Effect of drug treatment for lymphoma on male reproductive capacity. Ann Intern Med 1973;79:216-20.
19. Lendon M, Palmer MK, Hann IM, Shalet SM, Jones PHM. Testicular histology after combination chemotherapy in childhood for acute lymphoblastic leukaemia. Lancet 1978;2:439-41.
20. Johns DG, Rutherford LD, Keighton PC, Vogel CL. Secretion of methotrexate into human milk. Am J Obstet Gynecol 1972;112:978-80.

Name: **METHOXAMINE**

Class: **Sympathomimetic (Adrenergic)**   Risk Factor: **D**

Fetal Risk Summary

Methoxamine is a sympathomimetic used in emergency situations to treat hypotension. It has been recently discontinued by the manufacturer. Because of the nature of its indications, experience in pregnancy with methoxamine is limited. Uterine vessels are normally maximally dilated and they have only α-adrenergic receptors (1). Use of the predominantly α-adrenergic stimulant, methoxamine, could cause constriction of these vessels and reduce uterine blood flow, thereby producing fetal hypoxia (bradycardia). Methoxamine may also interact with oxytocics or ergot derivatives to produce severe persistent maternal hypertension (1). Rupture of a cerebral vessel is possible. If a pressor agent is indicated, other drugs such as ephedrine should be considered.

Breast Feeding Summary

No data available.

Reference

1. Smith NT, Corbascio AN. The use and misuse of pressor agents. Anesthesiology 1970;33:58–101.

Name: **METHSCOPOLAMINE**

Class: **Parasympatholytic (Anticholinergic)**   Risk Factor: **C**

Fetal Risk Summary

Methscopolamine is an anticholinergic quaternary ammonium bromide derivative of scopolamine (see also Scopolamine). In a large prospective study, 2,323 patients were exposed to this class of drugs during the 1st trimester, 2 of whom took methscopolamine (1). A possible association was found between the total group and minor malformations.

Breast Feeding Summary

No data available (see also Atropine).

Reference

1. Heinonen OP, Slone D, Shapiro S. *Birth Defects and Drugs in Pregnancy.* Littleton: Publishing Sciences Group, 1977:346–53.

Name: **METHSUXIMIDE**

Class: **Anticonvulsant**   Risk Factor: **C**

Fetal Risk Summary

Methsuximide is a succinimide anticonvulsant used in the treatment of petit mal epilepsy. The use of methsuximide during the 1st trimester has been reported in only 5 pregnancies (1, 2). No evidence of adverse fetal effects was found. Methsuximide has a much lower teratogenic potential than the oxazolidinedione class of anticonvulsants (see Trimethadione) (3, 4). The succinimide anticonvulsants should be considered the anticonvulsants of choice for the treatment of petit mal epilepsy during the 1st trimester (see Ethosuximide).

Breast Feeding Summary

No data available.

References

1. Annegers JF, Elveback LR, Hauser WA, Kurland LT. Do anticonvulsants have a teratogenic effect? Arch Neurol 1974;31:364–73.
2. Heinonen OP, Slone D, Shapiro S. *Birth Defects and Drugs in Pregnancy.* Littleton: Publishing Sciences Group, 1977:358–9.
3. Fabro S, Brown NA. Teratogenic potential of anticonvulsants. N Engl J Med 1979;300:1280–1.
4. The National Institutes of Health. Anticonvulsants found to have teratogenic potential. JAMA 1981;241:36.

Name: **METHYCLOTHIAZIDE**

Class: **Diuretic**   Risk Factor: **D**

Fetal Risk Summary

See Chlorothiazide.

Breast Feeding Summary

See Chlorothiazide.

Name: **METHYLDOPA**

Class: **Antihypertensive**   Risk Factor: **C**

Fetal Risk Summary

Methyldopa crosses the placenta and achieves fetal concentrations similar to the maternal serum (1–3). The Collaborative Perinatal Project monitored only 1 mother-child pair in which 1st trimester exposure to methyldopa was recorded (4). No abnormalities were found. A decrease in intracranial volume has been reported after 1st trimester exposure to methyldopa (5, 6). Infants evaluated at 4 years of age showed no association between small head size and retarded mental development (7). Review of 1,157 hypertensive pregnancies demonstrated no adverse effects from methyldopa administration (8–20). A reduced systolic blood pressure of 4 to 5 mm Hg in 24 infants for the first 2 days after delivery has been reported (21). This mild reduction in blood pressure was not considered significant. An infant born with esophageal atresia with fistula, congenital heart disease, absent left kidney and hypo-systolic blood pressure of 4 to 5 mm Hg in 24 infants for the first 2 days after delivery has been reported (21). This mild reduction in blood pressure was not considered significant. An infant born with esophageal atresia with fistula, congenital heart disease, absent left kidney and hypospadias was exposed to methyldopa throughout gestation (22). The mother also took clomiphene early in the 1st trimester.

Breast Feeding Summary

Methyldopa is excreted into breast milk in small amounts. A milk:plasma ratio of 1 has been reported (1).

References

1. Jones HMR, Cummings AJ. A study of the transfer of α-methyldopa to the human foetus and newborn infant. Br J Clin Pharmacol 1978;6:432-4.
2. Jones HMR, Cummings AJ, Setchell KDR, Lawson AM. Pharmacokinetics of methyldopa in neonates. Br J Clin Pharmacol 1979;8:433-40.
3. Cummings AJ, Whitelaw AGL. A study of conjugation and drug elimination in the human neonate. Br J Clin Pharmacol 1981;12:511-5.
4. Heinonen OP, Slone D, Shapiro S. *Birth Defects and Drugs in Pregnancy*. Littleton: Publishing Sciences Group, 1977:372.
5. Myerscough PR. Infant growth and development after treatment of maternal hypertension. Lancet 1980;1:883.
6. Moar VA, Jefferies MA, Mutch LMM, Dunsted MK, Redman CWG. Neonatal head circumference and the treatment of maternal hypertension. Br J Obstet Gynaecol 1978;85:933-7.
7. Dunsted M, Moar VA, Redman CWG. Infant growth and development following treatment of maternal hypertension. Lancet 1980;1:705.
8. Redman CWG, Bonnar J, Ounsted MK. Fetal outcome in the t8ial of antihypertensive treatment in pregnancy. Lancet 1976;2:754-6.
9. Hamilton M, Kopelman H. Treatment of severe hypertension with methyldopa. Br Med J 1963;1:151-5.
10. Abramowsky CR, Vegas ME, Swinehart G, Gyves MT. Decidual vasculopathy of the placenta in lupus erythematosus. N Engl J Med 1980;303:668-72.
11. Gallery EDM, Sounders DM, Hunyor SN, Gyory AZ. Randomised comparison of methyldopa and oxprenolol for treatment of hypertension in pregnancy. Br Med J 1979;1:1591-4.
12. Gyory AZ, Gallery ED, Hunyor SN. Effect of treatment of maternal hypertension with oxprenolol and α-methyldopa on plasma volume, placental and birth weights. Eighth World Congress of Cardiology, Tokyo, 1978; abstract No. 1098.
13. Arias F, Zamora J. Antihypertensive treatment and pregnancy outcome in patients with mild chronic hypertension. Obstet Gynecol 1979;53:489-94.
14. Redman CWG, Beilin LJ, Bonnar J. A trial of hypotensive treatment in pregnancy. Clin Sci Mol Med 1975;49:3-4.
15. Tcherdakoff P, Milliez P. Traitement de l'hypertension arterielle par alphamethyldopa au cours de lo grossesse. Proc Premier Symposium National, Hypertension Arterielle, Cannes, 1970:207-9.
16. Lselve A, Berger R, Vial JY, Gaillard MF. Alpha-methyldopa/aldomet and reserpine/serpasil: treatment of pregnancy hypertensions. J Med Lyon 1968;1369-75.
17. Leather HM, Humphreys DM, Baker P, Chadd MA. A controlled trial of hypotensive agents in hypertension in pregnancy. Lancet 1968;2:488-90.
18. Hamilton H. Some aspects of the long-term treatment of severe hypertension with methyldopa. Postgrad Med J 1968;44:66-9.
19. Skacel K, Sklendvsky A, Gazarek F, Matlocha Z, Mohapl M. Lecebne pouziti alfo-methyldopa u pozdni gestozy (therapeutic use of alpha-methyldopa in cases of late toxemia of pregnancy). Cesk Gynekol 1967;32:78-80.
20. Kincaid-Smith P, Bullen M. Prolonged use of methyldopa in severe hypertension in pregnancy. Br Med J 1966;1:274-6.
21. Whitelaw A. Maternal methyldopa treatment and neonatal blood pressure. Br Med J 1981;283:471.
22. Ylikorkala O. Congenital anomalies and clomiphene. Lancet 1975;2:1262-3.

Name: **METHYLENE BLUE**

Class: **Urinary Germicide/Diagnostic Dye**   Risk Factor: **C***

Fetal Risk Summary

Methylene blue may be administered orally for its weak urinary germicide properties or injected into the amniotic fluid to diagnose premature rupture of the membranes. For oral dosing, 9 exposures in the 1st trimester have been reported (1). No congenital abnormalities were observed. For use anytime during pregnancy, 46 exposures were reported (2). A possible association with malformations was found, but the statistical significance is not known.

Diagnostic intra-amniotic injection of methylene blue has resulted in hemolytic anemia and hyperbilirubinemia in the newborn (3–5). Doses of the dye ranged from 10 to 50 mg. One author suggested that smaller doses, such as 1.6 mg, would be adequate to confirm the presence of ruptured membranes without causing hemolysis (3). Inadvertent intrauterine injection in the 1st trimester has been reported (6). No adverse effects were reported in the full term neonate.

[* Risk Factor D if injected intra-amniotically.]

Breast Feeding Summary

No data available.

References

1. Heinonen OP, Slone D, Shapiro S. *Birth Defects and Drugs in Pregnancy.* Littleton: Publishing Sciences Group, 1977:299.
2. *Ibid*, 434–5.
3. Plunkett GD. Neonatal complications. Obstet Gynecol 1973;41:476–7.
4. Cowett RM, Hakanson DO, Kocon RW, Oh W. Untoward neonatal effect of intraamniotic administration of methylene blue. Obstet Gynecol 1976;48:74s–5s.
5. Kirsch IR, Cohen HJ. Heinz body hemolytic anemia from the use of methylene blue in neonates. J Pediatr 1980;96:276–8.
6. Katz Z, Lancet M. Inadvertent intrauterine injection of methylene blue in early pregnancy. N Engl J Med 1981;304:1427.

Name: **METHYLPHENIDATE**

Class: **Central Stimulant**   Risk Factor: **C**

Fetal Risk Summary

No reports linking the use of methylphenidate with congenital defects have been located. The Collaborative Perinatal Project monitored 3,082 mother-child pairs with sympathomimetic drugs, 11 of which were exposed to methylphenidate (1). No evidence for an increased malformation rate was found.

Breast Feeding Summary

No data available.

Reference

1. Heinonen OP, Slone D, Shapiro S. *Birth Defects and Drugs in Pregnancy*. Littleton: Publishing Sciences Group, 1977:346–7.

Name: **METOLAZONE**

Class: **Diuretic** Risk Factor: **D**

Fetal Risk Summary

Metolazone is structurally related to the thiazide diuretics. See Chlorothiazide.

Breast Feeding Summary

See Chlorothiazide.

Name: **METRONIDAZOLE**

Class: **Trichomonacide/Antibiotic** Risk Factor: **C**

Fetal Risk Summary

Two infants with midline facial defects were reported whose mothers were treated with metronidazole in the 1st trimester for amebiasis (1). Use of this drug at various stages of gestation without fetal harm has also been reported in over 800 pregnancies, including almost 300 in the 1st trimester (2–4). Based on this data, the teratogenic risk from metronidazole, if it exists, must be small.

Carcinogenicity in rodents and mutagenicity in bacteria have been observed and because of this, one publication suggested that metronidazole is potentially dangerous in humans and should not be used in pregnant women (5). However, a 20-year survey to assess the oncogenic effects in humans failed to discover a relationship with metronidazole (6).

Author (Ref)	No. Pts.	Indication	Gestational Age	Dose	Other Drugs	Fetal Effects	Comments
Cantu (1)	1	Amebiasis	1st trimester	Not stated (10 days)	Diiodohydroxyquino-line	Midline facial defect	
	1	Amebiasis	1st trimester	750 mg/day 3 days	Not stated	Midline facial defect	

Breast Feeding Summary

Metronidazole is excreted into breast milk. Peak milk concentrations of 1 to 7.7 µg/ml after a 200-mg dose and 45.8 µg/ml after a 2-g dose occurred at

2 to 4 hours (7, 8). Following the 2-g dose (for vaginitis due to *Trichomonas vaginalis*), the nursing infant could consume about 25 mg of metronidazole over 48 hours (8). Milk levels after metronidazole rectal suppositories (1 g every 8 hours for 7 doses) have been reported to range from 10 to 25 $\mu g/ml$ (9). One report described diarrhea and a secondary lactose intolerance in a nursing male infant whose mother was taking the drug (10). Although other reports of adverse effects in the nursing infant have not been located, three problems may exist for the infant: modification of bowel flora, direct effects on the infant and interference with the interpretation of culture results if a fever work-up is required.

References

1. Cantu JM, Garcia-Cruz D. Midline facial defect as a teratogenic effect of metronidazole. Birth Defects 1982;18:85–8.
2. Shepard TH. *Catalog of Teratogenic Agents*. Baltimore: Johns Hopkins University Press, 1980:228.
3. Robinson SC, Mirchandani G. Trichomonas vaginalis. V. Further observations on metronidazole (including infant follow-up). Am J Obstet Gynecol 1965;93:502–5.
4. Morgan I. Metronidazole treatment in pregnancy. Int J Gynaecol Obstet 1978;15:501–2.
5. Anonymous. Is Flagyl dangerous? Med Lett Drugs Ther 1975;17:53–4.
6. Goldman P. Metronidazole: proven benefits and potential risks. Johns Hopkins Med J 1980;147:1–9.
7. Gray MS, Kane DO, Squires S. Further observations on metronidazole. Br J Vener Dis 1961;37:278–9.
8. Erickson SH, Oppenheim GL, Smith GH. Metronidazole in breast milk. Obstet Gynecol 1981;57:48–50.
9. Moore B, Collier J. Drugs and breast-feeding. Br Med J 1979;2:211.
10. Clements CJ. Metronidazole and breast feeding. NZ Med J 1980;92:329.

Name: **MICONAZOLE**

Class: **Antifungal Antibiotic**　　　　　　　　　　　　　　Risk Factor: **B**

Fetal Risk Summary

Miconazole is normally used as a topical antifungal agent. Small amounts are absorbed from the vagina (1). Use in pregnant patients with vulvovaginal candidiasis (moniliasis) has not been associated with an increase in congenital malformations (1–5). Effects following intravenous use are not known.

Breast Feeding Summary

No data available.

References

1. Product information. *Physicians' Desk Reference*. Oradell, N.J.: Medical Economics Company, 1981:1304.
2. Culbertson C. Monistat: a new fungicide for treatment of vulvovaginal candidiasis. Am J Obstet Gynecol 1974;120:973–6.
3. Wade A, ed. *Martindale. The Extra Pharmacopoeia*, ed. 27. London: Pharmaceutical Press, 1977:648.

4. Davis JE, Frudenfeld JH, Goddard JL. Comparative evaluation of Monistat and Mycostatin in the treatment of vulvovaginal candidiasis. Obstet Gynecol 1974;44:403–6.
5. Wallenburg HCS, Wladimiroff JW. Recurrence of vulvovaginal candidosis during pregnancy. Comparison of miconazole vs nystatin treatment. Obstet Gynecol 1976;48:491–4.

Name: **MINERAL OIL**

Class: **Laxative**   Risk Factor: **C**

Fetal Risk Summary

Mineral oil is an emollient laxative. The drug is generally considered nonabsorbable. Chronic use may lead to decreased absorption of fat-soluble vitamins.

Breast Feeding Summary

No data available.

Name: **MINOCYCLINE**

Class: **Antibiotic**   Risk Factor: **D**

Fetal Risk Summary

See Tetracycline.

Breast Feeding Summary

See Tetracycline.

Name: **MINOXIDIL**

Class: **Antihypertensive**   Risk Factor: **C**

Fetal Risk Summary

No data available.

Breast Feeding Summary

No data available.

Name: **MITHRAMYCIN**

Class: **Antineoplastic**   Risk Factor: **D**

Fetal Risk Summary

No data available.

Breast Feeding Summary

No data available.

Name: **MOLINDONE**

Class: **Tranquilizer**   Risk Factor: **C**

Fetal Risk Summary

Molindone is an antipsychotic drug. The only reported use of it in pregnancy was in a woman who gave birth at term to normal twin boys (1). The mother had ingested 9800 mg of molindone during her 9-month pregnancy. No abnormalities in physical or mental development were noted in their first 20 years of life.

Breast Feeding Summary

No data available.

Reference

1. Ayd FJ Jr. Moban: the first of a new class of neuroleptics. In Ayd FJ Jr., ed. *Rational Psychopharmacotherapy and the Right to Treatment.* Baltimore: Ayd Medical Communications, 1975:91–106.

Name: **MORPHINE**

Class: **Narcotic Analgesic**   Risk Factor: **B***

Fetal Risk Summary

No reports linking the therapeutic use of morphine with major congenital defects have been located. Bilateral horizontal nystagmus persisting for 1 year was reported in one addicted newborn (1). Like all narcotics, placental transfer of morphine is very rapid (2, 3). Maternal addiction with subsequent neonatal withdrawal is well known following illicit use (see also Heroin) (1, 4, 5). Morphine was widely used in labor until the 1940's when it was largely displaced by meperidine. Clinical impressions that meperidine caused less respiratory depression in the newborn were apparently confirmed (6, 7). Other

·linicians reported no difference between narcotics in the degree of neonatal ¹epression when equianalgesic intravenous doses were used (3). The drug is ₁ow rarely used in labor.

The Collaborative Perinatal Project monitored 50,282 mother-child pairs, ˜0 of which had 1st trimester exposure to morphine (8). For use anytime ¹uring pregnancy, 448 exposures were recorded (9). No evidence was found ₒ suggest a relationship to large categories of major or minor malformations. ₁ possible association with inguinal hernia (10 cases) after anytime use was ₒbserved (10). The statistical significance of this association is unknown and ₁dependent confirmation is required.

* Risk Factor D if used for prolonged periods or in high doses at term.]

³reast Feeding Summary

Ɔnly trace amounts of morphine enter breast milk. The significance is unknown 11–13).

Author (ref)	No. Pts.	Dose	Concentrations (μg/ml)		M:P Ratio	Effect on Infant
			Serum	Milk		
erwilliger (11)	1	128 mg/day	Not stated	0	—	Infant exhibited signs of narcotic withdrawal not relieved by breast feeding.
	1	16 mg	Not stated	Trace	—	—
₃wit (12)	1	16 mg	Not stated	Less than 6 μg/ml	—	—

³eferences

1. Perlstein MA. Congenital morphinism. A rare cause of convulsions in the newborn. JAMA 1947;135:633.
2. Fisher DE, Paton JB. The effect of maternal anesthetic and analgesic drugs on the fetus and newborn. Clin Obstet Gynaecol 1974;17:275–87.
3. Bonica JJ. *Principles and Practice of Obstetric Analgesia and Anesthesia.* Philadelphia: FA Davis, 1967:247.
4. McMullin GP, Mobarak AN. Congenital narcotic addiction. Arch Dis Child 1970;45:140–1.
5. Cobrinik RW, Hodd RT Jr, Chusid E. The effect of maternal narcotic addiction on the newborn infant. Pediatrics 1959;24:288–304.
6. Gilbert G, Dixon AB. Observations on Demerol as an obstetric analgesic. Am J Obstet Gynecol 1943;45:320–6.
7. Way WL, Costley EC, Way EL. Respiratory sensitivity of the newborn infant to meperidine and morphine. Clin Pharmacol Thera 1965;6:454–61.
8. Heinonen OP, Slone D, Shapiro S. *Birth Defects and Drugs in Pregnancy.* Littleton: Publishing Sciences Group, 1977:287–95.
9. *Ibid*, 434.
₁0. *Ibid*, 484.
₁1. Terwilliger WG, Hatcher RA. The elimination of morphine and quinine in human milk. Surg Gynecol Obstet 1934;58:823–6.
₁2. Kwit NT, Hatcher RA. Excretion of drugs in milk. Am J Dis Child 1935;49:900–4.
₁3. Anonymous. Drugs in breast milk. Med Lett Drugs Ther 1979;21:21–4.

Name: **NADOLOL**

Class: **Antihypertensive**   Risk Factor: **C_M**

Fetal Risk Summary

Nadolol is a β-adrenergic blocking agent used for hypertension and angina pectoris. No information on its use in pregnancy has been located. The manufacturer states that nadolol should only be used in pregnancy if the expected benefits outweigh the unknown potential risks to the fetus (1).

Breast Feeding Summary

No data available.

Reference

1. Product information. Corgard. Squibb, 1981.

Name: **NAFCILLIN**

Class: **Antibiotic**   Risk Factor: **B**

Fetal Risk Summary

Nafcillin is a pencillin antibiotic (see also Pencillin G). No reports linking its use with congenital defects have been located. The Collaborative Perinatal Project monitored 50,282 mother-child pairs, 3,546 of which had 1st trimester exposure to pencillin derivatives (1). For use anytime during pregnancy, 7,171 exposures were recorded (2). In neither case was evidence found to suggest a relationship to large categories of major or minor malformations or to individual defects.

Breast Feeding Summary

No data available (see Pencillin G).

References

1. Heinonen OP, Slone D, Shapiro S. *Birth Defects and Drugs in Pregnancy*. Littleton: Publishing Sciences Group, 1977:297–313.
2. *Ibid*, 435.

238

Name: **NALBUPHINE**
Class: **Analgesic**   Risk Factor: **B***

Fetal Risk Summary

No congenital defects have been reported in humans or in laboratory animals
(1). Nalbuphine has both narcotic agonist and antagonist effects. Prolonged
use during pregnancy could theoretically result in fetal addiction with subsequent withdrawal in the newborn (see also Pentazocine). Use of the drug in
labor produces neonatal respiratory depression comparable to meperidine (1).
* Risk Factor D if used for prolonged periods or if high doses given at term.]

Breast Feeding Summary

No data available.

Reference

1. Miller RR. Evaluation of nalbuphine hydrochloride. Am J Hosp Pharm 1980;37:942–9.

Name: **NALIDIXIC ACID**   Risk Factor: **B**
Class: **Urinary Germicide**

Fetal Risk Summary

No reports linking the use of nalidixic acid with congenital defects have been
located. Chromosome damage was not observed in human leukocytes cultured
with varying concentrations of the drug (1). One author cautioned that the
drug should be avoided in late pregnancy since it may produce hydrocephalus
(2). However, a subsequent report examined the newborns of 63 patients
treated with nalidixic acid at various stages of gestation (3). No defects
attributable to the drug or intracranial hypertension were observed.

Breast Feeding Summary

Nalidixic acid is excreted into breast milk in low concentrations. Hemolytic
anemia was reported in one infant whose mother was taking 1 g four times a
day (4). Milk levels were not measured in this case, but the author noted data
from the manufacturer where milk levels from 4 women taking a similar dose
were found to be 4 μg/ml. The milk:plasma ratio has been reported as 0.08 to
0.13 (5). These quantities are normally considered insignificant (6).

References

1. Stenchever MA, Powell W, Jarvis JA. Effect of nalidixic acid on human chromosome integrity.
   Am J Obstet Gynecol 1970;107:329–30.
2. Asscher AW. Diseases of the urinary system. Urinary tract infections. Br Med J 1977;1:1332.
3. Murray EDS. Nalidixic acid in pregnancy. Br Med J 1981;282:224.

4. Belton EM, Jones RV. Hemolytic anemia due to nalidixic acid. Lancet 1965;2:691.
5. Wilson JT. Milk/plasma ratios and contraindicated drugs. In Wilson JT, ed. *Drugs in Breas Milk.* Australia: ADIS Press, 1981:78–9.
6. Takyi BE. Excretion of drugs in human milk. J Hosp Pharm 1970;28:317–25.

Name: **NALORPHINE**

Class: **Narcotic Antagonist**   Risk Factor: **C**

Fetal Risk Summary

Nalorphine is a narcotic antagonist that is used to reverse respiratory depression from narcotic overdose. It has been used either alone or in combination with meperidine or morphine during labor to reduce neonatal depression (1–6). Nalorphine has also been given to the newborn to prevent neonatal asphyxia (3, 7). Although some benefits were initially claimed, caution in the use of nalorphine during labor has been advised for the following reasons (8)

1. A statistically significant reduction in neonatal depression has not been demonstrated;
2. The antagonist also reduces analgesia; and
3. The antagonist may increase neonatal depression if an improper narcotic-narcotic antagonist ratio is used.

An adverse effect on fetal cord blood pH, pCO_2 and base deficit was shown when nalorphine was given in combination with meperidine during labor (9). As indicated above, nalorphine may cause respiratory depression in the absence of narcotics or if the critical ratio is exceeded (8). Because of these considerations, the use of nalorphine either alone or in combination therapy in pregnancy should be discouraged. If a narcotic antagonist is indicated, other agents that do not cause respiratory depression, such as naloxone, are preferred.

Breast Feeding Summary

No data available.

References

1. Cappe BE, Himel SZ, Grossman F. Use of a mixture of morphine and N-allynormorphine as an analgesic. Am J Obstet Gynecol 1953;66:1231–4.
2. Echenhoff JE, Hoffman GL, Funderburg LW. N-allynormorphine: an antagonist to neonatal narcosis produced by sedation of the parturient. Am J Obstet Gynecol 1953;65:1269–75.
3. Echenhoff JE, Funderburg LW. Observations in the use of the opiate antagonists nalorphine and levallorphan. Am J Med Sci 1954;228:546–53.
4. Baker FJ. Pethidine and nalorphine in labor. Anaesthesia 1957;12:282–92.
5. Gordon DWS, Pinker GD. Increased pethidine dosage in obstetrics associated with the use of nalorphine. J Obstet Gynaecol Br Commonw 1958;65:606–11.
6. Bullough J. Use of premixed pethidine and antagonists in obstetrical analgesia with special reference to cases in which levallorphan was used. Br Med J 1959;2:859–62.
7. Paterson S, Prescott F. Nalorphine in prevention of neonatal asphyxia due to maternal sedation with pethidine. Lancet 1954;1:490–3.

8. Bonica JJ. *Principles and Practice of Obstetric Analgesia and Anesthesia*. Philadelphia: FA Davis, 1967:254–9.
9. Hounslow D, Wood C, Humphrey M, Chang A. Intrapartum drugs and fetal blood pH and gas status. J Obstet Gynaecol Br Commonw 1973;80:1007–12.

Name: **NALOXONE**

Class: **Narcotic Antagonist**   Risk Factor: **C**

Fetal Risk Summary

Naloxone is a narcotic antagonist that is used to reverse the effects of narcotic overdose. The drug has no intrinsic respiratory depressive actions or other narcotic effects of its own (1). Naloxone has been shown to cross the placenta, appearing in fetal blood 2 minutes after a maternal dose and gradually increasing over 10 to 30 minutes (2). In 3 reports, naloxone was given to mothers in labor after the administration of meperidine (3–5). Clark found that 18 to 40 μg/kg (maternal weight) intravenously provided the best results in comparison with controls that did not receive meperidine or naloxone (4). In measurements of newborn neurobehavior, groups treated in labor with either meperidine or meperidine plus naloxone (0.4 mg) were compared with a non-treated control group (5). The control group scored better in the 1st 24 hours than either of the treated groups and, after 2 hours, no difference was found between meperidine or meperidine plus naloxone-treated patients. Naloxone has been given safely to newborns within a few minutes of delivery (6–10).

Naloxone has been used at term to treat fetal heart rate baselines with low beat-to-beat variability not due to maternally administered narcotics (11). This use was based on the assumption that the heart rate patterns were due to elevated fetal endorphins. In one case, however, naloxone may have enhanced fetal asphyxia leading to fatal respiratory failure in the newborn (11). Based on the above data, naloxone should not be given to the mother just prior to delivery to reverse the effects of narcotics in the fetus or newborn. It is the drug of choice, however, for the reversal of toxic narcotic effects in pregnancy or the newborn. Information on its fetal effects during pregnancy, other than labor, are not available.

Breast Feeding Summary

No data available.

References

1. Jaffe JH, Martin WR. Opoid analgesics and antagonists. In Gilman AG, Goodman LS, Gilman A, eds. *The Pharmacological Basis of Therapeutics*, ed. 6. New York: MacMillan, 1980:522–5.
2. Finster M, Gibbs C, Dawes GS, et al. Placental transfer of meperidine (Demerol) and naloxone (Narcan). Presented at the annual meeting of the American Society of Anesthesiologists, Boston, October 4, 1972. In: Clark RB, Beard AG, Greifenstein FE, Barclay DL. S Med J 1976;69:570–5.

3. Clark RB. Transplacental reversal of meperidine depression in the fetus by naloxone. J Arkansas Med Soc 1971;68:128–30.
4. Clark RB, Beard AG, Greifenstein FE, Barclay DL. Naloxone in the parturient and her infant. S Med J 1976;69:570–5.
5. Hodgkinson R, Bhatt M, Grewal G, Marx GF. Neonatal neurobehavior in the first 48 hours of life: effect of the administration of meperidine with and without naloxone in the mother. Pediatrics 1978;62:294–8.
6. Evans JM, Hogg MIJ, Rosen M. Reversal of narcotic depression in the neonate by naloxone. Br Med J 1976;2:1098–1100.
7. Wiener PC, Hogg MIJ, Rosen M. Effects of naloxone on pethidine-induced neonatal depression. II. Intramuscular naloxone. Br Med J 1977;2:229–31.
8. Wiener PC, Hogg MIJ, Rosen M. Effects of naloxone on pethidine-induced neonatal depression. I. Intravenous naloxone. Br Med J 1977;2:228–9.
9. Gerhardt T, Bancalari E, Cohen H, Rocha LF. Use of naloxone to reverse narcotic respiratory depression in the newborn infant. J Pediatr 1977;90:1009–12.
10. Bonta BW, Gagliardi JV, Williams V, Warshaw JB. Naloxone reversal of mild neurobehavioral depression in normal newborn infants after routine obstetric analgesia. J Pediatr 1979;94:102–5.
11. Goodlin RC. Naloxone and its possible relationship to fetal endorphin levels and fetal distress. Am J Obstet Gynecol 1981;139:16–9.

Name: **NAPROXEN**

Class: **Nonsteroidal Anti-inflammatory**   Risk Factor: **B*_M**

Fetal Risk Summary

Naproxen is a potent inhibitor of prostaglandin synthetase. Drugs in this class have been shown to inhibit labor and to prolong the length of pregnancy (1). Naproxen readily crosses the placenta to the fetal circulation (2, 3). In a mother treated with 250 mg of naproxen every 8 hours for 4 doses, cord blood levels in twins 5 hours after the last dose were 59.5 and 68 μg/ml, respectively (3). Prostaglandin synthetase inhibitors may cause constriction of the ductus arteriosus *in utero*, which may result in persistent pulmonary hypertension of the newborn (PPHN) (4, 5). The dose and duration of drug administration are important determinants of these effects. Three fetuses (1 set of twins) were exposed to naproxen early in the 3rd trimester (30 weeks) in an unsuccessful attempt to halt premature labor (3, 6). Plasma concentrations of prostaglandin E in the three infants were markedly depressed in comparison to levels measured in preterm infants of similar age but without cardiopulmonary disease. PPHN with severe hypoxemia, increased blood clotting times, hyperbilirubinemia and impaired renal function were observed in the newborns. One infant died four days after birth, probably due to subarachnoid hemorrhage. Autopsy revealed a short and constricted ductus arteriosus. Based on this data, naproxen should not be used in late pregnancy or near delivery (2, 3, 7).

[* Risk Factor D if used in 3rd trimester or near delivery.]

Breast Feeding Summary

Naproxen passes into breast milk in very small quantities. The milk:plasma ratio is approximately 0.01 (2). Following 250 or 375 mg twice daily, maximum milk levels were found 4 hours after a dose and ranged from 0.7 to 1.25 μg/ml and 1.76 to 2.37 μg/ml, respectively (8). The total amount of naproxen excreted in the infant's urine was 0.26% of the mother's dose. The effect on the infant from these amounts is not known.

References

1. Fuchs F. Prevention of prematurity. Am J Obstet Gynecol 1976;126:809–20.
2. Product information. Naprosyn. Syntex Laboratories, 1982.
3. Wilkinson AR. Naproxen levels in preterm infants after maternal treatment. Lancet 1980;2:591–2.
4. Levin DL. Effects of inhibition of prostaglandin synthesis on fetal development, oxygenation, and the fetal circulation. Semin Perinatol 1980;4:35–44.
5. Rudolph AM. The effects of nonsteroidal antiinflammatory compounds on fetal circulation and pulmonary function. Obstet Gynecol 1981;58 (Suppl):63s–7s.
6. Wilkinson AR, Aynsley-Green A, Mitchell MD. Persistent pulmonary hypertension and abnormal prostaglandin E levels in preterm infants after maternal treatment with naproxen. Arch Dis Child 1979;54:942–5.
7. Anonymous. PG-synthetase inhibitors in obstetrics and after. Lancet 1980;2:185–6.
8. Jamali F, Tam YK, Stevens RD. Naproxen excretion in breast milk and its uptake by suckling infant (Abstract). Drug Intell Clin Pharm 1982;16:475.

Name: **NEOMYCIN**

Class: **Antibiotic**

Risk Factor: **C**

Fetal Risk Summary

Neomycin is an aminoglycoside antibiotic. No reports describing its passage across the placenta to the fetus have been located, but this should be expected (see other aminoglycosides Amikacin, Gentamicin, Kanamycin, Streptomycin and Tobramycin).

Ototoxicity, which is known to occur after oral, topical and parenteral neomycin therapy, has not been reported as an effect of *in utero* exposure. However, eighth cranial nerve toxicity in the fetus is well known following exposure to kanamycin and streptomycin and may potentially occur with neomycin.

Oral neomycin therapy, 2 g daily, depresses urinary estrogen excretion apparently by inhibiting steroid conjugate hydrolysis in the gut (1). The fall in estrogen excretion resembles the effect produced by ampicillin but occurs about 2 days later. Urinary estriol was formerly used to assess the condition of the fetoplacental unit, depressed levels being associated with fetal distress. This assessment is now made by measuring plasma conjugated estriol, which is not usually affected by neomycin.

No reports linking the use of neomycin to congenital defects have been located. The Collaborative Perinatal Project monitored 50,282 mother-child pairs, 30 of which had 1st trimester exposure to neomycin (2). No evidence was found to suggest a relationship to large categories of major or minor malformations or to individual defects.

Breast Feeding Summary

No data available.

References

1. Pulkkinen M, Willman K. Reduction of maternal estrogen excretion by neomycin. Am J Obstet Gynecol 1973;115:1153.
2. Heinonen OP, Slone D, Shapiro S. *Birth Defects and Drugs in Pregnancy.* Littleton: Publishing Sciences Group, 1977:297–301.

Name: **NEOSTIGMINE**

Class: **Parasympathomimetic (Cholinergic)**   Risk Factor: **C**

Fetal Risk Summary

Neostigmine is a quaternary ammonium compound with anticholinesterase activity used in the diagnosis and treatment of myasthenia gravis. Because it is ionized at physiologic pH, it would not be expected to cross the placenta in significant amounts. One study reported 22 exposures to neostigmine in the 1st trimester (1). No relationship to congenital defects was found. A 1973 study described the use of 0.5 mg orally per day for 3 days in 27 pregnant patients (5 to 14 weeks) (2). One patient aborted and 26 went to term without complications. McNall considers neostigmine to be one of the drugs of choice for pregnant patients with myasthenia gravis (3). She also cautioned that intravenous anticholinesterases should not be used in pregnancy for fear of inducing premature labor and suggests that intramuscular neostigmine be used in place of intravenous edrophonium for diagnostic purposes. Other investigators have reported the safe use of neostigmine for myasthenia gravis in pregnancy (4–6). Although apparently safe for the fetus, cholinesterase inhibitors may affect the condition of the newborn (3, 7). Transient muscular weakness has been observed in about 20% of newborns whose mothers were treated for myasthenia gravis during pregnancy. While the exact cause of the neonatal myasthenia is unknown, anticholinesterases may contribute to the condition (7).

Breast Feeding Summary

Because it is ionized at physiologic pH, neostigmine would not be expected to be excreted into breast milk (8).

References

1. Heinonen OP, Slone D, Shapiro S. *Birth Defects and Drugs in Pregnancy.* Littleton: Publishing Sciences Group, 1977:345–56.
2. Brunclik V, Hauser GA. Short-term therapy in secondary amenorrhea. Ther Umsch 1973;30:496–502.
3. McNall PG, Jafarnia MR. Management of myasthenia gravis in the obstetrical patient. Am J Obstet Gynecol 1965;92:518–25.
4. Foldes FF, McNall PG. Myasthenia gravis: a guide for anesthesiologists. Anesthesiology 1962;23:837–72.
5. Chambers DC, Hall JE, Boyce J. Myasthenia gravis and pregnancy. Obstet Gynecol 1967;29:597–603.
6. Hay DM. Myasthenia gravis and pregnancy. J Obstet Gynaecol Br Commonw 1969;76:323–9.
7. Blackhall MI, Buckley GA, Roberts DV, Roberts JB, Thomas BH, Wilson A. Drug-induced neonatal myasthenia. J Obstet Gynaecol Br Commonw 1969;76:157–62.
8. Wilson JT. Pharmacokinetics of drug excretion. In Wilson JT, ed. *Drugs in Breast Milk.* Australia: ADIS Press, 1981:17.

Name: **NIALAMIDE**

Class: **Antidepressant**   Risk Factor: **C**

Fetal Risk Summary

No data available (see Phenelzine).

Breast Feeding Summary

No data available (see Phenelzine).

Name: **NICOTINYL ALCOHOL**

Class: **Vasodilator**   Risk Factor: **C**

Fetal Risk Summary

Nicotinyl alcohol is converted in the body to niacin, the active form. Only one report of its use in pregnancy has been located. The Collaborative Perinatal Project recorded one 1st trimester exposure to nicotinyl alcohol plus 14 other patients exposed to other vasodilators (1). From this small group of 15 patients, 4 malformed children were produced, a statistically significant incidence ($p < 0.02$). It was not stated if nicotinyl alcohol was taken by a mother of one of the affected infants. Although the data serves as a warning, the number of patients is so small that conclusions as to the relative safety of this drug in pregnancy cannot be made.

Breast Feeding Summary

No data available.

Reference

1. Heinonen OP, Slone D, Shapiro S. *Birth Defects and Drugs in Pregnancy*. Littleton: Publishing Sciences Group, 1977:371–3.

Name: **NICOUMALONE**

Class: **Anticoagulant**   Risk Factor: **D**

Fetal Risk Summary

See Coumarin Derivatives.

Breast Feeding Summary

See Coumarin Derivatives.

Name: **NITROFURANTOIN**

Class: **Urinary Germicide**   Risk Factor: **B**

Fetal Risk Summary

No reports linking the use of nitrofurantoin with congenital defects have been located. One manufacturer (Norwich-Eaton Laboratories) has collected over 1,700 case histories describing the use of this drug during various stages of pregnancy (95 references) (personal communication, 1981). None of the reports observed deleterious effects on the fetus. Nitrofurantoin is capable of inducing hemolytic anemia in glucose-6-phosphate dehydrogenase (G-6-PD) deficient patients and in patients whose red blood cells are deficient in reduced glutathione (1). Since the red blood cells of newborns are deficient in reduced glutathione, the manufacturer's package insert (Norwich-Eaton) carries a warning against use of the drug at term. However, hemolytic anemia in the newborn as a result of in utero exposure to nitrofurantoin has not been reported.

Nitrofurantoin has been reported to cause discoloration of the primary teeth when given to an infant, and by implication, could occur from *in utero* exposure (2). However, the fact that the baby was also given a 14-day course of tetracycline and the lack of other confirming reports makes the likelihood for a causal relationship remote (3). When given orally in high doses of 10 mg/kg/day to young males, nitrofurantoin may produce slight to moderate transient spermatogenic arrest (4). The lower doses used clinically do not seem to have this effect.

Breast Feeding Summary

Nitrofurantoin is excreted into breast milk in very low concentrations. The drug could not be detected in 20 samples from mothers receiving 100 mg four times daily (5). In a second study, 9 mothers were given 100 mg every 6 hours for 1 day, then either 100 mg or 200 mg the next morning (6). Only 2 of the 4 patients receiving the 200-mg dose excreted measurable amounts of nitrofurantoin, 0.3 to 0.5 μg/ml. Although these amounts are negligible, the authors cautioned that infants with G-6-PD deficiency may develop hemolytic anemia from this exposure.

References

1. Powell RD, DeGowin RL, Alving AS. Nitrofurantoin-induced hemolysis. J Lab Clin Med 1963;62:1002–3.
2. Ball JS, Ferguson AN. Permanent discoloration of primary dentition by nitrofurantoin. Br Med J 1962;2:1103.
3. Duckworth R, Swallow JN. Nitrofurantoin and teeth. Br Med J 1962;2:1617.
4. Nelson WO, Bunge RG. The effect of therapeutic dosages of nitrofurantoin (Furadantin) upon spermatogenesis in man. J Urol 1957;77:275–81.
5. Hosbach RE, Foster RB. Absence of nitrofurantoin from human milk. JAMA 1967;202:1057.
6. Varsano I, Fischl J, Shochet SB. The excretion of orally ingested nitrofurantoin in human milk. J Pediatr 1973;82:886–7.

Name: **NITROGLYCERIN**

Class: **Vasodilator**   Risk Factor: **C**

Fetal Risk Summary

Nitroglycerin is a rapid acting, short duration vasodilator used primarily for the treatment or prevention of angina pectoris. Due to the nature of its indication, experience in pregnancy is limited. The drug has been used to control severe hypertension during cesarean section (1). No hypotension or other effects of the drug were observed in the newborn infant. The Collaborative Perinatal Project recorded 7 1st trimester exposures to nitroglycerin and amyl nitrite plus 8 other patients exposed to other vasodilators (2). From this small group of 15 patients, 4 malformed children were produced, a statistically significant incidence ($p < 0.02$). It was not stated if nitroglycerin was taken by any of the mothers of the affected infants. Although the data serves as a warning, the number of patients is so small that conclusions as to the relative safety of nitroglycerin in pregnancy cannot be made.

Breast Feeding Summary

No data available.

References

1. Snyder SW, Wheeler AS, James FM III. The use of nitroglycerin to control severe hypertension of pregnancy during cesarean section. Anesthesiology 1979;51:563–4.

2. Heinonen OP, Slone D, Shapiro S. *Birth Defects and Drugs in Pregnancy*. Littleton: Publishing Sciences Group, 1977:371–3.

Name: **NITROPRUSSIDE**

Class: **Antihypertensive**   Risk Factor: **D**

Fetal Risk Summary

No reports linking the use of nitroprusside with congenital defects have been located. Nitroprusside has been used in 7 pregnant patients to produce deliberate hypotension during aneurysm surgery or to treat severe hypertension (1–3). Transient fetal bradycardia was the only adverse effect noted (1). Nitroprusside crosses the placenta and produces fetal cyanide concentrations higher than maternal levels in animals (4). This effect has not been studied in humans. Avoidance of prolonged maternal use and monitoring serum cyanide and/or thiocyanate levels in newborns exposed near term are recommended.

Breast Feeding Summary

No data available.

References

1. Donchin Y, Amirav B, Sahar A, Yarkoni S. Sodium nitroprusside for aneurysm surgery in pregnancy. Br J Anaesth 1978;50:849–51.
2. Paull J. Clinical report of the use of sodium nitroprusside in severe pre-eclampsia. Anesth Intensive Care 1975;3:72.
3. Rigg D, McDonogh A. Use of sodium nitroprusside for deliberate hypotension during pregnancy. Br J Anaesth 1981;53:985–7.
4. Lewis PE, Cefalo RC. Naulty JS, Rodkey RL. Placental transfer and fetal toxicity of sodium nitroprosside. Gynecol Invest 1977;8:46.

Name: **NORETHINDRONE**

Class: **Progestogenic Hormone**   Risk Factor: **D**

Fetal Risk Summary

Norethindrone is a progestogen derived from 19-nortestosterone. It is used in oral contraceptives and as hormonal pregnancy tests (no longer available in the United States). Masculinization of the female fetus has been associated with norethindrone (1–3). Jacobson observed an 18% incidence of masculinization of the female infants born to mothers given norethindrone (2). A more conservative estimate for the incidence of masculinization due to synthetic progestogens has been reported as 0.3% (4). The Collaborative Perinatal

Project monitored 866 mother-child pairs with 1st trimester exposure to progestational agents (including 132 with exposure to norethindrone) (5). Evidence of an increased risk of malformation was found for norethindrone. An increase in the expected frequency of cardiovascular defects and hypospadias was observed for progestational agents as a group (6). Dillion observed 2 infants with malformations exposed to norethindrone (7). The congenital defects included spina bifida and hydrocephalus. Both estrogens and progestogens have been associated with the occurrence of congenital heart defects but because of overlap, the data is not sufficient to adequately separate their effects (8).

Breast Feeding Summary

Norethindrone exhibits a dose-dependent suppression of lactation (9). Lower infant weight gain, decreased milk production and decreased composition of nitrogen and protein content of human milk have been associated with norethindrone and estrogenic agents (10–13). The magnitude of these changes is low. However, the changes in milk production and composition may be of nutritional importance in malnourished mothers. If breast feeding is desired, the lowest dose of oral contraceptives should be chosen. Monitoring of infant weight gain and the possible need for nutritional supplementation should be considered.

References

1. Hagler S, Schultz A, Hankin H, Kunstadter RN. Fetal effects of steroid therapy during pregnancy. Am J Dis Child 1963;106:586–90.
2. Jacobson BD. Hazards of norethindrone therapy during pregnancy. Am J Obstet Gynecol 1962;84:962–8.
3. Wilson JG, Brent RL. Are female sex hormones teratogenic? Am J Obstet Gynecol 1981;141:567–80.
4. Bongiovanni AM, McFadden AJ. Steroids during pregnancy and possible fetal consequences. Fertil Steril 1960;11:181–4.
5. Heinonen OP, Slone D, Shapiro S. *Birth Defects and Drugs in Pregnancy.* Littleton: Publishing Sciences Group, 1977:389, 391.
6. *Ibid,* 394.
7. Dillon S. Congenital malformations and hormones in pregnancy. Br Med J 1976;2:1446.
8. Heinonen OP, Slone D, Monson RR, Hook EB, Shapiro S. Cardiovascular birth defects and antenatal exposure to female sex hormones. N Engl J Med 1977;296:67–70.
9. Guiloff E, Ibarra-Polo A, Zanartu J, Toscanini C, Mischler TW, Gomez-Rogers C. Effect of contraception on lactation. Am J Obstet Gynecol 1974;118:42–5.
10. Karim M, Ammarr R, El-Mahgoubh S, El-Ganzoury B, Fikri F, Abdou I. Injected progestogen and lactation. Br Med J 1971;1:200–3.
11. Kora SJ. Effect of oral contraceptives on lactation. Fertil Steril 1969;20:419–23.
12. Miller GH, Hughes LR. Lactation and genital involution effects of a new low-dose oral contraceptive on breast-feeding mothers and their infants. Obstet Gynecol 1970;35:44–50.
13. Lonnerdal B, Forsum E, Hambraeus L. Effect of oral contraceptives on composition and volume of breast milk. Am J Clin Nutr 1980;33:816–24.

Name: **NORETHYNODREL**

Class: **Progestogenic Hormone**   Risk Factor: **D**

Fetal Risk Summary

Norethynodrel is a progestogen derived from 19-nortestosterone. It is used in oral contraceptive agents and as hormonal pregnancy tests (no longer available in the United States). Masculinization of the female infant has been associated with norethynodrel (1, 2). The Collaborative Perinatal Project monitored 866 mother-child pairs with 1st trimester exposure to progestational agents (including 154 with exposure to norethynodrel) (3). Fetuses exposed to norethynodrel were not at an increased risk for malformation. However, an increase in the expected frequency of cardiovascular defects and hypospadias was observed for progestational agents as a group (4). Dillion observed 3 infants who were exposed to norethynodrel and mestranol during the 1st trimester (5). The congenital defects reported included atrial and ventricular septal defects (1 infant), hypospadias (1 infant), and inguinal hernias (2 infants). Both estrogens and progestogens have been associated with the occurrence of congenital heart disease, but because of overlap, the data is not sufficient to adequately separate their effects (6).

Breast Feeding Summary

Norethynodrel exhibits a dose-dependent suppression of lactation (7). Lower infant weight gain, decreased milk production and decreased composition of nitrogen and protein content of human milk have been associated with similar synthetic progestogens with estrogen products (see Norethindrone, Mestranol, Ethinyl Estradiol, Oral Contraceptives) (8-10). The magnitude of these changes is low. However, the changes in milk production and composition may be of nutritional importance in malnourished mothers. If breast feeding is desired, the lowest dose of oral contraceptives should be chosen. Monitoring of infant weight gain and the possible need for nutritional supplementation should be considered.

References

1. Wilson JG, Brent RL. Are female sex hormones teratogenic? Am J Obstet Gynecol 1981;141:567–80.
2. Hagler S. Schultz A, Hankin H, Kunstadter RN. Fetal effects of steroid therapy during pregnancy. Am J Dis Child 1963;106:586–90.
3. Heinonen OP, Slone D, Shapiro S. *Birth Defects and Drugs in Pregnancy*. Littleton: Publishing Sciences Group, 1977:389, 391.
4. *Ibid*, 394.
5. Dillion S. Congenital malformations and hormones in pregnancy. Br Med J 1976;2:1446.
6. Heinonen OP, Slone D, Monson RR, Hook EB, Shapiro S. Cardiovascular birth defects and antenatal exposure to female hormones. N Engl J Med 1977;296:67–70.
7. Guiloff E, Ibarra-Polo A, Zanartu J, Toscanini C, Mischler TW, Gomez-Rogers C. Effect of contraception on lactation. Am J Obstet Gynecol 1974;118:42–5.
8. Kora SJ. Effect of oral contraceptives on lactation. Fertil Steril 1969;20:419–23.
9. Miller GH, Hughes LR. Lactation and genital involution effects of a new low-dose oral contraceptive on breast-feeding mothers and their infants. Obstet Gynecol 1970;35:44–50.

10. Lonnerdal B, Forsum E, Hambraeus L. Effect of oral contraceptives on composition and volume of breast milk. Am J Clin Nutr 1980;33:816–24.

Name: **NORGESTREL**

Class: **Progestogenic Hormone**   Risk Factor: **D**

Fetal Risk Summary

Norgestrel is commonly used as an oral contraceptive either alone or in combination with estrogens (see Oral Contraceptives).

Breast Feeding Summary

No data available (see Oral Contraceptives).

Name: **NORTRIPTYLINE**

Class: **Antidepressant**   Risk Factor: **D**

Fetal Risk Summary

Limb reduction anomalies have been reported with nortriptyline (1, 2). One child was not exposed until after the critical period for limb development (3). The second infant was also exposed to sulfamethizole and heavy cigarette smoking (1). Evaluation of 86 patients with 1st trimester exposure to amitriptyline, the active precursor of nortriptyline, do not support the drug as a major cause of congenital limb deformities (see also Amitriptyline). Urinary retention in the neonate has been associated with maternal use of nortriptyline (4).

Breast Feeding Summary

Nortriptyline is excreted into breast milk in low concentrations (5–7). The significance of these low amounts are not known (see also Amitriptyline).

Author (ref)	No. Pts.	Dose	Concentrations (μg/ml)		M:P Ratio	Effect on Infant
			Serum	Milk		
Bader (5)	1		0.086	0.059	0.7	No drug detected in infant serum
Erickson (6)	—		0.146	—	—	No drug detected in infant serum

References

1. Bourke GM. Antidepressant teratogenicity? Lancet 1974;1:98.
2. McBride WG. Limb deformities associated with iminobenzyl hydrochloride. Med J Aust 1972;1:492.

3. Australian Drug Evaluation Committee. Tricyclic antidepressants and limb reduction deformities. Med J Aust 1973;1:768–9.
4. Shearer WT, Schreiner RL, Marshall RE. Urinary retention in a neonate secondary to maternal ingestion of nortriptyline. J Pediatr 1972;81:570–2.
5. Bader TF, Newman K. Amitriptyline in human breast milk and the nursing infant's serum. Am J Psychiatry 1980;137:855–6.
6. Erickson SH, Smith GH, Heidrich F. Tricyclics and breast feeding. Am J Psychiatry 1979;136:1483.
7. Brixen-Rasmussen L, Halgrener J, Jorgensen A. Amitriptyline and nortriptyline excretion in human breast milk. Psychopharmacology (Berlin) 1982;76:94–5.

Name: **NOVOBIOCIN**

Class: **Antibiotic**   Risk Factor: **C**

Fetal Risk Summary

No reports linking the use of novobiocin with congenital defects have been located. One study listed 21 patients exposed to the drug in the 1st trimester (1). No association with malformations was found. Since novobiocin may cause jaundice due to inhibition of glucuronyl transferase, its use near term is not recommended (2).

Breast Feeding Summary

Novobiocin is excreted into breast milk. Concentrations up to 7 μg/ml have been reported with milk:plasma ratios of 0.1 to 0.25 (3, 4). While adverse effects have not been reported, 3 potential problems exist for the nursing infant: modification of bowel flora, direct effects on the infant and interference with the interpretation of culture results if a fever work-up is required.

References

1. Heinonen OP, Slone D, Shapiro S. *Birth Defects and Drugs in Pregnancy.* Littleton: Publishing Sciences Group, 1977:297, 301.
2. Weistein L. Antibiotics. IV. Miscellaneous antimicrobial, antifungal, and antiviral agents. In Goodman LS, Gilman A, eds. *The Pharmacological Basis of Therapeutics*, ed. 4. New York: MacMillan, 1970:1292.
3. Knowles JA. Excretion of drugs in milk—a review. J Pediatr 1965;66:1068–82.
4. Anderson PO. Drugs and breast feeding—a review. Drug Intell Clin Pharm 1977;11:208–23.

Name: **NYLIDRIN**

Class: **Vasodilator**   Risk Factor: **C**

Fetal Risk Summary

Nylidrin is a β-adrenergic receptor stimulant used as a vasodilator in the United States. The drug has been studied in Europe as a tocolytic agent for premature labor and for the treatment of hypertension in pregnancy (1–7). Systolic blood pressure is usually unchanged, with a fall in total peripheral resistance greater than the decrease in diastolic pressure (8, 9). Although maternal hyperglycemia has been observed, especially in diabetic patients, this or other serious adverse effects were not reported in the above studies in mothers or in newborns.

Breast Feeding Summary

No data available.

References

1. Neubuser D. Comparative investigation of two inhibitors of labour (TV 399 and buphenin). Geburtshilfe Fraunheilkd 1972;32:781–6.
2. Castren O, Gummerus M, Saarikoski S. Treatment of imminent premature labour. Acta Obstet Gynecol Scand 1975;54:95–100.
3. Gummerus M. Prevention of premature birth with nylidrin and verapamil. Z Geburtshilfe Perinatol 1975;179:261–6.
4. Wolff F, Bolte A, Berg R. Does an additional administration of acetylsalicylic acid reduce the requirement of betamimetics in tocolytic treatment? Geburtshilfe Fraunheilkd 1981;41:293–6.
5. Hofer U, Ammann K. The oral tocolytic longtime therapy and its effects on the child. Ther Umsch 1978;35:417–21.
6. Retzke VU, Schwarz R, Lanckner W, During R. Dilatol for hypertension therapy in pregnancy. Zentralbl Gynaekol 1979;101:1034–8.
7. During VR, Mauch I. Effects of nylidrine (Dilatol) on blood pressure of hypertensive patients in advanced pregnancy. Zentralbl Gynaekol 1980;102:193–8.
8. Retzke VU, Schwarz R, Barten G. Cardiovascular effects of nylidrin (Dilatol) in pregnancy. Zentralbl Gynaekol 1976;98:1059–65.
9. During VR, Reincke R. Action of nylidrin (Dilatol) on utero-placental blood supply. Zentralbl Gynaekol 1981;103:214–9.

Name: **NYSTATIN**

Class: **Antifungal Antibiotic**   Risk Factor: **B**

Fetal Risk Summary

Nystatin is poorly absorbed after oral administration and from intact skin and mucous membranes. The Collaborative Perinatal Project found a possible association with congenital malformations after 142 1st trimester exposures, but this was probably due to its use as an adjunct to tetracycline therapy (1). No association was found following 230 exposures anytime in pregnancy (2). Other investigators have reported its safe use in pregnancy (3–5).

Breast Feeding Summary

Since nystatin is poorly absorbed, if at all, serum and milk levels would not occur.

References

1. Heinonen OP, Slone D, Shapiro S. *Birth Defects and Drugs in Pregnancy.* Littleton: Publishing Sciences Group, 1977:313.
2. *Ibid*, 435.
3. Culbertson C. Monistat: a new fungicide for treatment of vulvovaginal candidiasis. Am J Obstet Gynecol 1974;120:973–6.
4. David JE, Frudenfeld JH, Goddard JL. Comparative evaluation of Monistat and Mycostatin in the treatment of vulvovaginal candidiasis. Obstet Gynecol 1974;44:403–6.
5. Wallenburg HCS, Wladimiroff JW. Recurrence of vulvovaginal candidosis during pregnancy. Comparison of miconazole vs nystatin treatment. Obstet Gynecol 1976;48:491–4.

Name: **OLEANDOMYCIN**

Class: **Antibiotic**   Risk Factor: **C**

Fetal Risk Summary

No reports linking the use of oleandomycin or its triacetyl ester, troleando-mycin, with congenital defects have been located. One study listed 9 patients exposed to the drugs in the 1st trimester (1). No association with malformations was found.

Breast Feeding Summary

No data available.

Reference

1. Heinonen OP, Slone D, Shapiro S. *Birth Defects and Drugs in Pregnancy*. Littleton: Publishing Sciences Group, 1977:297, 301.

Name: **OPIPRAMOL**

Class: **Antidepressant**   Risk Factor: **D**

Fetal Risk Summary

No data available (see Imipramine).

Breast Feeding Summary

No data available (see Imipramine).

Name: **OPIUM**

Class: **Narcotic Antidiarrheal**   Risk Factor: **B***

Fetal Risk Summary

The effects of opium are due to morphine (see Morphine). The Collaborative Perinatal Project monitored 50,282 mother-child pairs, 36 of which had 1st trimester exposure to opium (1). For use anytime during pregnancy, 181 exposures were recorded (2). Although these numbers are small, a possible relationship may exist between the use of this drug and major and minor malformations. Further, a possible association with inguinal hernia (7 cases) after anytime use was observed (3). The statistical significance of these associations is unknown and independent confirmation is required.

Narcotic withdrawal was observed in a newborn whose mother was treated for regional ileitis with deodorized tincture of opium during the 2nd and 3rd trimesters (4). Symptoms of withdrawal in the infant began at 48 hours of age.

[* Risk Factor D if used for prolonged periods or in high doses at term.]

Breast Feeding Summary

See Morphine.

References

1. Heinonen OP, Slone D, Shapiro S. *Birth Defects and Drugs in Pregacy.* Littleton: Publishing Sciences Group, 1977:287–295.
2. *Ibid*, 424.
3. *Ibid*, 485.
4. Fisch GR, Henley WL. Symptoms of narcotic withdrawal in a newborn infant secondary to medical therapy of the mother. Pediatrics 1961;28:852–3.

Name: **ORAL CONTRACEPTIVES**

Class: **Estrogenic/Progestogenic Hormones**   Risk Factor: **D**

Fetal Risk Summary

Oral contraceptives contain a 19-nortestosterone progestin and a synthetic estrogen (see Mestranol, Norethindrone, Norethynodrel, Ethinyl Estradiol, Progesterone, Hydroxyprogesterone, Ethisterone). Because oral contraceptives are primarily combination products it is difficult to separate entirely the fetal effects of progestogens and estrogens. Ambani in 1977 and Wilson in 1981 reviewed the effects of these hormones on the fetus (133 references) (1, 2). Several potential problems were discussed: congenital heart defects, central nervous system defects, limb reduction malformations, general malformations and modified development of sexual organs. Except for the latter category, no firm evidence has appeared that establishes a causal relationship between oral contraceptives and various congenital anomalies. The acronym VACTERL (Vertebral, Anal, Cardiac, Tracheal, Esophageal, Renal or Radial, and Limb) has been used to describe the fetal malformations produced by oral contraceptives or the related hormonal pregnancy test preparations (no longer available in the United States) (2, 3). The use of this acronym should probably be abandoned in favor of more conventional terminology as a large variety of malformations have been reported with estrogen-progestogen containing products (1–11). The Population Council estimates that even if the study findings for VACTERL malformations are accurate, such abnormalities would occur in only 0.07% of the pregnancies exposed to oral contraceptives (12). Finally, Wilson concluded from his review that the risk to the fetus for nongenital malformations after *in utero* exposure to these agents is small, if indeed it exists at all (2).

In contrast to the above, the effect of estrogens and some synthetic progestogens on the development of the sexual organs is well established (2). Masculinization of the female infant has been associated with norethindrone, norethynodrel, hydroxyprogesterone, medroxyprogesterone and diethylstilbestrol (2, 13, 14). Bongiovanni reported that the incidence of masculinization of female infants exposed to synthetic progestogens is 0.3% (15). Pseudohermaphroditism in the male infant is not a problem, due to the low doses of estrogen employed in oral contraceptives (14).

McConnell reported increased serum bilirubin in neonates of mothers taking oral contraceptives or progestogens before and after conception (16). Icterus occasionally reached clinically significant levels in infants whose mothers were exposed to the progestogens.

Concern that oral contraceptives may act as a risk factor for preeclampsia has been suggested on the basis of the known effects of oral contraceptives on blood pressure (16 references) (17). In a retrospective controlled review of 341 patients, no association was found between this effect and oral contraceptives.

Possible interactions between oral contraceptives and tetracycline, rifampin, ampicillin or chloramphenicol resulting in pregnancy have been reported (18–25). The mechanism for this interaction may involve the interruption of the enterhepatic circulation of contraceptive steroids by inhibiting gut hydrolysis of steroid conjugates, resulting in lower concentrations of circulating steroids.

Breast Feeding Summary

Use of oral contraceptives during lactation has been associated with shortened duration of lactation, decreased infant weight gain, decreased milk production and decreased composition of nitrogen and protein content of milk (26–29). The American Academy of Pediatrics has reviewed this subject (37 references) (30). Although the magnitude of these changes are low, the changes in milk production and composition may be of nutritional importance in malnourished mothers.

In general, progestin-only contraceptives demonstrate no consistent alteration of breast milk composition, volume or duration of lactation (30). The composition and volume of breast milk will vary considerably even in the absence of steroidal contraceptives (29). Both estrogens and progestins cross into milk. An infant consuming 600 ml of breast milk daily from a mother using contraceptives containing 50 μg of ethinyl estradiol will probably receive a daily dose in the range of 10 ng (30). This is in the same range as the amount of natural estradiol received by infants of mothers not using oral contraceptives. Progestins also pass into breast milk, although naturally occurring progestins have not been identified. One study estimated 0.03 μg, 0.15 μg and 0.3 μg of d-norgestrel per 600 ml of milk from mothers receiving 30 μg, 150 μg and 250 μg of the drug, respectively (31). A milk:plasma ratio of 0.15 for norgestrel was calculated by the authors (31). A ratio of 0.16 has been calculated for lynestrol (31, 32).

Reports of adverse effects are lacking except for one child with mild breast tenderness and hypertrophy who was exposed to large doses of estrogen (30). If breast feeding is desired, the lowest effective dose of oral contraceptives should be chosen. Infant weight gain should be monitored and the possible need for nutritional supplements should be considered.

References

1. Ambani LM, Joshi NJ, Vaidya RA, Devi PK. Are hormonal contraceptives teratogenic? Fertil Steril 1977;28:791–7.
2. Wilson JG, Brent RL. Are female sex hormones teratogenic? Am J Obstet Gynecol 1981;141:567–80.
3. Corcoran R, Entwistle GC. VACTERL congenital malformations and the male fetus. Lancet 1975;2:981–2.
4. Nora JJ, Nora AH. Can the pill cause birth defects. N Engl J Med 1974;294:731–2.
5. Kasan PN, Andrews J. Oral contraceptives and congenital abnormalities. Br J Obstet Gynaecol 1980;87:545–51.
6. Kullander S, Kallen B. A prospective study of drugs and pregnancy. Acta Obstet Gynecol Scand 1976;55:221–4.
7. Oakley GP, Flynt JW. Hormonal pregnancy test and congenital malformations. Lancet 1973; 2:256–7.
8. Savolainen E, Saksela E, Saxen L. Teratogenic hazards of oral contraceptives analyzed in a national malformation register. Am J Obstet Gynecol 1981;140:521–4.
9. Frost O. Tracheo-oesophageal fistula associated with hormonal contraception during pregnancy. Br Med J 1976;3:978.
10. Redline RW, Abramowsky CR. Transposition of the great vessels in an infant exposed to massive doses of oral contraceptives. Am J Obstet Gynecol 1981;141:468–9.
11. Farb HF, Thomason J, Carandang FS, Sampson MB, Spellacy WH. Anencephaly twins and HLA-B27. J Reprod Med 1980;25:166–9.
12. Department of Medical and Public Affairs. *Population Reports.* The George Washington University Medical Center, Washington. 1975;2:A 29–51.
13. Bongiovanni AM, DiGeorge AM, Grumbach MM. Masculinization of the female infant associated with estrogenic therapy alone during gestation: four cases. J Clin Endocrinol Metab 1959;19:1004–11.
14. Hagler S, Schultz A, Hankin H, Kunstadter RH. Fetal effects of steroid therapy during pregnancy. Am J Dis Child 1963;106:586–90.
15. Bongiovanni AM, McFadden AJ. Steroids during pregnancy and possible fetal consequences. Fertil Steril 1960;11:181–4.
16. McConnell JB, Glasgow JF, McNair R. Effect on neonatal jaundice of oestrogens and progestogens taken before and after conception. Br Med J 1973;3:605–7.
17. Bracken MB, Srisuphan W. Oral contraception as a risk factor for preeclampsia. Am J Obstet Gynecol 1982;142:191–6.
18. Bacon JF, Shenfield GM. Pregnancy attributable to interaction between tetracycline and oral contraceptives. Br Med J 1980;1:283.
19. Stockley I. Interactions with oral contraceptives. Pharm J 1976;216:140.
20. Reiners D, Nockefinck L, Breurer H. Rifampin and the "pill" do not go well together. JAMA 1974;227:608.
21. Dosseter EJ. Drug interactions with oral contraceptives. Br Med J 1975;1:1967.

22. Pullskinnen MO, Williams K. Reduced maternal plasma and urinary estriol during ampicillin treatment. Am J Obstet Gynecol 1971;109:895–6.
23. Friedman GI, Huneke AL, Kim MH, Powell J. The effect of ampicillin on oral contraceptive effectiveness. Obstet Gynecol 1980;55:33–7.
24. Back DJ, Breckenridge AM. Drug interactions with oral contraceptives. IPFF Med Bull 1978; 12:1–2.
25. Orme ML, Back DJ. Therapy with oral contraceptive steroids and antibiotics J Antimicrob Chemother 1979;5:124–6.
26. Miller GH, Hughes LR. Lactation and genital involution effects of a new low-dose oral contraceptive on breast-feeding mothers and their infants. Obstet Gynecol 1970;35:44–50.
27. Kora SJ. Effect of oral contraceptives on lactation. Fertil Steril 1969;20:419–23.
28. Guiloff E, Ibarra-Polo A, Zanartu J, Tuscanini C, Mischler TW, Gomez-Rodgers C. Effect of contraception on lactation. Am J Obstet Gynecol 1974;118:42–5.
29. Lonnerdal B, Forsum E. Hambraeus L. Effect of oral contraceptives on consumption and volume of breast milk. Am J Clin Nutr 1980;33:816–24.
30. Committee on Drugs. American Academy of Pediatrics. Breast-feeding and contraception. Pediatrics 1981;68:138–40.
31. Nilsson S, Nygren KC, Johansson EDB. D-norgestrel concentrations in maternal plasma, milk, and child plasma during administration of oral contraceptives to nursing women. Am J Obstet Gynecol 1977;129:178–83.
32. van der Molen HJ, Hart PG, Wijmenga HG. Studies with 4-^{14}C-lynestrol in normal and lactating women. Acta Endocrinol 1969;61:255–74.

Name: ORPHENADRINE

Class: **Parasympatholytic**   Risk Factor: **C**

Fetal Risk Summary

Orphenadrine is an anticholinergic agent used in the treatment of parkinsonism. No reports of its use in pregnancy have been located (see also Atropine).

Breast Feeding Summary

No data available (see also Atropine).

Name: OUABAIN

Class: **Cardiac Glycoside**   Risk Factor: **B**

Fetal Risk Summary
See Digitalis.

Breast Feeding Summary
See Digitalis.

Name: **OXACILLIN**

Class: **Antibiotic**   Risk Factor: **B**

Fetal Risk Summary

Oxacillin is a penicillin antibiotic (see also Penicillin G). The drug crosses the placenta in low concentrations. Cord serum and amniotic fluid levels were less than 0.3 µg/ml in 15 of 18 patients given 500 mg orally 0.5 to 4 hours prior to cesarian section (1). No effects were seen in the infants.

No reports linking the use of oxacillin with congenital defects have been located. The Collaborative Perinatal Project monitored 50,282 mother-child pairs, 3,546 of which had 1st trimester exposure to penicillin derivatives (2). For use anytime during pregnancy, 7,171 exposures were recorded (3). In neither case was evidence found to suggest a relationship to large categories of major or minor malformations or to individual defects.

Breast Feeding Summary

Oxacillin is excreted in breast milk in low concentrations. Although no adverse effects have been reported, three potential problems exist for the nursing infant: modification of bowel flora, direct effects on the infant (e.g., allergic response) and interference with the interpretation of culture results if a fever work-up is required.

References

1. Prigot A, Froix C, Rubin E. Absorption, diffusion, and excretion of new penicillin, oxacillin, Antimicrob Agents Chemother 1962:402–10.
2. Heinonen OP, Slone D, Shapiro S. *Birth Defects and Drugs in Pregnancy.* Littleton: Publishing Sciences Group, 1977:297–313.
3. *Ibid*, 435.

Name: **OXAZEPAM**

Class: **Sedative**   Risk Factor: **C**

Fetal Risk Summary

Oxazepam is an active metabolite of diazepam (see also Diazepam). It is a member of the benzodiazepine group. The drug, both free and conjugated forms, crosses the placenta achieving average cord:maternal serum ratios during the 2nd trimester of 0.6 and at term of 1.1 (1). Large variations between patients for placental transfer have been observed (1–3). Passage of oxazepam is slower than diazepam but the clinical significance of this is unknown (4). No reports linking the use of oxazepam with congenital defects have been located. Other drugs in this group have been suspected of causing fetal malformations (see also Diazepam or Chlordiazepoxide). Two reports have suggested that the use of oxazepam in preeclampsia would be safer for the newborn infant than diazepam (5, 6).

Breast Feeding Summary

Specific data relating to oxazepam usage in lactating women has not been located. Oxazepam has been detected in the urine of an infant exposed to high doses of diazepam during lactation (7). The infant was lethargic and demonstrated an EEG pattern compatible with sedative medication (see Diazepam).

References

1. Kangas L, Erkkola R, Kanto J, Eronen M. Transfer of free and conjugated oxazepam across the human placenta. Eur J Clin Pharmacol 1980;17:301–4.
2. Kanto J, Erkkola R, Sellman R. Perinatal metabolism of diazepam. Br Med J 1974;1:641–2.
3. Mandelli M, Morselli PL, Nordio S, et al. Placental transfer of diazepam and its disposition in the newborn. Clin Pharmacol Ther 1975;17:564–72.
4. Kanto JH. Use of benzodiazepines during pregnancy, labour and lactation, with particular reference to pharmacokinetic considerations. Drugs 1982;23:354–80.
5. Gillberg C. "Floppy infant syndrome" and maternal diazepam. Lancet 1977;2:612–3.
6. Drury KAD, Spalding E, Donaldson D, Rutherford D. Floppy-infant syndrome: is oxazepam the answer? Lancet 1977;2:1126–7.
7. Patrick MJ, Tilstone WJ, Reavey P. Diazepam and breast-feeding. Br Med J 1972; 1:542–3.

Name: OXTRIPHYLLINE

Class: **Spasmolytic/Vasodilator**   Risk Factor: **C**

Fetal Risk Summary

Oxtriphylline is a methylxanthine which is metabolized to theophylline. Theophylline has been found in cord blood but not in the serum of an infant whose mother had taken oxtriphylline during pregnancy (1). No adverse effects in the infant were observed (see also Theophylline).

Breast Feeding Summary

No data available (see also Theophylline).

Reference

1. Labovitz E, Spector S. Placental theophylline transfer in pregnant asthmatics. JAMA 1982;247:786–8.

Name: **OXYCODONE**

Class: **Narcotic Analgesic**   Risk Factor: **B***

Fetal Risk Summary

No reports linking the use of oxycodone with congenital defects have been located. The drug is rarely used in pregnancy.

[*Risk Factor D if used for prolonged periods or in high doses at term.]

Breast Feeding Summary

No data available.

Name: **OXYMORPHONE**

Class: **Narcotic Analgesic**   Risk Factor: **B***

Fetal Risk Summary

No reports linking the use of oxymorphone with congenital defects have been located. Use of this drug during labor produces neonatal respiratory depression to the same degree as other narcotic analgesics (1–4).

[*Risk Factor D if used for prolonged periods or in high doses at term.]

Breast Feeding Summary

No data available.

References

1. Simeckova M, Shaw W, Pool E, Nichols EE. Numorphan in labor—a preliminary report. Obstet Gynecol 1960;16:119–23.
2. Sentnor MH, Solomons E, Kohl SG. An evaluation of oxymorphone in labor. Am J Obstet Gynecol 1962;84:956–61.
3. Eames GM, Pool KRS. Clinical trial of oxymorphone in labor. Br Med J 1964; 2:353–5.
4. Ransom S. Oxymorphone as an obstetric analgesic—a clinical trial. Anesthesia 1966;21:464–71.

Name: **OXYPHENBUTAZONE**

Class: **Nonsteroidal Anti-inflammatory**   Risk Factor: **D**

Fetal Risk Summary

See Phenylbutazone.

Breast Feeding Summary

See Phenylbutazone.

Name: **OXYPHENCYCLIMINE**

Class: **Parasympatholytic (Anticholinergic)** Risk Factor: **C**

Fetal Risk Summary

Oxyphencyclimine is an anticholinergic agent. In a large prospective study, 2,323 patients were exposed to this class of drugs during the 1st trimester, 1 of whom took oxyphencyclimine (1). A possible association was found between the total group and minor malformations.

Breast Feeding Summary

No data available (see also Atropine).

Reference

1. Heinonen OP, Slone D, Shapiro S. *Birth Defects and Drugs in Pregnancy*. Littleton: Publishing Sciences Group, 1977:346–53.

Name: **OXYPHENONIUM**

Class: **Parasympatholytic (Anticholinergic)** Risk Factor: **C**

Fetal Risk Summary

Oxyphenonium is an anticholinergic quaternary ammonium bromide. No reports of its use in pregnancy have been located (see also Atropine).

Breast Feeding Summary

No data available (see also Atropine).

Name: **OXYTETRACYCLINE**

Class: **Antibiotic** Risk Factor: **D**

Fetal Risk Summary

See Tetracycline.

Breast Feeding Summary

See Tetracycline.

Name: **PARAMETHADIONE**

Class: **Anticonvulsant**   Risk Factor: **X**

Fetal Risk Summary

Paramethadione is an oxazolidinedione anticonvulsant used in the treatment of petit mal epilepsy. There have been three families (10 pregnancies) in which an increase in spontaneous abortion or abnormalities have been reported (1, 2). Paramethadione is considered equivalent to trimethadione in regard to its fetal effects. In fact, one of the families described by German was included in the fetal trimethadione syndrome (see Trimethadione) (3). This patient had one normal infant after anticonvulsant medications were withdrawn. Malformations reported in two additional families by Rutman are consistent with fetal paramethadione/trimethadione syndrome (2). The malformations included: tetralogy of Fallot, mental retardation, failure to thrive and increased incidence of spontaneous abortions (2). Because paramethadione has demonstrated both clinical and experimental fetal risk greater than other anticonvulsants, its use should be abandoned in favor of other anticonvulsants for the treatment of petit mal epilepsy (see also Ethosuximide, Phensuximide, Methsuximide) (4–6).

Breast Feeding Summary

No data available.

References

1. German J, Ehlers KH, Kowal A, DeGeorge PU, Engle MA, Passarge E. Possible teratogenicity of trimethadione and paramethadione. Lancet 1970;2:261–2.
2. Rutman JT. Anticonvulsants and fetal damage. N Engl J Med 1973;189:696–7.
3. German J, Kowal A, Ehlers KH. Trimethadione and human teratogenesis. Teratology 1970;3:349–62.
4. National Institute of Health. Anticonvulsants found to have teratogenic potential. JAMA 1981;245:36.
5. Fabro S, Brown NA. Teratogenic potential of anticonvulsants. N Engl J Med 1979;300:1280–1.
6. Hill RM. Managing the epileptic patient during pregnancy. Drug Therapy 1976:204–5.

Name: **PAREGORIC**

Class: **Antidiarrheal**   Risk Factor: **B***

Fetal Risk Summary

Paregoric is a mixture of opium powder, anise oil, benzoic acid, camphor, glycerin and ethanol. Its action is mainly due to morphine (see also Morphine). The Collaborative Perinatal Project monitored 50,282 mother-child pairs, 90 of which had 1st trimester exposure to paregoric (1). For use anytime during pregnancy, 562 exposures were recorded (2). No evidence was found to suggest a relationship to large categories of major or minor malformations or to individual defects.

[* Risk Factor D if used for prolonged periods or in high doses at term.]

Breast Feeding Summary

See Morphine.

References

1. Heinonen OP, Slone D, Shapiro S. *Birth Defects and Drugs in Pregnancy*. Littleton: Publishing Sciences Group, 1977:287–95.
2. *Ibid*, 434.

Name: **PARGYLINE**

Class: **Antihypertensive**   Risk Factor: **C**

Fetal Risk Summary

No data available.

Breast Feeding Summary

No data available.

Name: **PENICILLAMINE**

Class: **Heavy Metal Antagonist**   Risk Factor: **D**

Fetal Risk Summary

The use of penicillamine during pregnancy has been reported in 88 pregnancies (1–10). The authors have personal knowledge of one additional infant exposed to penicillamine throughout gestation (11). In each case, the mother had been treated for rheumatoid arthritis, cystinuria or Wilsons's disease. From these 89 pregnancies, anomalies were observed in 3 infants, apparently all related to penicillamine (see table below). A small ventricular septal defect (VSD) was observed in a fourth newborn but this was probably not associated with penicillamine. Although the evidence is incomplete, maintaining the daily dose at 500 mg or less may reduce the incidence of penicillamine-induced toxicity in the newborn (5, 10).

Author (ref)	No. Pts.	Indication	Gestational Age	Dose	Other Drugs	Fetal Effects	Comments
Mjolnerod (2)	1	Cystinuria	Through-out	2 g/day	Not stated	Cutis laxa Hypotonia Hyperflexion of hips and shoulders Pyloric stenosis Vein fragility Varicosities Impaired wound healing Death	
Solomon (6)	1	Rheumatoid arthritis	Through-out	0.9 g/day	Not stated	Cutis laxa Growth retardation Hernia Simian crease Perforated bowel Death	Bowel perforation was terminal event.
Lyle (8)	27	Rheumatoid arthritis (19) Cystinuria (8)	Through-out	Not stated	Not stated	1 VSD	Probably not drug related.
Linares (9)	1	Wilson's disease	Through-out	2 g/day	Not stated	Cutis laxa	Normal elasticity developed at 4 months of age.

Breast Feeding Summary

No data available.

References

1. Crawhall JC, Scowen EF, Thompson CJ, Watts RWE. Dissolution of cystine stones during d-penicillamine treatment of a pregnant patient with cystinuria. Br Med J 1967;2:216–8.
2. Mjolnerod OK, Rasmussen K, Dommerud SA, Gjeruldsen ST. Congenital connective-tissue defect probably due to d-penicillamine treatment in pregnancy. Lancet 1971;1:673–5.
3. Laver M, Fairley KF. D-penicillamine treatment in pregnancy. Lancet 1971;1:1019–20.
4. Scheinberg IH, Sternlieb I. Pregnancy in penicillamine-treated patients with Wilson's disease. N Engl J Med 1975; 293:1300–3.
5. Marecek Z, Graf M. Pregnancy in penicillamine-treated patients with Wilson's disease. N Engl J Med 1976; 295:841–2.
6. Solomon L, Abrams G, Dinner M, Berman L. Neonatal abnormalities associated with d-penicillamine treatment during pregnancy. N Engl J Med 1977;296:54–5.
7. Walshe JM. Pregnancy in Wilson's disease. Q J Med 1977;46:73–83.
8. Lyle WH. Penicillamine in pregnancy. Lancet 1978;1:606–7.
9. Linares A, Zarranz JJ, Rodriguez-Alarcon J, Diaz-Perez JL. Reversible cutis laxa due to maternal d-penicillamine treatment. Lancet 1979;2:43.
10. Endres W. D-penicillamine in pregnancy—to ban or not to ban? Klin Wochenschr 1981;59:535–7.
11. Briggs GG. Unpublished data, 1982.

Name: **PENICILLIN G**

Class: **Antibiotic**   Risk Factor: **B**

Fetal Risk Summary

Penicillin G is used routinely for maternal infections during pregnancy. Several investigators have documented its rapid passage into the fetal circulation and amniotic fluid (1–5). Therapeutic levels are reached in both sites except for the amniotic fluid during the 1st trimester (5). At term, maternal serum and amniotic fluid concentrations are equal 60 to 90 minutes after intravenous (IV) administration (2). Continuous IV infusions (10,000 units/hour) produced equal concentrations of penicillin G at 20 hours in maternal serum, cord serum and amniotic fluid (2).

The early use of penicillin G was linked to increased uterine activity and abortion (6–10). It is not known if this was due to impurities in the drug or to penicillin itself. No reports of this effect have appeared since a reference in 1950 (10). An anaphylactic reaction in a pregnant patient reportedly led to the death of her fetus *in utero* (11).

Only one reference has linked the use of penicillin G with congenital abnormalities (12). An examination of hospital records indicated that in 3 of 4 cases the administration of penicillin G had been followed by the birth of a malformed baby. A retrospective review of additional patients exposed to antibiotics in the 1st trimester indicated an increase in congenital defects. Unfortunately, the authors did not analyze their data for each antibiotic, so no causal relationship to penicillin G could be shown (12, 13). In another case, a patient was treated in early pregnancy with high doses of penicillin G procaine IV (?), cortisone and sodium salicylate (14). A cyclopic male was delivered at term but died 5 minutes later. The defect was attributed to salicylates, cortisone or maternal viremia. (Penicillin G procaine should not be given IV. The Editors are assuming the drug was either given intramuscularly (IM) or the procaine form was not used. We have not been able to contact the authors to clarify these assumptions.)

In a controlled study, 110 patients received 1 to 3 antibiotics during the 1st trimester for a total of 589 weeks (15). Penicillin G was given for a total of 107 weeks. The incidence of birth defects was no different than in a non-treated control group.

The Collaborative Perinatal Project monitored 50,282 mother-child pairs, 3,546 of which had 1st trimester exposure to penicillin derivatives (16). For use anytime during pregnancy, 7,171 exposures were recorded (17). In neither case was evidence found to suggest a relationship to large categories of major or minor malformations or to individual defects. Based on this data, it is unlikely that penicillin G is teratogenic.

Breast Feeding Summary

Penicillin G is excreted into breast milk in low concentrations. Milk:plasma ratios following IM doses of 100,000 units in 11 patients varied between 0.02 to 0.13 (18). The maximum concentration measured in milk was 0.6 units/ml after this dose. Although no adverse effects were reported, three potential problems exist for the nursing infant: modification of bowel flora, direct effects on the infant (e.g., allergic response) and interference with the interpretation of culture results if a fever work-up is required.

References

1. Herrel W, Nichols D, Heilman D. Penicillin. Its usefulness, limitations, diffusion and detection, with analysis of 150 cases in which it was employed. JAMA 1944;125:1003–11.
2. Woltz J, Zintel H. The transmission of penicillin to amniotic fluid and fetal blood in the human. Am J Obstet Gynecol 1945;50:338–40.
3. Hutter A, Parks J. The transmission of penicillin through the placenta. A preliminary report. Am J Obstet Gynecol 1945;49:663–5.
4. Woltz J, Wiley M. The transmission of penicillin to the previable fetus. JAMA 1946;131:969–70.
5. Wasz-Hockert O, Nummi S, Vuopala S, Jarvinen P. Transplacental passage of azidocillin, ampicillin and penicillin G during early and late pregnancy. Acta Paediatr Scand (Suppl) 1970;206:109–10.
6. Lentz J, Ingraham N Jr, Beerman H. Stokes J. Penicillin in the prevention and treatment of congenital syphilis. JAMA 1944;126:408–13.
7. Leavitt H. Clinical action of penicillin on the uterus. J Vener Dis Inf 1945;26:150–3.
8. McLachlan A, Brown D. The effects of penicillin administration on menstrual and other sexual functions. Br J Vener Dis 1947;23:1–10.
9. Mazingarbe A. Le pencilline possede-t-elle une action abortive? Gynecol Obstet 1946;45:487.
10. Perin L, Sissmann R, Detre F, Chertier A. La pencilline a-t-elle une action abortive? Bull Soc Fr Dermatol 1950;57:534–8.
11. Kosim H. Intrauterine fetal death as a result of anaphylactic reaction to penicillin in a pregnant woman. Dapim Refuiim 1959;18:136–7.
12. Carter M, Wilson F. Antibiotics and congenital malformations. Lancet 1963;1:1267–8.
13. Carter M, Wilson F. Antibiotics in early pregnancy and congenital malformations. Dev Med Child Neurol 1965;7:353–9.
14. Khudr G, Olding L. Cyclopia. Am J Dis Child 1973;125:120–2.
15. Ravid R, Toaff R. On the possible teratogenicity of antibiotic drugs administered during pregnancy—a prospective study. In Klingberg M, Abramovici A, Chemki J, eds. *Drugs and Fetal Development*. New York: Plenum Press, 1972:505–10.
16. Heinonen OP, Slone D, Shapiro S. *Birth Defects and Drugs in Pregnancy*. Littleton: Publishing Sciences Group, 1977:297–313.
17. *Ibid*, 435.
18. Greene H, Burkhart B, Hobby G. Excretion of penicillin in human milk following parturition. Am J Obstet Gynecol 1946;51:732–3.

Name: **PENICILLIN G, BENZATHINE**

Class: **Antibiotic**   Risk Factor: **B**

Fetal Risk Summary

Benzathine penicillin G is a combination of an ammonium base and penicillin G suspended in water. See Penicillin G.

Breast Feeding Summary

See Penicillin G.

Name: **PENICILLIN G, PROCAINE**

Class: **Antibiotic**   Risk Factor: **B**

Fetal Risk Summary

Procaine penicillin G is an equal molar combination of procaine and penicillin G suspended in water (1). The combination is broken down *in vivo* into the two components. See also Penicillin G.

A case report described the use of high doses of penicillin G procaine intravenously (IV) (?), cortisone and sodium salicylate in early pregnancy followed by the delivery at term of a cyclopic male infant (2). The lethal defect was attributed to salicylates, cortisone or maternal viremia. (Note: Penicillin G procaine should not be given IV. The Editors are assuming the drug was either given intramuscularly or the procaine form was not used. We have been unable to contact the authors of the paper to clarify these assumptions.)

Breast Feeding Summary

See Penicillin G.

References

1. Mandel G, Sande M. Antimicrobial agents (continued). Penicillins and cephalosporins. In Gilman AG, Goodman LS, Gilman A, eds. *The Pharmacological Basis of Therapeutics*, ed 6. New York: MacMillan, 1980:1137.
2. Khudr G, Olding L. Cyclopia. Am J Dis Child 1973;125:120–2.

Name: **PENICILLIN V**

Class: **Antibiotic**   Risk Factor: **B**

Fetal Risk Summary

No reports linking the use of penicillin V with congenital defects have been located. The Collaborative Perinatal Project monitored 50,282 mother-child pairs , 3,546 of which had 1st trimester exposure to penicillin derivatives (1). For use anytime during pregnancy, 7,171 exposures were recorded (2). In neither case was evidence found to suggest a relationship to large categories of major or minor malformations or to individual defects.

Penicillin V depresses both plasma-bound and urinary excreted estriol (3). Urinary estriol was formerly used to assess the condition of the fetoplacental unit, depressed levels being associated with fetal distress. This assessment is now made by measuring plasma-unconjugated estriol, which is not usually affected by penicillin V.

Breast Feeding Summary

No data available (see Penicillin G).

References

1. Heinonen OP, Slone D, Shapiro S. *Birth Defects and Drugs in Pregnancy.* Littleton: Publishing Sciences Group, 1977:297–313.
2. *Ibid*, 435.
3. Pulkkinen M, Willman K. Maternal oestrogen levels during penicillin treatment. Br Med J 1971;4:48.

Name: **PENTAERYTHRITOL TETRANITRATE**

Class: **Vasodilator**   Risk Factor: **C**

Fetal Risk Summary

Pentaerythritol tetranitrate is a long acting agent used for the prevention of angina pectoris. Due to the nature of its indication, experience in pregnancy is limited. The Collaborative Perinatal Project recorded 3 1st trimester exposures to pentaerythritol tetranitrate plus 12 other patients exposed to other vasodilators (1). From this small sample, 4 malformed children were produced, a statistically significant incidence ($p < 0.02$). It was not reported if pentaerythritol tetranitrate was taken by any of the mothers of the affected infants. Although this data serves as a warning, the number of patients is so small that conclusions as to the relative safety of this drug cannot be made.

Breast Feeding Summary

No data available.

Reference

1. Heinonen OP, Slone D, Shapiro S. *Birth Defects and Drugs in Pregnancy.* Littleton: Publishing Sciences Group, 1977:371–3.

Name: **PENTAZOCINE**

Class: **Analgesic**   Risk Factor: **B***

Fetal Risk Summary

No reports linking the use of pentazocine with congenital defects have been located. The drug rapidly crosses the placenta resulting in cord blood levels of 40 to 70% of maternal serum (1). Withdrawal has been reported in infants exposed *in utero* to chronic maternal ingestion of pentazocine (2–4). Symptoms, presenting within 24 hours of birth, consist of trembling and jitteriness, marked hyperirritability, hyperactivity with hypertonia, high-pitched cry, diaphoresis, diarrhea, vomiting and opisthotonic posturing.

During labor, increased overall uterine activity has been observed after pentazocine, but without changes in fetal heart rate (5). In equianalgesic doses, most studies report no significant differences between meperidine and pentazocine in pain relief, length of labor or Apgar scores (6–11). However, meperidine in one study was observed to produce significantly lower Apgar scores than pentazocine, especially in repeated doses (12). Severe neonatal respiratory depression may also occur with pentazocine (6, 12).

[* Risk Factor D if used for prolonged periods or in high doses at term.]

Breast Feeding Summary

No data available.

References

1. Beckett AH, Taylor JF. Blood concentrations of pethidine and pentazocine in mother and infant at time of birth. J Pharm Pharmacol 1967;19 (Suppl):50s–2s.
2. Goetz RL, Bain RV. Neonatal withdrawal symptoms associated with maternal use of pentazocine. J Pediatr 1974;84:887–8.
3. Scanlon JW. Pentazocine and neonatal withdrawal symptoms. J Pediatr 1974;85:735–6.
4. Kopelman AE. Fetal addiction to pentazocine. Pediatrics 1975;55:888–9.
5. Filler WW, Filler NW. Effect of a potent non-narcotic analgesic agent (pentazocine) on uterine contractility and fetal heart rate. Obstet Gynecol 1966;28:224–32.
6. Freedman H, Tafeen CH, Harris H. Parenteral Win 20,228 as analgesic in labor. NY State J Med 1967;67:2849–51.
7. Duncan SLB, Ginsburg J, Morris NF. Comparison of pentazocine and pethidine in normal labor. Am J Obstet Gynecol 1969;105:197–202.
8. Moore J, Hunter RJ. A comparison of the effects of pentazocine and pethidine administered during labor. J Obstet Gynaecol Br Commonw 1970;77:830–6.
9. Mowat J, Garrey MM. Comparison of pentazocine and pethidine in labour. Br Med J 1970;2:757–9.
10. Levy DL. Obstetric analgesia. Pentazocine and meperidine in normal primiparous labor. Obstet Gynecol 1971;38:907–11.
11. Moore J, Ball HG. A sequential study of intravenous analgesic treatment during labour. Br J Anaesth 1974;46:365–72.
12. Refstad SO, Lindbaek E. Ventilatory depression of the newborn of women receiving pethidine or pentazocine. Br J Aneasth 1980;52:265–70.

Name: **PENTOBARBITAL**

Class: **Sedative/Hypnotic**   Risk Factor: **C**

Fetal Risk Summary

No reports linking the use of pentobarbital with congenital defects have been located. The Collaborative Perinatal Project monitored 50,282 mother-child pairs, 250 of which had 1st trimester exposure to pentobarbital (1). No evidence was found to suggest a relationship to large categories of major or minor malformations or to individual defects. Hemorrhagic disease of the newborn and barbiturate withdrawal are theoretical possibilities (see also Phenobarbital).

Breast Feeding Summary

Pentobarbital is excreted into breast milk (2). Breast milk levels of 0.17 μg/ml have been detected 19 hours after a dose of 100 mg daily for 32 days. The effects of this amount on the nursing infant are not known.

References

1. Heinonen OP, Slone D, Shapiro S. *Birth Defects and Drugs in Pregnancy.* Littleton: Publishing Sciences Group, 1977:336–7.
2. Wilson JT, Brown RD, Cherek DR, et al. Drug excretion in human breast milk: principles, pharmacokinetics and projected consequences. Clin Pharmacokinet 1980;5:1–66.

Name: **PERPHENAZINE**

Class: **Tranquilizer**   Risk Factor: **C**

Fetal Risk Summary

Perphenazine is a piperazine phenothiazine in the same group as prochlorperazine (see Prochlorperazine). The phenothiazines readily cross the placenta (1). The Collaborative Perinatal Project monitored 50,282 mother-child pairs, 63 of which had 1st trimester exposure to perphenazine (2). For use anytime during pregnancy, 166 exposures were recorded. No evidence was found in either group to suggest a relationship to malformations, nor an effect on perinatal mortality rates, birth weight or intelligence quotient scores at 4 years of age. Although occasional reports have attempted to link various phenothiazine compounds with congenital defects, the bulk of the evidence indicates that these drugs are safe for the mother and fetus (see also Chlorpromazine).

Breast Feeding Summary

No data available.

References

1. Moya F, Thorndike V. Passage of drugs across the placenta. Am J Obstet Gynecol 1962;84:1778–98.
2. Slone D, Siskind V, Heinonen OP, Monson RR, Kaufman DW, Shapiro S. Antenatal exposure to the phenothiazines in relation to congenital malformations, perinatal mortality rate, birth weight, and intelligence quotient score. Am J Obstet Gynecol 1977;128:486–8.

Name: **PHENACETIN**

Class: **Analgesic/Antipyretic**   Risk Factor: **B**

Fetal Risk Summary

Phenacetin, in combination products, is routinely used during pregnancy. It is metabolized mainly to acetaminophen (see also Acetaminophen). The Collaborative Perinatal Project monitored 50,282 mother-child pairs, 5,546 of which had 1st trimester exposure to phenacetin (1). Although no evidence was found to suggest a relationship to large categories of major or minor malformations, possible associations were found with several individual defects (2). The statistical significance of these associations is unknown and independent confirmation is required. Further, phenacetin is rarely used alone, being consumed usually in combination with aspirin and caffeine.

Craniosynostosis (6 cases)
Adrenal syndromes (5 cases)
Anal atresia (7 cases)
Accessory spleen (5 cases)

For use anytime during pregnancy, 13,031 exposures were recorded (3). With the same qualifications, possible associations with individual defects were found (4).

Musculoskeletal (6 cases)
Hydronephrosis (8 cases)
Adrenal anomalies (8 cases)

Breast Feeding Summary

Phenacetin is excreted into breast milk, appearing along with its major metabolite, acetaminophen (5). Data from 2 patients who consumed 2 tablets of Empirin Compound with Codeine No. 3 (aspirin-phenacetin-caffeine-codeine) are presented below.

Author (ref)	No. Pts.	Dose	Concentrations (μg/ml)		M:P Ratio	Effect on Infant
			Serum	Milk		
Findlay (5)	2	324 mg	0.85 (peak) (0.5 hr)	0.071 (avg)	0.4–0.9 (avg: 0.7)	—
			3.45 (1.0 hr)	Not stated	0.16–0.39	—

References

1. Heinonen OP, Slone D, Shapiro S. *Birth Defects and Drugs in Pregnancy*. Littleton: Publishing Sciences Group, 1977:286–95.
2. *Ibid*, 471.
3. *Ibid*, 434.
4. *Ibid*, 483.
5. Findlay JWA, DeAngelis RL, Kearney MF, Welch RM, Findlay JM. Analgesic drugs in breast milk and plasma. Clin Pharmacol Ther 1981;29:625–33.

Name: **PHENAZOCINE**

Class: **Narcotic Analgesic**   Risk Factor: **B***

Fetal Risk Summary

No reports linking the use of phenazocine with congenital defects have been located. The drug is not commercially available in the United States. Withdrawal could theoretically occur in infants exposed *in utero* to prolonged maternal ingestion of phenazocine. Phenazocine may cause neonatal respiratory depression when used in labor (1, 2).

[* Risk Factor D if used for prolonged periods or if high doses given at term.]

Breast Feeding Summary

No data available.

References

1. Sadove M, Balagot R, Branion J Jr, Kobak A. Report on the use of a new agent, phenazocine, in obstetric analgesia. Obstet Gynecol 1960;16:448–53.
2. Corbit J, First S. Clinical comparison of phenazocine and meperidine in obstetric analgesia. Obstet Gynecol 1961;18:488–91.

Name: **PHENAZOPYRIDINE**

Class: **Urinary Tract Analgesic**   Risk Factor: **C**

Fetal Risk Summary

No reports linking the use of phenazopyridine with congenital defects have been located. The Collaborative Perinatal Project monitored 50,282 mother-child pairs, 219 of which had 1st trimester exposure to phenazopyridine (1). For use anytime during pregnancy, 1,109 exposures were recorded (2). In neither case was evidence found to suggest a relationship to large categories of major or minor malformations or to individual defects.

Breast Feeding Summary

No data available.

References

1. Heinonen OP, Slone D, Shapiro S. *Birth Defects and Drugs in Pregnancy.* Littleton: Publishing Sciences Group, 1977:299–308.
2. *Ibid*, 435.

Name: **PHENCYCLIDINE**

Class: **Hallucinogenic**   Risk Factor: **X**

Fetal Risk Summary

Phencyclidine (PCP) is an illicit drug used for its hallucinogenic effects. Placental transfer has been demonstrated in animals and humans (1–3). Qualitative analysis of the urine from two newborns discovered phencyclidine levels of 75 ng/ml or greater up to three days after birth (3). Relatively few studies have appeared on the use of phencyclidine during pregnancy, but fetal exposure may be more common than this lack of reporting indicates. During a 9-month period of 1980 to 1981 in a Cleveland hospital, 30 of 519 (5.8%) consecutively screened pregnant patients admitted PCP use (4). In this study, 70% of the PCP users also consumed other abuse drugs, with or without excessive alcohol intake.

Most pregnancies in which the mother used phencyclidine apparently end with healthy newborns (5). However, case reports involving four newborns indicate the use of this agent may result in long term damage (3, 5, 6). Irritability, jitteriness, hypertonicity, and poor feeding were common features in the affected infants. In three of the neonates, most of the symptoms had persisted at the time of the report. In the case wiht the malformed child, no causal relationship with PCP could be established. Marijuana is a known teratogen in some animal species (7). Human teratogenicity secondary to marijuana has been suspected but the evidence is weak, since the case reports also involved exposure to lysergic acid diethylamide (LSD) (8, 9).

Author (ref)	No. Pts.	Indication	Gestational Age	Dose	Other Drugs	Fetal Effects	Comments
Strauss (3)	2	Illicit	Through-out	Not stated	Marijuana	Depressed at birth Jittery Hypertonic Poor feeding	Hyperreflexia and hypertonicity still evident at 2 weeks in one; fine tremors still evident at 8 days in one
Lerner (5)	1	Illicit	Through-out	Not stated	Not stated	Irritable Poor feeding and sucking reflex	
Golden (6)	1	Illicit	Through-out	6 marijuana cigarettes dusted with PCP daily	Marijuana	Triangular shaped face with pointed chin; narrow mandibular angle; antimongoloid slanted eyes Poor head control Nystagmus Inability to track visually Respiratory distress Hypertonic Jitteriness	Roving eye movements, coarse tremors and spasticity still evident at 2 months

Breast Feeding Summary

Data on the excretion of phencyclidine into human milk is lacking. In mice, milk concentrations of PCP were ten times that of plasma (2). Women consuming PCP should not breast feed.

References

1. Cooper JE, Cummings AJ, Jones H. The placental transfer of phencyclidine in the pig: plasma levels in the sow and its piglets. J Physiol (Lond) 1977;267:17p–8p.
2. Nicholas JM, Lipshitz J, Schreiber EC. Phencyclidine: its transfer across the placenta as well as into breast milk. Am J Obstet Gynecol 1982;143:143–6.
3. Strauss AA, Modanlou HD, Bosu SK. Neonatal manifestations of maternal phencyclidine (PCP) abuse. Pediatrics 1981;68:550–2.

4. Golden NL, Sokol RJ, Martier S, Miller SI. A practical method for identifying angel dust abuse during pregnancy. Am J Obstet Gynecol 1982;142:359–61.
5. Lerner SE, Burns RS. Phencyclidine use among youth: history, epidemiology, and acute and chronic intoxication. In Petersen R, Stillman R, eds. *Phencyclidine (PCP) Abuse: An Appraisal.* National Institute on Drug Abuse Research Monograph No. 21, US Government Printing Office, 1978.
6. Golden NL, Sokol RJ, Rubin IL. Angel dust: possible effects on the fetus. Pediatrics 1980;65:18–20.
7. Persaud TVN, Ellington AC. Teratogenic activity of cannabis resin. Lancet 1968;2:406–7.
8. Hecht F, Beals RK, Lees MH, Jolly H, Roberts P. Lysergic-acid-diethylamide and cannabis as possible teratogens in man. Lancet 1968;2:1087.
9. Carakushansky G, Neu RL, Gardner LI. Lysergide and cannabis as possible teratogens in man. Lancet 1969;1:150–1.

Name: **PHENDIMETRAZINE**

Class: **Central Stimulant/Anorectant**   Risk Factor: **C**

Fetal Risk Summary

No data available (see Phentermine or Dextroamphetamine).

Breast Feeding Summary

No data available.

Name: **PHENELZINE**

Class: **Antidepressant**   Risk Factor: **C**

Fetal Risk Summary

Phenelzine is a monoamine oxidase inhibitor. The Collaborative Perinatal Project monitored 21 mother-child pairs exposed to these drugs during the 1st trimester, 3 of which were exposed to phenelzine (1). An increased risk of malformations was found. Details of the 3 cases with phenelzine exposure are not available.

Breast Feeding Summary

No data available.

Reference

1. Heinonen OP, Slone D, Shapiro S. *Birth Defects and Drugs in Pregnancy.* Littleton: Publishing Sciences Group, 1977:336–7.

Name: **PHENINDIONE**

Class: **Anticoagulant**   Risk Factor: **D**

Fetal Risk Summary

See Coumarin Derivatives.

Breast Feeding Summary

See Coumarin Derivatives.

Name: **PHENOBARBITAL**

Class: **Sedative/Anticonvulsant**   Risk Factor: **B**

Fetal Risk Summary

Phenobarbital has been used widely in clinical practice as a sedative and anticonvulsant since 1912 (1). The potential teratogenic effects of phenobarbital were recognized in 1964 along with phenytoin (2). It is clear that the epileptic patient on anticonvulsant medication is at a higher risk for having a child with congenital defects than the general population (3–9). The difficulty in evaluating the increased malformation rate in epileptic patients lies in attempting to disentangle the effects of multiple drug therapy, the effects of the disease itself on fetal outcome, and any pattern of malformations associated with the drug. The phenotype described for the fetal hydantoin syndrome is discussed under phenytoin. Many of these case reports mention phenobarbital or other anticonvulsants in combinatioin with phenytoin. Differences in study design and conflicting results for an association between 1st trimester usage of phenobarbital with congenital defects do not support a phenotype for a fetal phenobarbital syndrome.

The Collaborative Perinatal Project monitored 50,282 mother-child pairs, 1,415 of which had 1st trimester exposure to phenobarbital (10). For use anytime during pregnancy, 8,037 exposures were recorded (11). In neither case was evidence found to suggest a relationship to large categories of major or minor malformations. A possible association with Down's syndrome was shown statistically. Other reports linking the use of phenobarbital alone with congenital malformations have been found for 21 infants exposed during the 1st trimester (6, 8, 12–19). Malformations frequently associated with phenobarbital are difficult to confirm as other drugs are usually taken in combination, especially by the epileptic patient. Malformations described in 102 infants exposed to phenobarbital and other anticonvulsants during the 1st trimester are summarized in the table below (6, 8, 13–24). Barbiturates as a group have also been associated with congenital anomalies, but phenobarbital was not specifically identified in these reports (25, 26).

Malformation*	Phenobarbital Only (N=21)	Phenobarbital with Other Anticonvulsants (N=102)
Growth		
Prenatal deficiency		2
Postnatal deficiency	2	2
Performance		
Mental retardation	2	2
Defective speech		1
Craniofacial		
Cleft lip/palate	2	23
Hydrocephalus	1	2
Microcephalus	1	2
Large fontanel		2
Anencephaly		3
High arched palate		1
Trigoncephaly		1
Micrognathia		1
Minor facial anomalies		7
Chest		
Congenital heart defects		15
Pulmonary hypoplasia	1	
Skeletal/Limbs		
Abnormal digits/nails	3	2
Talipes	1	2
Metatarsus varus deformity	1	3
Skeletal defects (unspecified)	1	
Simian/palmar creases	1	3
Spina bifida		1
Polydactyly		4
Chrondrodystrophy		1
Dislocated hip		2
Clicking hip		3
Hyperlaxity of joints		1
Other:		
Malformations–not specified	3	5
Menngomyelocele	1	3
Hypospadius	1	2
Ureter duplication	1	
Ileal atresia	1	
Hernias	1	6
Tracheoesophageal fistula	1	
Meconium ileus		1
Ambiguous genitalia		3
Undescended testes		1
Calcifying epithelium		1
Benign tumors		4

* Not mutually exclusive.

In addition to congenital defects there are other potential complications with the use of phenobarbital during pregnancy. These complications include a barbiturate withdrawal syndrome and neonatal hemorrhage. Desmond described 15 addicted infants born to mothers receiving barbiturates during pregnancy (16). The dosage of phenobarbital varied from 64 mg to 300 mg daily (unknown amounts for 4 drug addicts). The symptomatology shown by these 15 infants included:

	No. Infants	%
Overactivity	15	100
Disturbed sleep	15	100
Excessive crying	15	100
Tremors	12	80
Hyperphagia	11	73
Hyperflexion	11	73
Vasomotor instability	9	60
Sneezing, hiccups,		
mouthing movements	5	33
Shrill cry	3	20
Excessive sweating	2	13
Vomiting	4	27
Diarrhea	3	20
Poor weight gain	3	20
Positional deformities		
(metatarsus varus)	4	27

The average onset of the withdrawal symptoms in these infants occurred at 6 days (range 3–14 days).

There are at least 31 case reports of neonatal hemorrhage associated with barbiturates alone or in combination with other anticonvulsants (18, 27–33). Suppression of vitamin K_1-dependent clotting factors II and VII is the proposed mechanism (29, 33–35). Barbiturates such as primidone, metharbital and amobarbital have also been implicated in these reports (27, 30, 31). Administration of parenteral vitamin K_1 to the mother prior to delivery and to the infant immediately after birth is recommended.

Breast Feeding Summary

Phenobarbital is excreted into breast milk (36–39). A milk:plasma ratio of approximately 0.5 has been reported (37). The amount of phenobarbital ingested by the nursing infant has been estimated to reach 2 to 4 mg/day (38). Sedative effects due to phenobarbital have been reported in three nursing infants possibly caused by accumulation of the drug (36). Patients that decide to breast feed should be instructed to watch for sedation in the infant.

Author (ref)	No. Pts.	Dose	Concentrations (μg/ml) Serum	Milk	M:P Ratio	Effect on Infant
Tyson (36)	20	120 mg/days for 4 days	Qualitative: 65% positive for pheno-barbital in breast milk (total of 77 samples)	—	—	None
	21	90 mg/day for 4 days	Qualitative: 80% positive for pheno-barbital in breast milk (total of 87 samples)	—	—	2 infants with sedation. Onset in one infant was on the 8th day of breast feeding. A third infant with sedative effects was cited from a 1926 paper.
Kaneko (37)	8	Not stated	19.3 (Range 2.5–42)	10.4 (Range 0.5–33)	0.46	—
Horning (38)	2	120 mg/day for 3.5 days	—	2.7	—	Not stated
Reith (39)	Not stated	75 mg/day	—	5–9	—	Not stated

References

1. Hauptmann A. Luminal bei epilepsie. Munchen Med Wochenschr 1912;59:1907–8.
2. Janz D, Fuchs V. Are anti-epileptic drugs harmful when given during pregnancy? German Medical Monographs 1964;9:20–3.
3. Hill RB. Teratogenesis and anti-epileptic drugs. N Engl J Med 1973;289:1089–90.
4. Bodendorfer TW. Fetal effects of anticonvulsant drugs and seizure disorders. Drug Intell Clin Pharm 1978;12:14–21.
5. Committee on Drugs, American Academy of Pediatrics. Anticonvulsants and pregnancy. Pediatrics 1977;63:331–3.
6. Nakane Y, Okoma T, Takahashe R et al. Multi-institutional study of the teratogenicity and fetal toxicity of anti-epileptic drugs: a report of a collaborative study group in Japan. Epilepsia 980;21:633–80.
7. Andermann E, Dansky L, Andermann F, Loughnan PM, Gibbons J. Minor congenital malformations and dermatoglyphic alterations in the offspring of epileptic women; a clinical investigation of the teratogenic effects of anticonvulsant medication. In *Epilepsy, Pregnancy and the Child*. Proceedings of a Workshop in Berlin, September 1980. New York: Raven Press, 1981 (in press).
8. Dansky L, Andermann E, Andermann F. Major congenital malformations in the offspring of epileptic patients. Ibid. In *Epilepsy, Pregnancy and the Child*. Proceedings of a Workshop in Berlin, September 1980. New York: Raven Press, 1981 (in press).
9. Janz D. The teratogenic risks of antiepileptic drugs. Epilepsia 1975;16:159–69.
10. Heinonen OP, Slone D, Shapiro S. *Birth Defects and Drugs in Pregnancy*. Littleton: Publishing Sciences Group, 1977:336–9.
11. *Ibid*, 438.
12. Seip M. Growth retardation, dysmorphic facies and minor malformations following massive exposure to phenobarbitone in utero. Acta Paediatr Scand 1976;65:617–21.
13. Fedrick J. Epilepsy and pregnancy. A report from the Oxford Record Linkage Study. Br Med J 1973;2:442–8.
14. Lowe CR. Congenital malformations among infants born to epileptic women. Lancet 1973;1:9–10.
15. Shapiro S, Hartz SC, Siskind V, et al. Anticonvulsants and parental epilepsy in the development of birth defects. Lancet 1976;1:272–5.
16. Desmond MM, Schwanecke RP, Wilson GS, Yasunaga S, Burgdorff I. Maternal barbiturate utilization and neonatal withdrawal symptomatology. J. Pediatr 1972;80:190–7.
17. Kuenssberg EV, Knox JDE. Teratogenic effect of anticonvulsants. Lancet 1973;1:198.
18. Spiedel BD, Meadow SR. Maternal epilepsy and abnormalities of the fetus and the newborn. Lancet 1972;2:839–43.

19. Annegers JF, Elveback LR, Hauser WA, Kurland LT. Do anticonvulsants have a teratogenic effect? Arch Neurol 1974;31:364–73.
20. Biale Y, Lewenthal H, Aderet NB. Congenital malformations due to anticonvulsive drugs. Obstet Gynecol 1975;45:439–42.
21. McMullin GP. Teratogenic effects of anticonvulsants. Br Med J 1971;4:430.
22. Starreveld-Zimmerman AAE, van Derkok WJ, Meinardi H, Elshove J. Are anticonvulsants teratogenic? Lancet 1973;2:48–9.
23. Loughnan PM, Gold H, Vance JC. Phenytoin teratogenicity in man. Lancet 1973;1:70–2.
24. Zellweger H. Anticonvulsants during pregnancy: a danger to the developing fetus? Clin Pediatr (Phila) 1979;13:338–46.
25. Annegers JF, Hauser WA, Elveback LR, Anderson WE, Kurland LT. Congenital malformations and seizure disorders in the offspring on parents with epilepsy. Int J Epidemiol 1978;7:241–7.
26. Nelson MM, Forfar JO. Associations between drugs administered during pregnancy and congenital abnormalities of the fetus. Br Med J 1971;1:523–7.
27. Bleyer WA, Skinner AL. Fatal neonatal hemorrhage after maternal anticonvulsant therapy. JAMA 1976;235:826–7.
28. Lawrence A. Anti-epileptic drugs and the foetus. Br Med J 1963;2:1267.
29. Kohler HG. Haemorrhage in the newborn of epileptic mothers. Lancet 1966;1:267.
30. Mountain KR, Hirsh J, Gallus AS. Neonatal coagulation defect due to anticonvulsant drug treatment in pregnancy. Lancet 1970;1:265–8.
31. Evans AR, Forrester RM, Discombe C. Neonatal haemorrhage during anticonvulsant therapy. Lancet 1970;1:517–8.
32. Margolin FG, Kantor NM. Hemorrhagic disease of the newborn. An unusual case related to maternal ingestion of an anti-epileptic drug. Clin Pediatr (Phila) 1972;11:59–60.
33. Srinivasan G, Seeler RA, Tiruvury A, Pildes RS. Maternal anticonvulsant therapy and hemorrhagic disease of the newborn. Obstet Gynecol 1982;59:250–2.
34. Solomon GE, Hilgartner MW, Kutt H. Coagulation defects caused by diphenylhydantoin. Neurology 1972;22:1165–71.
35. Keith PA, Gallop PM. Phenytoin, hemorrhage, skeletal defects and vitamin K in the newborn. Med Hypotheses 1979;5:1347–51.
36. Tyson RM, Shrader EA, Perlman HN. Drugs transmitted through breast-milk. II. Barbiturates. J Pediatr 1938;13:86–90.
37. Kaneko S, Sata T, Suzuki K. The levels of anticonvulsants in breast milk. Br J Clin Pharmacol 1979;7:624–7.
38. Horning MG, Stillwell WG, Nowlin J. Lertratanangkoon K, Stillwell RN, Hill RM. Identification and quantification of drugs and drug metabolites in human breast milk using GC-MS-COM methods. Mod Probl Paediatr 1975;15:73–9.
39. Reith H, Schafer H. Antiepileptic drugs during pregnancy and the lactation period. Pharma-cokinetic data. Dtsch Med Wochenschr 1979;104:818–23.

Name: PHENPROCOUMON

Class: **Anticoagulant**   Risk Factor: **D**

Fetal Risk Summary

See Coumarin Derivatives.

Breast Feeding Summary

See Coumarin Derivatives.

Name: **PHENSUXIMIDE**

Class: **Anticonvulsant**   Risk Factor: **C**

Fetal Risk Summary

The use of phensuximide, the first succinimide anticonvulsant used in the treatment of petit mal epilepsy, has been reported in 3 pregnancies (1, 2). Due to multiple drug therapy and difference in study methodology, conclusions linking the use of phensuximide with congenital defects are difficult. Fetal abnormalities identified with the three pregnancies include: ambiguous genitalia, inquinal hernia and pyloric stenosis. Phensuximide has a much lower teratogenic potential than the oxozolidinedione class of anticonvulsants (see Trimethadione) (3, 4). Due to a high incidence of toxic effects, the new succinimides should be considered in favor of phensuximide for the treatment of petit mal epilepsy (see Ethosuximide, Methsuximide) (5).

Breast Feeding Summary

No data available.

References

1. Fedrick J. Epilepsy and pregnancy: a report from the Oxford Record Linkage Study. Br Med J 1973;2:442–8.
2. McMullin GP. Teratogenic effects of anticonvulsants. Br Med J 1971;2:430.
3. Fabro S, Brown NA. Teratogenic potential of anticonvulsants. New Engl J Med 1979;300:1280–1.
4. The National Institutes of Health. Anticonvulsants found to have teratogenic potential. JAMA 1981;241:36.
5. Schmidt RP, Wilder BJ. Epilepsy. In *Contemporary Neurology Series*: No. 2. Philadelphia: FA Davis, 1968;159.

Name: **PHENTERMINE**

Class: **Central Stimulant**   Risk Factor: **C**

Fetal Risk Summary

No data available (see Diethylpropion or Dextroamphetamine).

Breast Feeding Summary

No data available.

Name: **PHENYLBUTAZONE**

Class: Nonsteroidal Anti-Inflammatory Analgesic   Risk Factor: **D**

Fetal Risk Summary

Two reports have been located that describe congenital defects in the offspring of mothers consuming phenylbutazone during pregnancy (1, 2). A cause-and-effect relationship was not established in either case. Possible embryotoxicity has been demonstrated in animals, and the drug crosses the placenta to the human fetus (3–5). Theoretically, phenylbutazone, a prostaglandin synthetase inhibitor, could cause constriction of the ductus arteriosus *in utero* (6). Persistent pulmonary hypertension of the newborn should also be considered (6). Drugs in this class have been shown to inhibit labor and prolong pregnancy (7). The manufacturer recommends that the drug not be used in pregnancy (3).

Author (ref)	No. Pts.	Indication	Gestational Age	Dose	Other Drugs	Fetal Effects	Comment
hmann-Duplessis (1)	1	Analgesic	22–32 days	2 tablets 3 times a day	Pyrethane Numerous other drugs 2nd and 3rd trimesters	Absence of usual 5 digits on hands/feet and their replacement with 2 single and opposed fingers and toes	Ethyl carbamate (urethane) is a component of pyrethane and is an animal teratogen
lander (2)	18	Analgesic	1st trimester	Not stated	Not stated	1 miscarriage 6 minor malformations 1 major malformation	Specific data on defects not given

Breast Feeding Summary

Phenylbutazone is excreted into breast milk in low concentrations, although some investigators failed to detect the drug 3 hours after maternal administration (6–8). The drug has been measured in infant serum after breast feeding, but no adverse effects in the nursing infant have been reported.

Author (ref)	No. Pts.	Dose	Concentrations (μg/ml)		M:P Ratio	Effect on Infant
			Serum	Milk		
Wilson (8)	—	—	—	—	0.1–0.3	—
Leuxner (4)	—	750 mg (IM)*	20–50	6.3	0.13	Serum levels in infants 3–20 μg/ml
Stobel (5)	20	600 mg (IM)	—	0 (0.5–3.0 hr)	—	—

* IM, intramuscular.

References

1. Tuchmann-Duplessis H. Medication in the course of pregnancy and teratogenic malformation. Concours Med 1967;89:2119–20.
2. Kullander S, Kallen B. A prospective study of drugs in pregnancy. Acta Obstet Gynecol Scand 1976;55:289–95.
3. Product information. Physicians' Desk Reference, ed. 34. Oradell, N.J.: Medical Economics Company, 1980.
4. Leuxner E, Pulver R. Verabreichung von irgapryin bei schwangeren und wochnerinnen. Munchen Med Wochenschr 1956;98:84–6.
5. Strobel S, Leuxner E. Uber die zullassigkeit der verabreichung von butazolidin bei schwangeren und wochnerinnen. Med Klin 1957;39:1708–10.
6. Levin DL. Effects of inhibition of prostaglandin synthesis on fetal development, oxygenation, and the fetal circulation. Semin Perinatol 1980;4:35–44.
7. Fuchs F. Prevention of prematurity. Am J Obstet Gynecol 1976;126:809–20.
8. Wilson JT. Milk/plasma ratios and contraindicated drugs. In Wilson JT, ed. Drugs in Breast Milk. Australia: ADIS Press, 1981:78–9.

Name: **PHENYLEPHRINE**

Class: **Sympathomimetic (Adrenergic)**   Risk Factor: **D**

Fetal Risk Summary

Phenylephrine is a sympathomimetic used in emergency situations to treat hypotension and to alleviate allergic symptoms of the eye and ear. Uterine vessels are normally maximally dilated and they have only α-adrenergic receptors (1). Use of the predominantly α-adrenergic stimulant, phenylephrine, could cause constriction of these vessels and reduce uterine blood flow, thereby producing fetal hypoxia (bradycardia). Phenylephrine may also interact with oxytocics or ergot derivatives to produce severe persistent maternal hypertension (1). Rupture of a cerebral vessel is possible. If a pressor agent is indicated, other drugs such as ephedrine should be considered. Sympathomimetic amines are teratogenic in some animal species, but human teratogenicity has not been suspected (2, 3). Recent data may require a reappraisal of this opinion. The Collaborative Perinatal Project monitored 50,282 mother-child pairs, 1,249 of which had 1st trimester exposure to phenylephrine (4). For use anytime during pregnancy, 4,194 exposures were recorded (5). An association was found between 1st trimester use of phenylephrine and malformations; minor defects greater than major (4). For individual malformations, several possible associations were found (4, 6, 7):

First trimester:
eye and ear (8 cases)
syndactyly (6 cases)
pre-auricular skin tag (4 cases)
clubfoot (3 cases)
Anytime use:
congenital dislocation of hip (15 cases)

other musculoskeletal (4 cases)

umbilical hernia (6) cases)

The statistical significance of these associations is not known. Independent confirmation is required. For the sympathomimetic class of drugs as a whole, an association was found between 1st trimester use and minor malformations (not life-threatening or major cosmetic defects), inguinal hernia and clubfoot (4).

Sympathomimetics are often administered in combination with other drugs to alleviate the symptoms of upper respiratory infections. Thus, the fetal effects of sympathomimetics, other drugs and viruses cannot be totally separated. However, indiscriminate use of this class of drugs, especially in the 1st trimester, is not without risk.

Breast Feeding Summary

No data available.

References

1. Smith NT, Corbascio AN. The use and misuse of pressor agents. Anesthesiology 1970;33:58–101.
2. Nashimura H, Tanimura T. *Clinical Aspects of the Teratogenicity of Drugs.* Amsterdam: Excerpta Medica, 1976:231.
3. Shepard TH. *Catalog of Teratogenic Agents,* ed. 3. Baltimore: Johns Hopkins University Press, 1980:134–5.
4. Heinonen OP, Slone D, Shapiro S. *Birth Defects and Drugs in Pregnancy.* Littleton: Publishing Sciences Group, 1977:345–56.
5. *Ibid,* 439.
6. *Ibid,* 476.
7. *Ibid,* 491.

Name: **PHENYLPROPANOLAMINE**

Class: **Sympathomimetic (Adrenergic)**   Risk Factor: **C**

Fetal Risk Summary

Phenylpropanolamine is a sympathomimetic used for anorexia and to alleviate the symptoms of allergic disorders or upper respiratory infections. Uterine vessels are normally maximally dilated and they have only α-adrenergic receptors (1). Use of the α- and β-adrenergic stimulant, phenylpropanolamine, could cause constriction of these vessels and reduce uterine blood flow, thereby producing fetal hypoxia (bradycardia). This drug is a common component of proprietary mixtures containing antihistamines and other drugs. Thus, it is difficult to separate the effects of phenylpropanolamine on the fetus from other drugs, disease states and viruses.

Sympathomimetic amines are teratogenic in some animal species, but human teratogenicity has not been suspected (2, 3). Recent data may require a reappraisal of this opinion. The collaborative Perinatal Project monitored 50,282 mother-child pairs, 726 of which had 1st trimester exposure to phenylpropanolamine (4). For use anytime during pregnancy, 2,489 exposures were recorded (5). An association was found between 1st trimester use of phenylpropanolamine and malformations; minor defects greater than major (4). For individual malformations, several possible associations were found (4, 6, 7).

First trimester:
 hypospadias (4 cases)
 eye and ear* (7 cases)
 polydactyly (6 cases)
 cataract (3 cases)
 pectus excavatum (7 cases)
Anytime use: congenital dislocation of hip (12 cases)

---

* Statistically significant

Except for the eye and ear defects, the statistical significance of these associations is not known. Independent confirmation is required. For the sympathomimetic class of drugs as a whole, an association was found between 1st trimester use and minor malformations (not life-threatening or major cosmetic defects), inguinal hernia and clubfoot (4). Indiscriminate use of this class of drugs, especially in the 1st trimester, is not without risk.

A case of infantile malignant osteopetrosis was described in a 4-month-old boy exposed *in utero* on several occasions to Contac (chlorpheniramine, phenylpropanolamine and belladonna alkaloids) but this is a known genetic defect (8). The boy also had a continual "stuffy" nose.

Breast Feeding Summary

No data available.

References:

1. Smith NT, Corbascio AN. The use and misuse of pressor agents. Anesthesiology 1970;33:58–101.
2. Nishimura H, Tanimura T. *Clinical Aspects of the Teratogenicity of Drugs.* Amsterdam: Excerpta Medica, 1976:231.
3. Shepard TH. *Catalog of Teratogenic Drugs*, 3rd ed. Baltimore: Johns Hopkins University Press, 1980:134–5.
4. Heinonen OP, Slone D, Shapiro S. *Birth Defects and Drugs in Pregnancy.* Littleton: Publishing Sciences Group, 1977:345–56.
5. *Ibid*, 439.
6. *Ibid*, 477.
7. *Ibid*, 491.
8. Golbus MS, Koerper MA, Hall BD. Failure to diagnose osteopetrosis in utero. Lancet 1976;2:1246.

Name: **PHENYLTOLOXAMINE**

Class: **Antihistamine**   Risk Factor: **C**

Fetal Risk Summary

No data available.

Breast Feeding Summary

No data available.

Name: **PHENYTOIN**

Class: **Anticonvulsant**   Risk Factor: **D**

Fetal Risk Summary

Phenytoin is a hydantoin anticonvulsant introduced in 1938. The teratogenic effects of phenytoin were recognized in 1964 (1). Since this report there has been a deluge of case reports, editorials, retrospective reviews and a few prospective studies on the teratogenic effects of anticonvulsants. It is clear that the epileptic patient on anticonvulsant medication is at a higher risk for having a child with congenital defects than the general population (2–8). The major difficulty in evaluating the increased malformation rate in epileptic patients lies in attempting to disentangle the effects of a particular anticonvulsant (multiple drug regimens are normal), the effects of the disease itself and any pattern of malformations associated with the drug.

The phenotype of fetal hydantoin syndrome (FHS) first appeared with reports of limb and skeletal abnormalities in 1973 (9, 10). The basic syndrome consists of variable degrees of hypoplasia and ossification of the distal phalanges and craniofacial abnormalities (11). Clinical features added recently include neuroblastoma, hemorrhagic diathesis, hirsutism, abnormal genitalia, acne vulgaris and optic nerve hypoplasia. The table summarizes the 118 cases of FHS (9–35).

Features of Fetal Hydantoin Syndrome (118 cases)

	No. Cases*	%
Growth:		
postnatal deficiency	25	21
prenatal deficiency	10	8
Chest:		
congenital heart disease	32	27
widespread hypoplastic nipples	6	5
rib/sternal abnormality	3	3
Performance:		
mental retardation	13	11
Craniofacial:		
broad nasal bridge	34	29
wide fontanel	23	19
low set hairline	17	14
broad alveolar ridge	16	14
metopic ridging	17	14
short neck	14	12
ocular hypertelorism	14	12
microcephaly	11	9
cleft lip/palate	9	8
abnormal or low set ears	9	8
epicanthal folds	8	7
ptosis of eyelids	6	5
coloboma	3	3
coarse scalp hair	1	1
Limbs:		
small or absent nails	38	32
hypoplasia of distal phalanges	36	31
altered palmar crease	29	25
digital thumb	17	14
dislocated hip	3	3
Other:		
pilonidal sinus	21	18
hernia (umbilical or inguinal)	19	16
optic nerve hypoplasia	7	6
abnormal genitalia	6	5
neuroblastoma	5	4
acne vulgaris	1	1
hemorrhagic disease	1	1
hirsutism	1	1
melanotic neuroectodermal tumor	1	1
retinoschisis	1	1

* Not mutually exclusive.

The phenotype of FHS may expand as more information becomes available. Hirschberger reported another set of malformations consisting of exstrophy of the bladder, omphalocele, imperforate anus, rectourethral fistula, solitary kidney and cutis marmorata (36). A single case of a baby with the VACTERL (Vertebral, Anal, Cardiac, Tracheal, Esophageal, Renal, Limb) combination of defects has also been reported (37).

Two features of the FHS which require additional comment are the development of neuroblastoma and hemorrhagic disease. Experimental information on the effects of phenytoin on chromosomes, depression of cellular and

humoral immunity and carcinogenesis had been primarily of academic interest. However, the five cases of neuroblastoma and a recently reported case
of a melanotic neuroectodermal tumor suggest that phenytoin or combination
of anticonvulsants with phenytoin are potential human transplacental carcin-
ogens (11, 20, 28, 32, 34, 37). The association of hemorrhagic disease and
FHS is not unexpected. There are 21 case reports of neonatal hemorrhage
associated with phenytoin alone or in combination with barbiturates (38–48)
(see also Phenobarbital). Suppression of vitamin K_1-dependent clotting factors, particularly factors II and VII, and thrombocytopenia are the proposed
mechanisms (38, 46–48). Administration of parenteral vitamin K_1 to the
mother prior to delivery and to the infant immediately after birth and monitoring
of platelet counts in the neonate are recommended.

The pharmacokinetics and placental transport of phenytoin have been
well studied (50–53). Plasma concentrations of phenytoin may fall during
pregnancy (50, 53–56). Animal studies and recent reports suggest a dose-
related teratogenic effect of phenytoin (56, 57). While these results are based
on a small series of patients with higher than average socioeconomic and
medical problems, it is reasonable to avoid excessively high plasma concentrations of phenytoin (58). Close monitoring of plasma phenytoin concentrations is recommended to maintain adequate seizure control and prevent
potential fetal hypoxia.

Breast Feeding Summary

Phenytoin is excreted into breast milk. The available studies involve only a
few patients. Milk:plasma ratios range from 0.18 to 0.54 (50, 53, 59–62).
Methemoglobin anemia, drowsiness and decreased sucking activity have
been reported in one infant (63). Patients that decide to breast feed should
be instructed to watch for potential sedative effects in the infant.

Author (ref)	No. Pts.	Dose	Concentrations (μg/ml)		M:P Ratio	Effect on Infant
			Serum	Milk		
Rane (61)	1	250 mg/day	0.58	0.26	0.45	—
Mirkin (50)	2	300 mg/day	2.7	1.4	0.54	—
			6.2	1.5	0.27	—
Kanelco (59)	Not stated	Not stated	4.5	0.8	0.18	—
Horning (60)	1	100 mg single dose	—	4.2 peak at 3 hr 1.7 average	—	—
Svensmark (62)	1	Not stated	28	6	0.21	—
Finch (63)	1	—	—	—	—	Methenoglo-bin ane-mia Drowsiness Decreased sucking

References

1. Janz D, Fuchs V. Are anti-epileptic drugs harmful when given during pregnancy? German Medical Monographs 1964;9:20–3.
2. Hill RB. Teratogenesis and antiepileptic drugs. N Engl J Med 1973;289:1089–90.
3. Janz D. The teratogenic risk of antiepileptic drugs. Epilepsia 1975;16:159–69.
4. Bodendorfer TW. Fetal effects of anticonvulsant drugs and seizure disorders. Drug Intell Clin Pharm 1978;12:14–21.
5. Committee on Drugs, American Academy of Pediatrics. Anticonvulsants and pregnancy. Pediatrics 1977;63:331–3.
6. Nakane Y, Okuma T, Takahashi R, et al. Multi-institutional study of the teratogenicity and fetal toxicity of antiepileptic drugs: a report of a collaborative study group in Japan. Epilepsia 1980;21:663–80.
7. Andermann E, Dansky L, Andermann F, Loughnan PM, Gibbons J. Minor congenital malformations and dermatoglyphic alterations in the offspring of epileptic women: a clinical investigation of the teratogenic effects of anticonvulsant medication. In *Epilepsy, Pregnancy and the Child*. Proceedings of a Workshop in Berlin, September 1980. New York: Raven Press, 1981 (in press).
8. Dansky L, Andermann E, Andermann F. Major congenital malformations in the offspring of epileptic patients. In *Epilepsy, Pregnancy and the Child*. Proceedings of a Workshop in Berlin, September 1980. New York: Raven Press, 1981 (in press).
9. Loughnan PM, Gold H, Vance JC. Phenytoin teratogenicity in man. Lancet 1973;1:70–2.
10. Hill RM, Horning MG, Horning EC. Antiepileptic drugs and fetal well-being. In Boreus L, ed. *Fetal Pharmacology*. New York: Raven Press, 1973:375–9.
11. Allen RW Jr, Ogden B, Bentley FL, Jung AL. Fetal hydantoin syndrome, neuroblastoma, and hemorrhagic disease in a neonate. JAMA 1980;244:1464–5.
12. Pinto W Jr, Gardner LI, Rosenbaum P. Abnormal genitalia as a presenting sign in two male infants with hydantoin embryopathy syndrome. Am J Dis Child 1977;131:452–5.
13. Hoyt CS, Billson FA. Maternal anticonvulsants and optic nerve hypoplasia. Br J Ophthalmol 1978;62:3–6.
14. Wilson RS, Smead W, Char F. Diphenylhydantoin teratogenicity: ocular manifestations and related deformities. J Pediatr Ophthalmol Strabismus 1970;15:137–40.
15. Dabee V, Hart AG, Hurley RM. Teratogenic effects of diphenylhydantoin. Can Med Assoc J 1975;112:75–7.
16. Taylor WF, Myers M, Taylor WR. Extrarenal Wilms' tumour in an infant exposed to intrauterine phenytoin. Lancet 1980;2:481–2.
17. Anderson RC. Cardiac defects in children of mothers receiving anticonvulsant therapy during pregnancy. J Pediatr 1976;89:318–9.
18. Hill RM, Verniaud WM, Horning MG, McCulley LB, Morgan NF. Infants exposed in utero to antiepileptic drugs. A prospective study. Am J Dis Child 1974;127:645–53.
19. Kousseff B. Subcutaneous vascular abnormalities in fetal hydantoin syndrome. Regional Genetic Program, South Illinois University, School of Medicine. Springfield, 1981 (unpublished data).
20. Seller RA, Israel JN, Royal JE, Kaye CL, Rao S, Abulaban M. Ganglioneuroblastoma and fetal hydantoin-alcohol syndromes. Pediatrics 1979;63:524–7.
21. Stankler L, Campbell AGM. Neonatal acne vulgaris: a possible feature of the fetal hydantoin syndrome. Br J Dermatol 1980;103:453–5.
22. Ringrose CAD. The hazard of neurotropic drugs in the fertile years. Can Med Assoc J 1972;106:1058.
23. Pettifor JM, Benson R. Congenital malformations associated with the administration of oral anticoagulants during pregnancy. J Pediatr 1975;86:459–61.
24. Hanson JW, Smith DW. The fetal hydantoin syndrome. J Pediatr 1975;87:285–90.
25. Barr M Jr, Poznanski AK, Schmickel RD. Digital hypoplasia and anticonvulsants during gestation: a teratogenic syndrome? J Pediatr 1974;84:254–6.
26. Biale Y, Lewenthal H, Aderet NB. Congenital malformations due to anticonvulsant drugs and congenital abnormalities. Obstet Gynecol 1975;45:439–42.
27. Aase JM. Anticonvulsant drugs and congenital abnormalities. Am J Dis Child 1974;127:758.

28. Pendergrass TW, Hanson JW. Fetal hydantoin syndrome and neuroblastoma. Lancet 1976;2:150.
29. Lewin PK. Phenytoin associated congenital defects with Y-chromosome variant. Lancet 1973 I:559.
30. Zellweger H. Anticonvulsants during pregnancy: a danger to the developing fetus. Clin Pediatr (Phila) 1974;13:338–46.
31. Yang TS, Chi CC, Tsai CJ, Chang MJ. Diphenylhydantoin teratogenicity in man. Obstet Gynecol 1978;52:682–4.
32. Sherman S, Roizen N. Fetal hydantoin syndrome and neuroblastoma. Lancet 1976;2:517.
33. Mallow DW, Herrick MK, Gathman G. Fetal exposure to anticonvulsant drugs. Arch Pathol Lab Med 1980;104:215–8.
34. Ramilo J, Harris VJ. Neuroblastoma in a child with the hydantoin and fetal alcohol syndrome. The radiographic features. Br J Radiol 1979;52:993–5.
35. Jiminez JF, Siebert RW, Char F, Brown RE, Seibert JJ. Melanotic neuroectodermal tumor of infancy and fetal hydantoin syndrome. Am J Pediatr Hematol Oncol 1981;3:9–15.
36. Hirschberger M, Kleinberg F. Maternal phenytoin ingestion and congenital abnormalities: report of a case. Am J Dis Child 1975;129:984.
37. Corcoran R, Rizk MW. VACTERL congenital malformation and phenytoin therapy? Lancet 1976;2:960.
38. Lawrence A. Antiepileptic drugs and the foetus. Br Med J 1963;2:1267.
39. Kohler HG. Haemorrhage in newborn of epileptic mothers. Lancet 1966;1:267.
40. Douglas H. Haemorrhage in the newborn. Lancet 1966;1:816–7.
41. Monnet P, Rosenberg D, Bovier-Lapierre M. Terapeutique anticomitale administree pendant la grosses et maladie hemorragique du nouveau-ne. In Bleyer WA, Skinner AL. Fetal neonatal hemorrhage after maternal anticonvulsant therapy. JAMA 1976;235:626–7.
42. Davis PP. Coagulation defect due to anticonvulsant drug treatment in pregnancy. Lancet 1970;1:413.
43. Evans AR, Forrester RM, Discombe C. Neonatal hemorrhage following maternal anticonvulsant therapy. Lancet 1970;1:517–8.
44. Stevensom MM, Bilbert EF. Anticonvulsants and hemorrhagic diseases of the newborn infant. J Pediatr 1970;77:516.
45. Speidel BD, Meadow SR. Maternal epilepsy and abnormalities of the fetus and newborn. Lancet 1972;2:839–40.
46. Hoyme HE, Page TE, Markarian M, Jones KL. Neonatal hemorrhage secondary to thrombocytopenia: an occasional manifestation of prenatal hydantoin exposure. Division of Dysmorphology, University California, San Diego, School of Medicine. La Jolla, 1981 (unpublished data).
47. Truog WE, Feusner JH, Baker DL. Association of hemorrhagic disease and the syndrome of persistent fetal circulation with the fetal hydantoin syndrome. J Pediatr 1980;96:112–4.
48. Solomon GE, Hilgartner MW, Kutt H. Coagulation defects caused by diphenylhydantoin. Neurology 1972;22:1165–71.
49. van der Klign E, Schobben F, Bree TB. Clinical pharmacokinetics of antiepileptic drugs. Drug Intell Clin Pharm 1980;14:674–85.
50. Mirkin BL. Diphenylhydantoin: placental transport, fetal localization, neonatal metabolism, and possible teratogenic effects. J Pediatr 1971;78:329–37.
51. Baughman FA, Randinitis EJ. Passage of diphenylhydantoin across the placenta. JAMA 1970;213:466.
52. Rane A. Urinary excretion of diphenylhydantoin metabolites in newborn infants. J Pediatr 1974;85:543–5.
53. Reith H, Schafer H. Antiepileptic drugs during pregnancy and the lactation period. Pharmacokinetic data. Dtsch Med Wochenschr 1979;22:818–23.
54. Kochenour NK, Emery MG, Sawchuk RJ. Phenytoin metabolism in pregnancy. Obstet Gynecol 1980;56:577–82.
55. Landon MJ, Kirkley M. Metabolism of diphenylhydantoin (phenytoin) during pregnancy. Br J Obstet Gynaecol 1979;86:125–32.
56. Dansky L, Andermann E, Sherwin AL, Andermann F. Plasma levels of phenytoin during pregnancy and the puerperium. In *Epilepsy, Pregnancy and the Child*. Proceedings of a

Workshop held in Berlin, September 1980. New York: Raven Press, 1981 (in press).

57. Dansky L, Andermann E, Andermann F, Sherwin AL, Kinch RA. Maternal epilepsy and congenital malformation: correlation with maternal plasma anticonvulsant levels during pregnancy. In *Epilepsy, Pregnancy and the Child.* Proceedings of a Workship held in Berlin, September 1980. New York: Raven Press, 1981 (in press).

58. Personal communication. L Dansky, Montreal Neurological Hospital, Montreal, Quebec, June, 1981.

59. Kaneko S, Sato T, Suzuke K. The levels of anticonvulsants in breast milk. Br J Clin Pharmacol 1979;7:624–7.

60. Horning MG, Stillwell WG, Nowling J, Lertratanangkoon K, Stillwell RN, Hill RM. Identification and quantification of drugs and drug metabolites in human breast milk using GC-MS-COM methods. Mod Probl Pediatr 1975;15:73–9.

61. Rane A, Garle M, Borga O. Sjoquist F. Plasma disappearance of transplacentally transferred diphenylhydantoin in the newborn studied by mass fragmentography. Clin Pharmacol Ther 1974;15:39–49.

62. Svensmark O, Schiller PJ. 5-5-Diphenylhydantoin (Dilantin) blood level after oral or intravenous dosage in man. Acta Pharmacol Toxicol 1960;16:331–46.

63. Finch E, Lorber J. Methaemoglobinaemia in the newborn. Probably due to phenytoin excreted in human milk. J Obstet Gynaecol Br Emp 1954;61:833.

Name: **PHTHALYLSULFACETAMIDE**

Class: **Anti-infective**   Risk Factor: **B***

Fetal Risk Summary

See Sulfonamides.

[* Risk Factor D if administered near term.]

Breast Feeding Summary

See Sulfonamides.

Name: **PHTHALYLSULFATHIAZOLE**

Class: **Anti-infective**   Risk Factor: **B***

Fetal Risk Summary

See Sulfonamides.

[* Risk Factor D if administered near term.]

Breast Feeding Summary

See Sulfonamides.

Name: **PHYSOSTIGMINE**

Class: **Parasympathomimetic (Cholinergic)**   Risk Factor: **C**

Fetal Risk Summary

Physostigmine is rarely used in pregnancy. No reports linking its use with congenital defects have appeared. One report described its use in 15 women at term to reverse scopolamine-induced twilight sleep (1). Apgar scores of 14 of the newborns ranged from 7 to 9 at 1 minute and 8 to 10 at 5 minutes. One infant was depressed at birth and required resuscitation, but the mother had also received meperidine and diazepam. No other effects in the infants were mentioned. Physostigmine is an anticholinesterase but it does not contain a quaternary ammonium element. It crosses the blood-brain barrier and should be expected to cross the placenta (2). Cholinesterase inhibitors may affect the condition of the newborn (3). Transient muscular weakness has been observed in about 20% of newborns whose mothers were treated for myasthenia gravis during pregnancy. While the exact cause of the neonatal myasthenia is unknown, anticholinesterases may contribute to the condition (4).

Breast Feeding Summary

No data available.

References

1. Smiller BG, Bartholomew EG, Sivak BJ, Alexander GD, Brown EM. Physostigmine reversal of scopolamine delirium in obstetric patients. Am J Obstet Gynecol 1973;116:326–9.
2. Taylor P. Anticholinesterase agents. In Gilman AG, Goodman LS, Gilman A, eds. *The Pharmacological Basis of Therapeutics*, ed. 6. New York: MacMillan, 1980:100–19.
3. McNall PG, Jafarnia MR. Management of myasthenia gravis in the obstetrical patient. Am J Obstet Gynecol 1965;92:518–25.
4. Blackhall MI, Buckley GA, Roberts DV, Roberts JB, Thomas BH, Wilson A. Drug-induced neonatal myasthenia. J Obstet Gynaecol Br Commonw 1969;76:157–62.

Name: **PILOCARPINE**

Class: **Parasympathomimetic (Cholinergic)**   Risk Factor: **C**

Fetal Risk Summary

Pilocarpine is used in the eye. No reports of its use in pregnancy have been located.

Breast Feeding Summary

No data available.

Name: **PIPERACETAZINE**

Class: **Tranquilizer**   Risk Factor: **C**

Fetal Risk Summary

Piperacetazine is a piperidyl phenothiazine. The phenothiazines readily cross the placenta (1). No specific information on the use of piperacetazine in pregnancy has been located. Although occasional reports have attempted to link various phenothiazine compounds with congential malformations, the bulk of the evidence indicates that these drugs are safe for the mother and fetus (see also Chlorpromazine).

Breast Feeding Summary

No data available.

Reference

1. Moya F, Thorndike V. Passage of drugs across the placenta. Am J Obstet Gynecol 1962;84:1778–98.

Name: **PIPERAZINE**

Class: **Anthelmintic**   Risk Factor: **B**

Fetal Risk Summary

No reports linking the use of piperazine with congenital defects have been located. Animal data has also failed to demonstrate any teratogenic effect. The Collaborative Perinatal Project monitored 50,282 mother-child pairs, 3 of which had 1st trimester exposure to piperazine. No evidence was found to suggest a relationship to malformations (1).

Breast Feeding Summary

No data available.

Reference

1. Heinonen OP, Slone D, Shapiro S. *Birth Defects and Drugs in Pregnancy*. Littleton: Publishing Sciences Group, 1977:299.

Name: **PIPERIDOLATE**

Class: **Parasympatholytic (Anticholinergic)**   Risk Factor: **C**

Fetal Risk Summary

Piperidolate is an anticholinergic agent. In a large prospective study, 2,323 patients were exposed to this class of drugs during the 1st trimester, 16 of whom took piperadolate (1). A possible association was found between the total group and minor malformations.

Breast Feeding Summary

No data available (see also Atropine).

Reference

1. Heinonen OP, Slone D, Shapiro S. *Birth Defects and Drugs in Pregnancy*. Littleton: Publishing Sciences Group, 1977:346–53.

Name: **POLYMYXIN B**

Class: **Antibiotic**   Risk Factor: **B**

Fetal Risk Summary

No reports linking the use of polymyxin B with congenital defects have been located. Although available for injection, polymyxin B is used almost exclusively by topical administration. In one study, 7 exposures were recorded in the 1st trimester (1). No association with congenital defects was observed.

Breast Feeding Summary

No data available.

Reference

1. Heinonen OP, Slone D, Shapiro S. *Birth Defects and Drugs in Pregnancy*. Littleton: Publishing Sciences Group, 1977:297.

Name: **POLYTHIAZIDE**

Class: **Diuretic**   Risk Factor: **D**

Fetal Risk Summary

See Chlorothiazide.

Breast Feeding Summary

See Chlorothiazide.

Name: **POTASSIUM CHLORIDE**

Class: **Electrolyte** Risk Factor: **A**

Fetal Risk Summary

Potassium chloride is a natural constituent of human tissues and fluids. Exogenous potassium chloride may be indicated as replacement therapy for pregnant women with low potassium serum levels, such as those receiving diuretics. Since high or low levels are detrimental to maternal and fetal cardiac function, serum levels should be closely monitored.

Breast Feeding Summary

Human milk is naturally low in potassium (1). If maternal serum levels are maintained in a physiologic range, no harm will result in the nursing infant from the administration of potassium chloride to the mother.

Reference

1. Wilson JT. Production and characteristics of breast milk. In Wilson JT, ed. *Drugs in Breast Milk*. Australia: ADIS Press, 1981:12.

Name: **POTASSIUM CITRATE**

Class: **Electrolyte** Risk Factor: **A**

Fetal Risk Summary

See Potassium Chloride.

Breast Feeding Summary

See Potassium Chloride.

Name: **POTASSIUM GLUCONATE**

Class: **Electrolyte** Risk Factor: **A**

Fetal Risk Summary

See Potassium Chloride.

Breast Feeding Summary

See Potassium Chloride.

Name: **PRAZOSIN**

Class: **Antihypertensive**   Risk Factor: **C**

Fetal Risk Summary

No data available.

Breast Feeding Summary

No data available.

Name: **PREDNISOLONE**

Class: **Corticosteroid**   Risk Factor: **B**

Fetal Risk Summary

Prednisolone is the biologically active form of prednisone (see Prednisone). The placenta can oxidize prednisolone to inactive prednisone or less active cortisone (see Cortisone).

Breast Feeding Summary

See Prednisone.

Name: **PREDNISONE**

Class: **Corticosteroid**   Risk Factor: **B**

Fetal Risk Summary

Prednisone is activated to prednisolone *in vivo*. There are a number of studies in which pregnant patients received prednisone or prednisolone (see also various antineoplastic agents for additional references) (1–14). These corticosteroids apparently have little, if any, effect on the developing fetus. Immunosuppression was observed in a newborn exposed to high doses of prednisone with azathioprine throughout gestation (15). The newborn had lymphopenia, decreased survival of lymphocytes in culture, absence of IgM, and reduced levels of IgG. Recovery occurred at 15 weeks of age. These effects were not observed in a larger group of similarly exposed newborns (16). A 1968 study reported an increase in the incidence of stillbirths following prednisone therapy during pregnancy (7). Increased fetal mortality has not been confirmed by other investigators.

In a 1970 case report, a female infant with multiple deformities was described (17). Her father had been treated several years prior to conception with prednisone, azathioprine and radiation for a kidney transplant. The authors speculated that the child's defects may have been related to the father's immunosuppressive therapy. A relationship to prednisone seems remote since previous studies have shown that the drug has no effect on chromosome number or morphology (18). High, prolonged doses of prednisolone (30 mg/day for at least 4 weeks) may damage spermatogenesis (19). Recovery may require six months after the drug is stopped.

Prednisone has been used to successfully prevent neonatal respiratory distress syndrome when premature delivery occurs between 28 and 36 weeks of gestation (20). Therapy between 16 and 25 weeks of gestation had no effect on lecithin/sphingomyelin ratios (21).

In summary, prednisone and prednisolone apparently pose a very small risk to the developing fetus. The available evidence supports their use to control various maternal diseases.

Author (ref)	No. Pts.	Indication	Gestational Age	Dose	Other Drugs	Fetal Effects	Comment
Kraus (1)	1	Regional enteritis	Through-out	15–60 mg/day	Cortisone	Cataracts	Consistent with reports of subcapsular cataracts in adults receiving corticosteroids

Breast Feeding Summary

Trace amounts of prednisone and prednisolone have been measured in breast milk (22, 23). Following a 10-mg oral dose of prednisone, milk concentrations of prednisone and prednisolone at 2 hours were 0.03 and 0.002 $\mu g/ml$, respectively (22). In a second study utilizing radioactive-labeled prednisolone in 7 patients, a mean of 0.14% of a 5-mg oral dose was recovered per liter of milk over 48 to 61 hours (23). This is equivalent to 0.007 $\mu g/ml$. Although nursing infants were not involved in either study, it is doubtful if these amounts are clinically significant. Reports of infants exposed *via* the breast milk to either corticosteroid have not been located.

References

1. Kraus AM. Congenital cataract and maternal steroid injection. J Pediatr Ophthalmol 1975;12:107–8.
2. Durie BGM, Giles HR. Successful treatment of acute leukemia during pregnancy: combination therapy in the third trimester. Arch Intern Med 1977;137:90–1.
3. Nolan GH, Sweet RL, Laros RK, Roure CA. Renal cadaver transplantation followed by successful pregnancies. Obstet Gynecol 1974;43:732–9.
4. Grossman JH III, Littner MR. Severe sarcoidosis in pregnancy. Obstet Gynecol 1977;50(Suppl):81s–4s.
5. Cutting HO, Collier TM. Acute lymphocytic leukemia during pregnancy: report of a case. Obstet Gynecol 1964;24:941–5.
6. Hanson GC, Ghosh S. Systemic lupus erythematosus and pregnancy. Br Med J 1965;2:1227–8.
7. Warrell DW, Taylor R. Outcome for the foetus of mothers receiving prednisolone during pregnancy. Lancet 1968;1:117–8.

8. Walsh SD, Clark FR. Pregnancy in patients on long-term corticosteroid therapy. Scott Med J 1967;12:302–6.
9. Zulman JI, Talal N, Hoffman GS, Epstein WV. Problems associated with the management of pregnancies in patients with systemic lupus erythematosus. J Rheumatol 1980;7:37–49.
10. Hartikainen-Sorri AL, Kaila J. Systemic lupus erythematosus and habitual abortion: case report. Br J Obstet Gynaecol 1980;87:729–31.
11. Minchinton RM, Dodd NJ, O'Brien H, Amess JAL, Waters AH. Autoimmune thrombocytopenia in pregnancy. Br J Haematol 1980;44:451–9.
12. Tozman ECS, Urowitz MB, Gladman DD. Systemic lupus erythematosus and pregnancy. J Rheumatol 1980;7:624–32.
13. Karpatkin M, Porges RF, Karpatkin S. Platelet counts in infants of women with autoimmune thrombocytopenia: effect of steroid administration to the mother. N Engl J Med 1981;305:936–9.
14. Pratt WR. Allergic diseases in pregnancy and breast feeding. Ann Allergy 1981;47:355–60.
15. Cote CJ, Meuwissen HJ, Pickering RJ. Effects on the neonate of prednisone and azathioprine administered to the mother during pregnancy. J Pediatr 1974;85:324–8.
16. Cederqvist LL, Merkatz IR, Litwin SD. Fetal immunogloblin synthesis following maternal immunosuppression. Am J Obstet Gynecol 1977;129:687–90.
17. Tallent MB, Simmons RL, Najarian JS. Birth defects in child of male recipient of kidney transplant.JAMA 1970;211:1854–5.
18. Jensen MK. Chromosome studies in patients treated with azathioprine and amethopterin. Acta Med Scand 1967;182:445–55.
19. Mancini RE, Larieri JC, Muller F, Andrada JA, Saraceni DJ. Effect of prednisolone upon normal and pathologic human spermatogenesis. Fertil Steril 1966;17:500–13.
20. Szabo I, Csaba I, Novak P, Drozgyik I. Single-dose glucocorticoid for prevention of respiratory-distress syndrome. Lancet 1977;2:243.
21. Szabo I, Csaba I, Bodis J, Novak P, Drozgyik J, Schwartz J. Effect of glucocorticoid on fetal lecithin and sphingomyelin concentrations. Lancet 1980;1:320.
22. Katz FH, Duncan BR. Entry of prednisone into human milk. N Engl J Med 1975;293:1154.
23. McKenzie SA, Selley JA, Agnew JE. Secretion of prednisone into breast milk. Arch Dis Child 1975;50:894–6.

Name: **PRIMAQUINE**

Class: **Plasmodicide**   Risk Factor: **C**

Fetal Risk Summary

No reports linking the use of primaquine with congenital defects have been located. Primaquine may cause hemolytic anemia in patients with glucose-6-phosphate dehydrogenase deficiency. Pregnant patients at risk for this disorder should be tested accordingly (1). If possible, the drug should be withheld until after delivery (2).

Breast Feeding Summary

No data available

References

1. Trenholme GM, Parson PE. Therapy and prophylaxis of malaria. JAMA 1978;240:2293–5.
2. Anonymous. Chemoprophylaxis of malaria. In Center for Disease Control Morbidity and Mortality Weekly Reports 1978;27:81–90.

Name: **PRIMIDONE**

Class: **Anticonvulsant**   Risk Factor: **D**

Fetal Risk Summary

Primidone, a structural analog of phenobarbital, is effective against generalized convulsive seizures and psychomotor attacks. It is clear that the epileptic patient on anticonvulsant medication is at a higher risk for having a child with congenital defects than the general population (1–7). The difficulty in evaluating the increased malformation rate in epileptic patients lies in attempting to disentangle the effects of multiple drug therapy, the effects of the disease itself on the fetal outcome and any pattern of malformations associated with the drug. The literature describes 323 infants who were exposed to primidone during the 1st trimester (4, 8–17). Of the 41 malformed infants described in these reports, only 3 infants were exposed to primidone and no other anticonvulsants during gestation (8, 15, 16). The table summarizes the clinical features described in the cases reviewed.

Feature	Primidone Only N = 3	Primidone with Other Anticonvulsants N = 320	Feature	Primidone Only	Primidone with other Anticonvulsants
Malformations (details not stated)	—	22	ventricular septal defect	2	4
Growth:			tetralogy of Fallot	—	1
postnatal deficiency	1	1	Skeletal/limbs:		
Performance:			abnormal palmar creases	—	3
mental retardation	0	1	hypoplastic nails	2	2
Craniofacial:			polydactyly	—	1
cleft/lip palate	0	10	congenital dislocation	—	3
abnormal or low set ears	2	2	of hip		
depressed/wide nasal bridge	2	2	Other:		
epicanthal folds	2	0	torticollis	—	3
hypertelorism	1	4	meningomyelocele	—	1
wide fontanel	0	1	hernias (inguinal)	1	4
short or webbed neck	1	1	coagulation or	1	5
anencephalus	0	1	hemorrhagic disease		
small mandible	2	—	hypospadias	—	1
Chest:			abnormal genitalia	—	2
congenital heart disease	2	5	accessory nipple	—	1
(not specific)			stomach tumor	—	1

* Cases not mutually exclusive.

There are other potential complications associated with the use of primidone during pregnancy. Neurologic manifestations in the newborn such as overactivity and tumors have been associated with use of primidone in pregnancy (16, 18). Neonatal hemorrhagic disease with primidone alone or in combination with other anticonvulsants has been reported (14, 19–23). Suppression of vitamin K_1-dependent clotting factors is the proposed mechanism of primidone's hemorrhagic effect (14, 19). Administration of parenteral vitamin K_1 to the mother prior to delivery and to the infant immediately after birth is recommended (see Phenytoin, Phenobarbital).

Breast Feeding Summary

Primidone is excreted into breast milk (24). Because primidone undergoes limited conversion to phenobarbital, breast milk concentrations of phenobarbital should also be anticipated (see Phenobarbital). A milk:plasma ratio of 0.8 for primidone has been reported (24). The amount of primidone available to the nursing infant is small with milk concentrations of 2.3 $\mu g/ml$. No reports linking adverse effects to the nursing infant have been located, however, patients that breast feed should be instructed to watch for potential sedative effects in the infant.

References

1. Hill RB. Teratogenesis and antiepileptic drugs. N Engl J Med 1973;289:1089–90.
2. Bodendorfer TW. Fetal effect of anticonvulsant drugs and seizure disorders. Drug Intell Clin Pharm 1978;12:14–21.
3. Committee on Drugs, American Academy of Pediatrics. Anticonvulsants and pregnancy. Pediatrics 1977;63:331–3.
4. Nakane Y, Okoma T, Takahashe R, et al. Multiple-institutional study of the teratogenicity and fetal toxicity of antiepileptic drugs: a report of a collaborative study group in Japan. Epilepsia 1980;21:663–80.
5. Andermann E, Dansky L, Andermann F, Loughnan PM, Gibbons J. Minor congenital malformations and dermatoglyphic alterations in the offspring of epileptic women: a clinical investigation of the teratogenic effects of anticonvulsant medication. In *Epilepsy, Pregnancy and the Child*. Proceedings of a Workshop held in Berlin September 1980. New York: Raven Press, 1981 (in press).
6. Danksy L, Andermann F. Major congenital malformations in the offspring of epileptic patients. In *Epilepsy, Pregnancy and the Child*. Proceedings of a Workshop held in Berlin September 1980. New York: Raven Press, 1981 (in press).
7. Janz D. The teratogenic risks of antiepileptic drugs. Epilepsia 1975;16:159–69.
8. Lowe CR. Congenital malformations among infants born to epileptic women. Lancet 1973;1:9–10.
9. Lander CM, Edwards BE, Eadie MJ, Tyrer JH. Plasma anticonvulsants concentrations during pregnancy. Neurology 1977;27:128–31.
10. Speidel BD, Meadow SR. Maternal epilepsy and abnormalities of the fetus and newborn. Lancet 1972;2:839–43.
11. McMullin GP. Teratogenic effects of anticonvulsants. Br Med J 1971;4:430.
12. Fedrick J. Epilepsy and pregnancy: a report from the Oxford Record Linkage Study. Br Med J 1973;2:442–8.
13. Biale Y, Lewenthal H, Aderet NB. Congenital malformations due to anticonvulsant drugs. Obstet Gynecol 1975;45:439–42.
14. Thomas P, Buchanan N. Teratogenic effect of anticonvulsants. J Pediatr 1981;99:163.
15. Myhree SA, Williams R. Teratogenic effects associated with maternal primidone therapy. J Pediatr 1981;99:160–2.
16. Rudd NL, Freedom RM. A possible primidone embryopathy. J Pediatr 1979;94:835–7.
17. Heinonen OP, Slone D, Shapiro S. *Birth Defects and Drugs in Pregnancy*. Littleton: Publishing Sciences Group, 1977:358.
18. Martinez G, Snyder RD. Transplacental passage of primidone. Neurology 1973;23:381–3.
19. Kohler HG. Haemorrhage in the newborn of epileptic mothers. Lancet 1966;1:267.
20. Bleyer WA, Skinner AL. Fatal neonatal hemorrhage after maternal anticonvulsant therapy. JAMA 1976;235:826–7.
21. Mountain KR, Hirsh J, Gallus AS. Neonatal coagulation defect due to anticonvulsant drug treatment in pregnancy. Lancet 1970;1:265–8.
22. Evans AR, Forrester RM, Discombe C. Neonatal hemorrhage following maternal anticonvulsant therapy. Lancet 1970;1:517–8.

23. Margolin DO, Kantor NM. Hemorrhagic disease of the newborn: an unusual case related to maternal ingestion of antiepileptic drug. Clin Pediatr (Phila) 1972;11:59-60.
24. Kaneko S, Sato T, Suzuki K. The levels of anticonvulsants in breast milk. Br J Clin Pharmacol 1979;7:624-7.

Name: **PROBENECID**

Class: **Uricosuric/Renal Tubular Blocking Agent**   Risk Factor: **B**

Fetal Risk Summary

No reports linking the use of probenecid with congenital defects have been located. Probenecid has been used during pregnancy without producing adverse effects in the fetus or in the infant (1-3).

Breast Feeding Summary

No data available.

Reference

1. Beidleman B. Treatment of chronic hypoparathyroidism with probenecid. Metabolism 1958;7:690-8.
2. Lee FI, Loeffler FE. Gout and pregnancy. J Obstet Gynaecol Br Commonw 1962;69:299.
3. Batt RE, Cirksena WJ, Lebhertz TB. Gout and salt-wasting renal disease during pregnancy. Diagnosis, management and follow-up. JAMA 1963;186:835-8.

Name: **PROCARBAZINE**

Class: **Antineoplastic**   Risk Factor: **D**

Fetal Risk Summary

The use of procarbazine during pregnancy has been described in 7 patients, 5 during the 1st trimester (1-6). One of the 1st trimester exposures was electively terminated, but no details on the fetus were given (5). Congenital malformations were observed in the remaining four 1st-trimester exposures (see table below) (1-4). A patient in the early 2nd trimester received procarbazine, 50 mg daily, in error for 30 days when she was given the drug instead of an iron/vitamin supplement (6). An apparently normal male infant was delivered. Long term studies of growth and mental development in offspring exposed to procarbazine during the 2nd trimester, the period of neuroblast multiplication, have not been conducted (7). Data from one review indicated that 40% of the infants exposed to anticancer drugs were of low birth weight (8). This finding was not related to the timing of exposure.

Procarbazine is mutagenic and carcinogenic in animals (9). In combination with other antineoplastic drugs, procarbazine may produce gonadal dysfunction in males and females (10–14). Ovarian and testicular function may return to normal, with successful pregnancies possible, depending on the patient's age at the time of therapy and the total dose of chemotherapy received (14).

Author (ref)	No. Pts.	Indication	Gestational Age	Dose	Other Drugs	Fetal Effects	Comments
Wells (1)	1	Hodgkin's	1st trimester	150 mg/M^2 orally	Isoniazid Pyridoxine	Multiple hemangiomas	
Garrett (2)	1	Hodgkin's	1st trimester	Not stated	Mechlorethamine	Spontaneous abortion at 24 weeks of gestation	
					Vinblastine	Oligodactyly of both feet with webbing of 3rd and 4th toes	
						4 metatarsals on left, 3 on right	
						Bowing of right tibia	
						Cerebral hemorrhage	
Mennuti (3)	1	Hodgkin's	1st trimester	200 mg/day	Mechlorethamine Vincristine	Elective abortion Malformed kidneys—markedly reduced size and malposition	
Thomas (4)	2	Hodgkin's	1st trimester	1–2 g total dose	Vinblastine Vincristine	1 elective abortion; details of fetus not given	
						1 1900-g male delivered at 37 weeks of gestation; developed fatal RDS; small secundum atrial septal defect	

Breast Feeding Summary

No data available.

References

1. Wells JH, Marshall JR, Carbone PP. Procarbazine therapy for Hodgkin's disease in early pregnancy. JAMA 1968;205:935–7.
2. Garrett MJ. Teratogenic effects of combination chemotherapy. Ann Intern Med 1974;80:667.
3. Mennuti MT, Shepard TH, Mellman WJ. Fetal renal malformation following treatment of Hodgkin's disease during pregnancy. Obstet Gynecol 1975;46:194–6.
4. Thomas PRM, Peckham MJ. The investigation and management of Hodgkin's disease in the pregnant patient. Cancer 1976;38:1443–51.
5. Daly H, McCann SR, Hanratty TD, Temperley IJ. Successful pregnancy during combination chemotherapy for Hodgkin's disease. Acta Haematol (Basel) 1980;64:154–6.
6. Daw EG. Procarbazine in pregnancy. Lancet 1970;2:984.
7. Dobbing J. Pregnancy and leukaemia. Lancet 1977;1:1155.
8. Nicholson HO. Cytotoxic drugs in pregnancy: review of reported cases. J Obstet Gynecol Br Commonw 1968;75:307–12.
9. Lee IP, Dixon RL. Mutagenicity, carcinogenicity and teratogenicity of procarbazine. Mutat Res 1978;55:1–14.
10. Sherins RJ, DeVita VT Jr. Effect of drug treatment for lymphoma on male reproductive capacity: studies of men in remission after therapy. Ann Intern Med 1973;79:216–20.
11. Sherins RJ, Olweny CLM, Ziegler JL. Gynecomastia and gonadal dysfunction in adolescent boys treated with combination chemotherapy for Hodgkin's disease. N Engl J Med 1978;299:12–6.
12. Johnson SA, Goldman JM, Hawkins DF. Pregnancy after chemotherapy for Hodgkin's disease. Lancet 1979;2:93.
13. Card RT, Holmes IH, Sugarman RG, Storb R, Thomas ED. Successful pregnancy after high

dose chemotherapy and marrow transplantation for treatment of aplastic anemia. Exp Hematol 1980;8:57–60.

14. Schilsky RL, Sherins RJ, Hubbard SM, Wesley MN, Young RC, DeVita VT Jr. Long-term follow-up of ovarian function in women treated with MOPP chemotherapy for Hodgkin's disease. Am J Med 1981;71:552–6.

Name: **PROCHLORPERAZINE**

Class: **Tranquilizer**   Risk Factor: **C**

Fetal Risk Summary

Prochlorperazine is a piperazine phenothiazine. The drug readily crosses the placenta (1). Prochlorperazine has been used to treat nausea and vomiting of pregnancy. Most studies have found the drug to be safe for this indication (see also Chlorpromazine) (2–4). The Collaborative Perinatal Project monitored 50,282 mother-child pairs, 877 of which had 1st trimester exposure to prochlorperazine (4). For use anytime during pregnancy, 2023 exposures were recorded. No evidence was found in either group to suggest a relationship to malformations, or an effect on perinatal mortality rate, birth weight or intelligence quotient scores at 4 years of age. Two reports of congenital defects in infants exposed to prochlorperazine are described in the table below (5, 6). A third report provided brief data on 14 infants, one half of whom were exposed to the drug before embryologic timing of their malformations (7). In summary, although there are isolated reports of congenital defects in children exposed to prochlorperazine *in utero*, the majority of the evidence indicates that this drug, and the general class of phenothiazines, is safe for both mother and fetus if used occasionally in low doses. Other reviewers have also concluded that the phenothiazines are not teratogenic (8, 9).

Author (ref)	No. Pts.	Indication	Gestational Age	Dose	Other Drugs	Fetal Effects	Comment
Ho (5)	1	Nausea and vomiting	1st trimester	10 mg/day 14 times	1st trimester: Estrogens Bendectin Excedrin 2nd trimester: Chlorpromazine Lomotil Excedrin	Cleft palate, micrognathia, congenital heart disease, skeletal defects	Relationship to drugs unclear; only prochlorperazine and estrogens taken during critical period
Farag (6)	1	Nausea and vomiting	1st trimester	10 mg intramuscular 8 times	Pyridoxine	Thanatophoric dwarfism (short limb anomaly)	Possible genetic defect

Breast Feeding Summary

No data available.

References

1. Moya F, Thornidke V. Passage of drugs across the placenta. Am J Obstet Gynecol 1962;84:1778–98.

2. Reider RO, Rosenthal D. Wender P, Blumenthal H. The offspring of schizophrenics. Fetal and neonatal deaths. Arch Gen Psychiatry 1975; 32:200–11.
3. Milkovich L, Van den Berg BJ. An evaluation of the teratogenicity of certain antinauseant drugs. Am J Obstet Gynecol 1976;125:244–8.
4. Slone D, Siskind V, Heinonen OP, Monson RR, Kaufman DW, Shapiro S. Antenatal exposure to the phenothiazines in relation to congenital malformations, perinatal mortality rate, birth weight, and intelligence quotient score. Am. J Obstet Gynecol 1977;128:486–8.
5. Ho CK, Kaufman RL, McAlister WH. Congenital malformations. Cleft palate, congenital heart disease, absent tibiae, and polydactyly. Am J Dis Child 1975;129:714–6.
6. Farag RA, Ananth J. Thanatophoric dwarfism associated with prochlorperazine administration. NY State J Med 1978;78:279–82.
7. Mellin GW. Report of prochlorperazine during pregnancy from the fetal life study bank. Teratology 1975;11:28A (Abstract).
8. Ayd FJ Jr. Children born of mothers treated with chlorpromazine during pregnancy. Clin Med 1964;71:1758–63.
9. Ananth J. Congenital malformations with psychopharmacologic agents. Compr Psychiatry 1975;16:437–45.

Name: **PROCYCLIDINE**

Class: **Parasympatholytic (Anticholinergic)**   Risk Factor: **C**

Fetal Risk Summary

Procyclidine is an anticholinergic agent used in the treatment of parkinsonism. No reports of its use in pregnancy have been located (see also Atropine).

Breast Feeding Summary

No data available (see also Atropine).

Name: **PROMAZINE**

Class: **Tranquilizer**   Risk Factor: **C**

Fetal Risk Summary

Promazine is a propylamino phenothiazine structurally related to chlorpromazine. The drug readily crosses the placenta (1, 2). A possible relationship between the use of promazine (100 mg or more) in labor and neonatal hyperbilirubinemia was reported in 1975 (3). The Collaborative Perinatal Project monitored 50,282 mother-child pairs, 50 of which had 1st trimester exposure to promazine (4). For use anytime during pregnancy, 347 exposures were recorded. No evidence was found in either group to suggest a relationship to malformations, or an effect on perinatal mortality rate, birth weight or intelligence quotient scores at 4 years of age. Although occasional reports have attempted to link various phenothiazine compounds with congenital defects, the bulk of the evidence indicates that these drugs are safe for mother and fetus (see also Chlorpromazine).

Breast Feeding Summary

No data available.

References

1. Moya F, Thorndike V. Passage of drugs across the placenta. Am J Obstet Gynecol 1962;84:1778–98.
2. O'Donoghue SEF. Distribution of pethidine and chlorpromazine in maternal, foetal and neonatal biological fluids. Nature 1971;229:124–5.
3. John E. Promazine and neonatal hyperbilirubinemia. Med J Aust 1975;2:342–4.
4. Slone D, Siskind V, Heinonen OP, Monson RR, Kaufman DW, Shapiro S. Antenatal exposure to the phenothiazines in relation to congenital malformations, perinatal mortality rate, birth weight, and intelligence quotient score. Am J Obstet Gynecol 1977;128:486–8.

Name: **PROMETHAZINE**

Class: **Antihistamine**   Risk Factor: **C**

Fetal Risk Summary

Promethazine is a phenothiazine antihistamine that is sometimes used as an antiemetic in pregnancy and as an adjunct to narcotic analgesics during labor. The Collaborative Perinatal Project monitored 50,282 mother-child pairs, 114 of which had promethazine exposure in the 1st trimester (1). For use anytime during pregnancy, 746 exposures were recorded (2). In neither case was evidence found to suggest a relationship to large categories of major or minor malformations or to individual defects. A 1964 report also failed to show an association between 165 cases of promethazine exposure in the 1st trimester and malformations (3). Finally, in a 1971 reference, infants of mothers who had ingested antiemetics during the 1st trimester actually had significantly fewer abnormalities when compared to controls (4). Promethazine was the most commonly used antiemetic in this latter study.

At term, the drug rapidly crosses the placenta, appearing in cord blood within 1½ minutes of an intravenous dose (5). Fetal and maternal blood concentrations are at equilibrium in 15 minutes with infant levels persisting for at least 4 hours.

Several investigators have studied the effect of promethazine on labor and the newborn (6–13). Significant neonatal respiratory depression was seen in a small group of patients (6). However, in 3 large series, no clinical evidence of promethazine-induced respiratory depression was found (7–9). In a series of 33 mothers at term, 28 received either promethazine alone (1 patient), or a combination of meperidine with promethazine or phenobarbital (27 patients). Transient behavioral and EEG changes, persisting for less than 3 days, were seen in all newborns (11).

Maternal tachycardia due to promethazine (mean increase 30 beats/minute) or promethazine-meperidine (mean increase 42 beats/minute) was observed in one series (10). The maximum effect occurred about 10 minutes after injection. The fetal heart rate did not change significantly.

Effects on the uterus have been mixed, with both increases and decreases in uterine activity reported (9, 10, 12).

Promethazine used during labor has been shown to markedly impair platelet aggregation in the newborn but not in the mother (13). While the clinical significance of this is unknown, the degree of impairment is comparable to those disorders associated with a definite bleeding state.

Promethazine has been used to treat hydrops fetalis in cases of anti-erythrocytic isoimmunization (14). Six patients were treated with 150 mg orally per day between the 26th and 34th week of gestation while undergoing intraperitoneal transfusions. No details on the infant's conditions were given except that all were born alive.

Two female anencephalic infants were born to mothers after ovulatory stimulation with clomiphene (15). One of the mothers had taken promethazine for morning sickness. No association between promethazine and this defect has been suggested.

Breast Feeding Summary

Available laboratory methods for the accurate detection of promethazine in breast milk are not clinically useful due to the rapid metabolism of phenothiazines (16).

References

1. Heinonen OP, Slone D, Shapiro S. *Birth Defects and Drugs in Pregnancy.* Littleton: Publishing Sciences Group, 1977:323–4.
2. *Ibid*, 437.
3. Wheatley D. Drugs and the embryo. Br Med J 1964;1:630.
4. Nelson MM, Forfar JO. Association between drugs administered during pregnancy and congenital abnormalities of the fetus. Br Med J 1971;1:523–7.
5. Moya F, Thorndike V. The effects of drugs used in labor on the fetus and newborn. Clin Pharmacol Ther 1963;4:628–53.
6. Crawford JS, as quoted by Moya F, Thorndike V. The effects of drugs used in labor on the fetus and newborn. Clin Pharmacol Ther 1963;4:628–53.
7. Powe CE, Kiem IM, Fromhagen C, Cavanagh D. Propiomazine hydrochloride in obstetrical analgesia. JAMA 1962;181:290–4.
8. Potts CR, Ullery JC. Maternal and fetal effects of obstetric analgesia. Am J Obstet Gynecol 1961;81:1253–9.
9. Carroll JJ, Moir RS. Use of promethazine (Phenergan) hydrochloride in obstetrics. JAMA 1958;168:2218–24.
10. Riffel HD, Nochimson DJ, Paul RH, Hon EH. Effects of meperidine and promethazine during labor. Obstet Gynecol 1973;42:738–45.
11. Borgstedt AD, Rosen MG. Medication during labor correlated with behavior and EEG of the newborn. Am J Dis Child 1968;115:21–4.
12. Zakut H, Mannor SM, Serr DM. Effect of promethazine on uterine contractions. Harefuah 1970;78:61–2. As reported in JAMA 1970; 211:1572.
13. Corby DG, Shulman I. The effects of antenatal drug administration on aggregation of platelets of newborn infants. J Pediatr 1971;79:307–13.
14. Bierme S, Bierme R. Antihistamines in hydrops foetalis. Lancet 1967;1:574.

15. Dyson JL, Kohler HC. Anecephaly and ovulation stimulation. Lancet 1973;1:1256–7.
16. Personal communication. M. Lipshutz, Assistant to Director, Medical Communications, Wyeth
    Laboratories, 1981.

Name: **PROPANTHELINE**

Class: **Parasympatholytic (Anticholinergic)**   Risk Factor: **C**

Fetal Risk Summary

Propantheline is an anticholinergic quaternary ammonium bromide. The Collaborative Perinatal Project monitored 50,282 mother-child pairs, 33 of which used propantheline in the 1st trimester (1). No evidence was found for an association with congenital malformations. However, when the group of parasympatholytics were taken as a whole (2,323 exposures), a possible association with minor malformations was found (1).

Breast Feeding Summary

No data available (see also Atropine).

Reference

1. Heinonen OP, Slone D, Shapiro S. *Birth Defects and Drugs in Pregnancy*. Littleton: Publishing
   Sciences Group, 1977:346–53.

Name: **PROPOXYPHENE**

Class: **Analgesic**   Risk Factor: **C***

Fetal Risk Summary

Two case reports, involving 3 patients, have linked the use of propoxyphene during pregnancy to congenital abnormalties (1, 2). In both reports, however, other drugs were used and any association may be fortuitous.

The Collaborative Perinatal Project monitored 50,282 mother-child pairs, 686 of which had 1st trimester exposure to propoxyphene (3). For use anytime during pregnancy, 2,914 exposures were recorded (4). No evidence was found in either case to suggest a relationship to large categories of major or minor malformations or, in the 1st trimester, to individual defects. Five possible associations with individual defects after anytime use were observed (5). The statistical significance of these associations is unknown and independent confirmation is required.

Microcephaly (6 cases)

Ductus arteriosus persistens (5 cases)

Cataract (5 cases)

Benign tumors (12 cases)
Clubfoot (18 cases)

Neonatal withdrawal has been reported in 4 infants (6–9). The relationship between heavy maternal ingestion of this drug and neontal withdrawal seems clear. The infants were asymptomatic, with normal Apgar scores, until 3½ to 14 hours after delivery. Withdrawal was marked by the onset of irritability, tremors, diarrhea, fever, high-pitched cry, hyperactivity, hypertonicity, diaphoresis and, in one case, seizures. Symptoms began to subside by day 4, usually without specific therapy. Examinations after 2 to 3 months were normal.

Propoxyphene has been used in labor without causing neonatal respiratory depression (10). However, a significant shortening of the first stage of labor occurred without an effect on uterine contractions.

Author (ref)	No. Pts.	Indication	Gestational Age	Dose	Other Drugs	Fetal Effects	Comment
Barrow (1)	1	Pain	Through-out	1.3–2.34 g/day	Antiemetics Phenytoin "Numerous other drugs"	Pierre Robin Syndrome Arthrogryposis Severe mental and growth retardation	Cause-and-effect relationship unclear
Ringrose (2)	1	Pain	Through-out	6.5 mg as needed	Diazepam APC Vitamins Iron	Congenital absence of left forearm and radial 2 digits Syndactyly of ulnar 3 digits and left 4th and 5th toes Hypoplastic left femur	
	1	Pain	Through-out	Not stated	Meprobamate	Omphalocele, defective anteior left wall, diaphragmatic defect CHD with partial ectopic cordis due to sternal cleft and dysplastic hips	

[* Risk Factor D if used for prolonged periods.]

Breast Feeding Summary

Propoxyphene passes into breast milk, but the amounts and clinical significance are unknown. In one case, a nursing mother attempted suicide with propoxyphene (11). The concentration of the drug in her breast milk was found to be 50% of her plasma level. By calculation, the authors predicted a mother consuming a maximum daily dose of the drug would provide her infant with 1 mg per day.

References

1. Barrow MV, Souder DE. Propoxyphene and congenital malformations. JAMA 1971;217: 1551–2.
2. Ringrose CAD. The hazard of neurotrophic drugs in the fertile years. Can Med Assoc J 1972;106:1058.
3. Heinonen OP, Slone D, Shapiro S. Birth Defects and Drugs in Pregnancy. Littleton: Publishing Sciences Group, 1977:287–95.
4. Ibid, 434.
5. Ibid, 484.

6. Tyson HK. Neonatal withdrawal symptoms associated with maternal use of propoxyphene hydrochloride (Darvon). J Pediatr 1974;85:684–5.
7. Klein RB, Blatman S, Little GA. Probable neonatal propoxyphene withdrawal: a case report. Pediatrics 1975;55:882–4.
8. Quillan WW, Dunn CA. Neonatal drug withdrawal from propoxyphene. JAMA 1976;235:2128.
9. Ente G, Mehra MC. Neonatal drug withdrawal from propoxyphene hydrochloride. NY State J Med 1978;78:2084–5.
10. Eddy NB, Friebel H, Hahn KJ, Halbach H. Codeine and its alternatives for pain and cough relief. 2. Alternates for pain relief. Bull WHO 1969;40:1–53.
11. Catz C, Guiacoia G. Drugs and breast milk. Pediatr Clin North Am 1972;19:151–66.

Name: **PROPRANOLOL**

Class: **Sympatholytic (β-adrenergic Blocker)**   Risk Factor: **C**

Fetal Risk Summary

Propranolol is a β-adrenergic blocking agent that has been used for various indications in pregnancy:

Maternal hyperthyroidism (1–7)
Pheochromocytoma (8)
Maternal cardiac disease (6,7,9–20)
Fetal tachycardia/arrhythmia (21,22)
Maternal hypertension (7,20,23–30)
Dysfunctional labor (31)
Termination of pregnancy (32)

The drug readily crosses the placenta (2,6,12,16,22,29). Cord serum levels varying between 19 and 127% of maternal serum have been reported (2,-16,22,29). Oxytocic effects have been demonstrated following intravenous and extra-amniotic injections and high oral dosing (17,31–34). Intravenous propranolol has been shown to block or decrease the marked increase in maternal plasma progesterone induced by vasopressin or theophyllamine (35).

A number of fetal/neonatal adverse effects have been reported following the use of propranolol in pregnancy. Whether these effects are due to propranolol, maternal disease, other drugs consumed concurrently, or a combination of these factors is not always clear. Daily doses of 160 mg per day or higher seem to produce the more serious complications but lower doses have also resulted in toxicity. Analysis of 26 reports involving 153 liveborn infants exposed to chronic propranolol *in utero* is shown below (1–4,6,7,9,11–14,20,22–24,26–29,36–38):

	No. Cases	%
Probably Related to Propranolol		
Intrauterine growth retardation	23	15
Hypoglycemia	14	9
Bradycardia	12	8
Respiratory depression at birth	6	4
Small placenta (size not always noted)	4	3
Probably Not Related to Propranolol		
Hyperbilirubinemia	6	4
Polycythemia	2	1
Thrombocytopenia ($40,000/mm^3$)	1	0.7
Hyperirritability	1	0.7
Hypocalcemia with convulsions	1	0.7
Blood coagulation defect	1	0.7

Two infants were reported to have anomalies (pyloric stenosis; crepitus of hip), but the authors did not relate these to propranolol (27, 36). In another case, a malformed fetus was spontaneously aborted from a 30-year-old woman with chronic renovascular hypertension (39). The patient had been treated with propranolol, amiloride and captopril for her severe hypertension. Malformations included absence of the left leg below the mid-thigh and no obvious skull formation above the brain tissue. The authors attributed the defect either to captopril alone, or to a combination effect of the three drugs.

Respiratory depression was noted in 4 of 5 infants whose mothers were given 1 mg of propranolol intravenously just prior to cesarean section (40). None of the 5 controls in the double-blind study were depressed at birth. The author suggested the mechanism may have been due to β-adrenergic blockade of the cervical sympathetic discharge which occurs at cord clamping.

Fetal bradycardia was observed in 2 of 10 patients treated with propranolol, 1 mg per minute for 4 minutes, for dysfunctional labor (31). No lasting effects were seen in the babies. In a retrospective study, 8 markedly hypertensive patients (9 pregnancies) treated with propranolol were compared with 15 hypertensive controls not treated with propranolol (25). Other antihypertensives were used in both groups. A significant difference was found between the perinatal mortality rates, with 7 deaths in the propranolol group (78%) and only 5 deaths in the controls (33%). However, a possible explanation for the difference may have been the more severe hypertension and renal disease in the propranolol group than in the controls (41).

Intrauterine growth retardation may be related to propranolol. Several possible mechanisms for this effect, if indeed it is associated with the drug, have been reviewed by Redmond (42). Premature labor has been suggested as a possible complication of propranolol therapy in patients with pregnancy-induced hypertension (PIH). (38). In 9 women treated with propranolol for PIH, 3 delivered prematurely. The author speculated that these patients were relatively hypovolemic and when a compensatory increase in cardiac output failed to occur, premature delivery resulted.

In summary, propranolol has been used during pregnancy for maternal and fetal indications. The drug is apparently not a teratogen but fetal and neonatal toxicity may occur.

Breast Feeding Summary

Propranolol is excreted into breast milk. Peak concentrations occur 2 to 3 hours after a dose (12,20,43). Since no adverse effects such as respiratory depression, bradycardia, or hypoglycemia have been reported, breast feeding during maternal propranolol therapy is probably safe.

Author (ref)	No. Pts.	Dose	Concentrations (ng/ml) Serum	Milk	M:P Ratio	Effect on Infant
Levitan (12)	1	40 mg once	60.8 (1 hr)	9.7	0.2	—
			— (2 hr)	30.0	—	
			43.8 (3 hr)	15.9	0.4	
Taylor (29)	1	40 mg/day	17	4	0.2	Calculated daily intake by infant
			16	11	0.7	= 3 µg
Karlberg (43)	2	20–160 mg (single doses)	10–110 (3 hr)	3–110	0.3–1.5	
			18–200 (3 hr)	10–120	0.6	
Bauer (20)	1	40 mg once (2 doses 5 days apart)	18–23 (peak 2–3 hr)	4–9 (Peak 2–3 hr)	0.2–0.5	
		160 mg/day	65 (3 hr)	42 (3 hr)	0.6	Calculated daily intake by infant consuming 500 ml of milk = 21 µg (after 160 mg/day);
		240 mg/day for 30 days	— —	26 (pre-dose) 64 (3 hr)	— —	32 µg after 240 mg/day

References

1. Jackson GL. Treatment of hyperthyroidism in pregnancy. Pa Med 1973;76:56–7.
2. Langer A, Hung CT, McA'Nulty JA, Harrigan JT, Washington E. Adrenergic blockade: a new approach to hyperthyroidism during pregnancy. Obstet Gynecol 1974;44:181–6.
3. Bullock JL, Harris RE, Young R. Treatment of thyrotoxicosis during pregnancy with propranolol. Am J Obstet Gynecol 1975;121:242–5.
4. Lightner ES, Allen HD, Loughlin G. Neonatal hyperthyroidism and heart failure: a different approach. Am J Dis Child 1977;131:68–70.
5. Levy CA, Waite JH, Dickey R. Thyrotoxicosis and pregnancy. Use of preoperative propranolol for thyroidectomy. Am J Surg 1977;133:319–21.
6. Habib A, McCarthy JS. Effects on the neonate of propranolol administered during pregnancy. J Pediatr 1977; 91:808–11.
7. Pruyn SC, Phelan JP, Buchanan GC. Long-term propranolol therapy in pregnancy: maternal and fetal outcome. Am J Obstet Gynecol 1979;135:485–9.
8. Leak D, Carroll JJ, Robinson DC, Ashworth EJ. Management of pheochromocytoma during pregnancy. Can Med Assoc J 1977;116:371–5.
9. Turner GM, Oakley CM, Dixon HG. Management of pregnancy complicated by hypertrophic obstructive cardiomyopathy. Br Med J 1968;4:281–4.
10. Barnes AB. Chronic propranolol administration during pregnancy: a case report. J Reprod Med 1970;5:79–80.
11. Schroeder JS, Harrison DC. Repeated cardioversion during pregnancy. Am J Cardiol 1971;27:445–6.
12. Levitan AA, Manion JC. Propranolol therapy during pregnancy and lactation. Am J Cardiol 1973;32:247.
13. Reed RL, Cheney CB, Fearon RE, Hook R, Hehre FW. Propranolol therapy throughout pregnancy: a case report. Anesth Analg (Cleve) 1974;53:214–8.
14. Fiddler GI. Propranolol pregnancy. Lancet 1974;2:722–3.
15. Kolibash AE, Ruiz DE, Lewis RP. Idiopathic hypertrophic subaortic stenosis in pregnancy. Ann Intern Med 1975;82:791–4.
16. Cottrill CM, McAllister RG Jr, Gettes L, Noonan JA. Propranolol therapy during pregnancy,

labor, and delivery: evidence for transplacental drug transfer and impaired neonatal drug disposition. J Pediatr 1977;91:812–4.

17. Datta S, Kitzmiller JL, Ostheimer GW, Schoenbaum SC. Propranolol and parturition. Obstet Gynecol 1978;51:577–81.

18. Diaz JH, McDonald JS. Propranolol and induced labor: anesthetic implications. Anesth Rev 1979;6:29–32.

19. Oakley GDG, McGarry K, Limb DG, Oakley CM. Management of pregnancy in patients with hypertrophic cardiomyopathy. Br Med J 1979;1:1749–50.

20. Bauer JH, Pape B, Zajicek J, Groshong T. Propranolol in human plasma and breast milk. Am J Cardiol 1979;43:860–2.

21. Eibschitz I, Abinader EG, Klein A, Sharf M. Intrauterine diagnosis and control of fetal ventricular arrhythmia during labor. Am J Obstet Gynecol 1975;122:597–600.

22. Teuscher A, Boss E, Imhof P, Erb E, Stocker FP, Weber JW. Effect of propranolol on fetal tachycardia in diabetic pregnancy. Am J Cardiol 1978;42:304–7.

23. Gladstone GR, Hordof A, Gersony WM. Propranolol administration during pregnancy: effects on the fetus. J Pediatr 1975;86:962–4.

24. Tcherdakoff PH, Colliard M, Berrard E, Kreft C, Dupry A, Bernaille JM. Propranolol in hypertension during pregnancy. Br Med J 1978;2:670.

25. Lieberman BA, Stirrat GM, Cohen SL, Beard RW, Pinker GD, Belsey E. The possible adverse effect of propranolol on the fetus in pregnancies complicated by severe hypertension. Br J Obstet Gynaecol 1978;85:678–83.

26. Eliahou HE, Silverberg DS, Reisin E, Romen I, Mashiach S, Serr DM. Propranolol for the treatment of hypertension in pregnancy. Br J Obstet Gynaecol 1978;85:431–6.

27. Bott-Kanner G, Schweitzer A, Schoenfeld A, Joel-Cohen J, Rosenfeld JB. Treatment with propranolol and hydralazine throughout pregnancy in a hypertensive patient: a case report. Is J Med Sci 1978;14:466–8.

28. Bott-Kanner G, Reisner SH, Rosenfeld JB. Propranolol and hydralazine in the management of essential hypertension in pregnancy. Br Obstet Gynaecol 1980;87:110–4.

29. Taylor EA, Turner P. Anti-hypertensive therapy with propranolol during pregnancy and lactation. Postgrad Med J 1981;57:427–30.

30. Serup J. Propranolol for the treatment of hypertension in pregnancy. Acta Med Scand 1979;206:333.

31. Mitrani A, Oettinger M, Abinader EG, Sharf M, Klein A. Use of propranolol in dysfunctional labour. Br J Obstet Gynaecol 1975;82:651–5.

32. Amy JJ, Karim SMM. Intrauterine administration of 1-noradrenaline and propranolol during the second trimester of pregnancy. J Obstet Gynaecol Br Commonw 1974;81:75–83.

33. Barden TP, Stander RW. Myometrial and cardiovascular effects of an adrenergic blocking drug in human pregnancy. Am J Obstet Gynecol 1968;101:91–9.

34. Wansbrough H, Nakanishi H, Wood C. The effect of adrenergic receptor blocking drugs on the human fetus. J Obstet Gynaecol Br Commonw 1968;75:189–98.

35. Fylling P. Dexamethasone or propranolol blockade of induced increase in plasma progesterone in early human pregnancy. Acta Endocrinol (Copenh) 1973;72:569–72.

36. O'Connor PC, Jick H, Hunter JR, Stergachis A, Madsen S. Propranolol and pregnancy outcome. Lancet 1981;2:1168.

37. Caldroney RD. Beta-blockers in pregnancy. N Engl J Med 1982;306:810.

38. Goodlin RC. Beta blocker in pregnancy-induced hypertension. Am J Obstet Gynecol 1982;143:237.

39. Duminy PC, Burger P du T. Fetal abnormaiity associated with the use of captopril during pregnancy. S Afr Med J 1981;60:805.

40. Tunstall ME. The effect of propranolol on the onset of breathing at birth. Br J Anaesth 1969;41:792.

41. Rubin PC. Beta-blockers in pregnancy. N Engl J Med 1981;305:1323–6.

42. Redmond GP. Propranolol and fetal growth retardation. Sem Perinatol 1982;6:142–7.

43. Karlberg B, Lundberg O, Aberg H. Excretion of propranolol in human breast milk. Acta Pharmacol Toxicol (Copenh) 1974;34:222–4.

Name: **PROTAMINE**

Class: **Antiheparin**   Risk Factor: **C**

Fetal Risk Summary

Protamine is used to neutralize the anticoagulant effect of heparin. No reports of its use in pregnancy have been located. Reproduction studies in animals have not been conducted (1).

Breast Feeding Summary

No data available.

Reference

1. Product information. Protamine sulfate. Eli Lilly and Company, 1981.

Name: **PROTRIPTYLINE**

Class: **Antidepressant**   Risk Factor: **C**

Fetal Risk Summary

No data available.

Breast Feeding Summary

No data available.

Name: **PSEUDOEPHEDRINE**

Class: **Sympathomimetic (Adrenergic)**   Risk Factor: **C**

Fetal Risk Summary

Pseudoephedrine is a sympathomimetic used to alleviate the symptoms of allergic disorders or upper respiratory infections. It is a common component of proprietary mixtures containing antihistamines and other ingredients. Thus, it is difficult to separate the effects of pseudoephedrine on the fetus from other drugs, disease states and viruses.

Sympathomimetic amines are teratogenic in some animal species, but human teratogenicity has not been suspected (1,2). Recent data may require a reappraisal of this opinion. The Collaborative Perinatal Project monitored 50,282 mother-child pairs, 3,082 of which had 1st trimester exposure to sympathomimetic drugs (3). For use anytime during pregnancy, 9,719 exposures were recorded (4). An association in the 1st trimester was found between the sympathomimetic class of drugs as a whole and minor malformations (not life-threatening or major cosmetic defects), inguinal hernia and clubfoot (3). This data is presented as a warning that indiscriminate use of pseudoephedrine, especially in the 1st trimester, is not without risk.

Breast Feeding Summary

No data available.

References

1. Nishimura H, Tanimura T. *Clinical Aspects of the Teratogenicity of drugs.* Amsterdam: Excerpta Medica, 1976:231.
2. Shepard TH. *Catalog of Teratogenic drugs*, ed. 3 Baltimore: Johns Hopkins University Press, 1980:134–5.
3. Heinonen OP, Slone D, Shapiro S. *Birth Defects and Drugs in Pregnancy.* Littleton: Publishing Sciences Group, 1977:345–56.
4. *Ibid*, 439.

Name: **PYRANTEL PAMOATE**

Class: **Anthelmintic**   Risk Factor: **C**

Fetal Risk Summary

No data available.

Breast Feeding Summary

No data available.

Name: **PYRIDOSTIGMINE**

Class: **Parasympathomimetic (Cholinergic)**   Risk Factor: **C**

Fetal Risk Summary

Pyridostigmine is a quaternary ammonium compound with anticholinesterase activity used in the treatment of myasthenia gravis. The drug has been used in pregnancy without producing fetal malformations (1–8). Because it is ionized at physiologic pH, pyridostigmine would not be expected to cross the placenta in significant amounts. Caution has been advised against the use in pregnancy of intravenous anticholinesterases since they may cause premature labor (1,3). This effect on the pregnant uterus increases near term. Although apparently safe for the fetus, cholinesterase inhibitors may affect the condition of the newborn (3,7). Transient muscular weakness has been observed in about 20% of newborns whose mothers were treated for myasthenia gravis during pregnancy. While exact cause of the neonatal myasthenia is unknown, anticholinesterases may contribute to the condition (7).

Breast Feeding Summary

Because it is ionized at physiologic pH, pyridostigmine would not be expected to be excreted into breast milk (9).

References

1. Foldes FF, McNall PG. Myasthenia gravis: a guide for anesthesiologists. Anesthesiology 1962;23:837–72.
2. Plauche WC. Myasthenia gravis in pregnancy. Am J Obstet Gynecol 1964;88:404–9.
3. McNall PG, Jafarnia MR. Management of myasthenia gravis in the obstetric patient. Am J Obstet Gynecol 1965;92:518–25.
4. Chambers DC, Hall JE, Boyce J. Myasthenia gravis and pregnancy. Obstet Gynecol 1967;29:597–603.
5. Hay DM. Myasthenia gravis and pregnancy. J Obstet Gynaecol Br Commonw 1969;76:323–9.
6. Heinonen OP, Slone D, Shapiro S. Birth Defects and Drugs in Pregnancy. Littleton: Publishing Sciences Group, 1977:345–56.
7. Blackhall MI, Buckley GA, Roberts DV, Roberts JB, Thomas BH, Wilson A. Drug-induced neonatal myasthenia. J Obstet Gynaecol Br Commonw 1969;76:157–62.
8. Robbin SH, Levinson G, Shnider SM, Wright RG. Anesthetic considerations for myasthenia gravis and pregnancy. Anesth Analg (Cleve) 1978;57:441–7.
9. Wilson JT. Pharmacokinetics of drug excretion. In Wilson JT, ed. Drugs in Breast Milk. Australia: ADIS Press, 1981:17.

Name: **PYRILAMINE**

Class: **Antihistamine**   Risk Factor: **C**

Fetal Risk Summary

Pyrilamine is used infrequently during pregnancy. The Collaborative Perinatal Project monitored 50,282 mother-child pairs, 121 of which had pyrilamine exposure in the 1st trimester (1). No evidence was found to suggest a relationship to large categories of major or minor malformations. For use anytime during pregnancy, 392 exposures were recorded (2). A possible association with malformations was found based on 12 defects, 6 of which involved benign tumors (3).

Breast Feeding Summary

No data available.

References

1. Heinonen OP, Slone D, Shapiro S. Birth Defects and Drugs in Pregnancy. Littleton: Publishing Sciences Group, 1977:323–4.
2. Ibid, 436–7.
3. Ibid, 489.

Name: **PYRIMETHAMINE**

Class: **Antimalarial**   Risk Factor: **C**

Fetal Risk Summary

No reports linking the use of pyrimethamine with congenital defects have been located. One study listed 2 patients exposed to the drug in the 1st trimester (1). No malformations were observed. Pyrimethamine is a folic acid antagonist. Since some folic acid antagonists may be teratogenic (e.g., see Methotrexate), pyrimethamine should be used with caution, if at all, in pregnancy.

Breast Feeding Summary

Pyrimethamine is excreted into breast milk. Mothers treated with 25 to 75 mg orally produced peak concentrations of 3.1 to 3.3 μg/ml at 6 hours (2). The drug was detectable up to 48 hours after a dose. Malaria parasites were completely eliminated in infants up to 6 months of age who were entirely breast fed.

References

1. Heinonen OP, Slone D, Shapiro. *Birth Defects and Drugs in Pregnancy.* Littleton: Publishing Sciences Group, 1977;299,302.
2. Clyde DF, Shute GT, Press J. Transfer of pyrimethamine in human milk. J Trop Med Hyg 1956;59:277–84.

Name: **PYRVINIUM PAMOATE**

Class: **Anthelmintic**   Risk Factor: **C**

Fetal Risk Summary

No data available.

Breast Feeding Summary

No data available.

Name: **QUINACRINE**
Class: **Antimalarial/Anthelmintic**

Risk Factor: **C**

Fetal Risk Summary

A newborn with renal agenesis, hydronephrosis, spina bifida, megacolon and hydrocephalus whose mother received quinacrine 0.1 g per day during the 1st trimester has been reported (1). Animal data does not support a teratogenic effect. Topical application of solutions containing 125 mg/ml of quinacrine directly into the uterine cavity have resulted in tubal occlusion and infertility (2).

Breast Feeding Summary

No data available.

References

1. Vevera J, Zatlovkal F. Pfipad uruzenych malformact zpusobenych pravdepodobne atebrinemym uranem tehotenstui. In Nishmura H, Tanimura T, eds. *Clinical Aspects of the Teratogenicity of Drugs.* New York: American Elsevier 1976:145.
2. Zipper JA, Stachetti E, Medel M. Human fertility control by transvaginal application of quinacrine on the fallopian tube. Fertil Steril 1970;21:581–9.

Name: **QUINETHAZONE**
Class: **Diuretic**

Risk Factor: **D**

Fetal Risk Summary

Quinethazone is structurally related to the thiazide diuretics. See Chlorothiazide.

Breast Feeding Summary

See Chlorothiazide.

Name: **QUINIDINE**

Class: **Antiarrthymic**

Risk Factor: **C**

Fetal Risk Summary

No reports linking the use of quinidine with congenital defects have been located. Eighth cranial nerve damage has been erroneously reported with high doses (1, 2). Quinine, the optical isomer of quinidine, was the actual drug suggested in the original reports (see Quinine) (3). Neonatal thrombocytopenia has been reported after maternal use of quinidine (4). Quinidine crosses the placenta and achieves fetal serum levels similar to maternal levels (1). Amniotic fluid levels may be in the toxic range (9–10 μg/ml) but the significance of this finding.

Quinidine has been in use as an antiarrhythmic drug since 1918. Based on the available literature, its use in pregnancy can be recommended. The oxytocic properties of quinidine have not been observed in gravid patients (5).

Breast Feeding Summary

Quinidine freely diffuses into the breast milk (1). The milk:plasma ratio is approximately 1, based on a study which demonstrated milk concentrations of 6.4 to 8.2 μg/ml and maternal serum concentrations of 9.0 μg/ml (1).

References

1. Hill LM, Malkasian GD Jr. The use of quinidine sulfate throughout pregnancy. Obstet Gynecol 1979;54:366–8.
2. Berkowitz RL, Coustan DR, Mochizuki TK. *Handbook for Prescribing Medications during Pregnancy*. Boston: Little, Brown, 1981:191.
3. Mendelson CL. Disorders of the heartbeat during pregnancy. Am J Obstet Gynecol 1956;72:1268–1301.
4. Domula VM, Weissach G, Lenk H. Uber die auswirkung medikamentoser behandlung in der schwangerschaft auf das gerennungspotential des neugeborenen. Zentralbl Gynaekol 1977;99:473.
5. Bigger JT, Hoffman BF. Antiarrythmic drugs. In Gilman AG, Goodman LS, Gilman A eds. *The Pharmacological Basis of Therapeutics ed 6*. New York: MacMillan, 1980:768.

Name: **QUININE**

Class: **Plasmodicide**

Risk Factor: **C**

Fetal Risk Summary

Nishimura summarized the human case reports of teratogenic effects linked with quinine ingestion (1). The malformations noted are varied, although CNS anomalies and limb defects were the most frequent. Auditory and optic nerve damage have been reported (1–5). These reports usually concern the use of quinine in toxic doses as an abortifacient. Epidemiologic observations do not support an increased teratogenic risk or increased risk of congenital deafness over non-quinine-exposed patients (1, 6). Neonatal and maternal thrombocytopenia purpura and hemolysis in glucose-6-phosphate dehydrogenase (G-6-PD)-deficient newborns has been reported (7, 8).

Quinine has effectively been replaced by newer agents for the treatment of malaria. Although no increased teratogenic risk can be documented, its use during pregnancy should be avoided except in the treatment of uncomplicated attacks of chloroquine-resistant *Plasmodium falciparum*.

Author (ref)	No. Pts.	Indication	Gestational Age	Dose	Other Drugs	Fetal Effects	Comment
Nishimura (1)	21	Abortifacient	1st trimester	1–4 g/day	Not stated	10 CNS anomalies (6 with hydrocephalus) 8 limb defects (3 dysmelias) 7 facial defects 6 heart defects 5 digestive organ anomalies 3 urogenital anomalies 3 hernias 1 vertebral anomaly	Animal data supports only auditory nerve damage.

Breast Feeding Summary

Quinine is excreted into breast milk. Following 300- and 640-mg oral doses in 6 patients, milk concentrations varied up to 2.2 μg/ml with an average level of 1 μg/ml at 3 hours (9). No adverse effects were reported in the nursing infants. Patients at risk for G-6-PD deficiency should not be breast fed until this disease can be ruled out.

References

1. Nishimura H, Tanimura T. *Clinical Aspects of the Teratogenicity of Drugs*. Amsterdam: Excerpta Medica, 1976:140–3.
2. Robinson GC, Brummitt JR, Miller JR. Hearing loss in infants and preschool children II. Etiological considerations. Pediatrics 1963;32:115–24.
3. West RA. Effect of quinine upon auditory nerve. Am J Obstet Gynecol 1938;36:241–8.
4. McKinna AJ. Quinine induced hypoplasia of the optic nerve. Can J Ophthalmol 1966;1:261.
5. Morgon A, Charachon D, Brinquier N. Disorders of the auditory apparatus caused by embryopathy or foetopathy. Prophylaxis and treatment. Acta Otolaryngol (Stockh) 1971;291(Suppl):5.
6. Heinonen OP, Slone D, Shapiro S. *Birth Defects and Drugs in Pregnancy*. Littleton: Publishing Sciences Group, 1977:299,302,333.
7. Mauer MA, DeVaux W, Lahey ME. Neonatal and maternal thrombocytopenic purpura due to quinine. Pediatrics 1957;19:84–7.
8. Glass L, Rajegowda BK, Bowne E, Evans HE. Exposure to quinine and jaundice in a glucose-6-phosphate dehydrogenase-deficient newborn infant. Pediatrics 1973;82:734–5.
9. Terwilliger WG, Hatcher RA. The elimination of morphine and quinine in human milk. Surg Gynecol Obstet 1934;58:823–6.

Name: **RESERPINE**

Class: **Antihypertensive**

Risk Factor: **D**

Fetal Risk Summary

The Collaborative Perinatal Project monitored 50,282 mother-child pairs, 48 of which had 1st trimester exposure to reserpine (1). There were 4 defects with 1st trimester use. Although this incidence (8%) is greater than the expected frequency of occurrence, no major category or individual malformations were identified. For use anytime in pregnancy, 475 exposures were recorded (2). Malformations included:

Microcephaly (7 cases)
Hydronephrosis (3 cases)
Hydroureter (3 cases)
Inguinal hernia (12 cases)

These latter malformations were not found to be statistically significant (3). Reserpine crosses the placenta. Use of reserpine near term has resulted in nasal discharge, retraction, lethargy and anorexia in the newborn (4). Concern over reserpine's ability to deplete catecholamine levels has appeared (5). The significance of this is not known.

Breast Feeding Summary

Reserpine is excreted into breast milk (6). No clinical reports of untoward effects in the nursing infant have been located.

References

1. Heinonen OP, Slone D, Shaprio S. *Birth Defects and Drugs in Pregnancy.* Littleton: Publishing Sciences Group, 1977:376.
2. *Ibid*, 441.
3. *Ibid*, 495.
4. Budnick IS, Leikin S, Hoeck LE. Effect in the newborn infant to reserpine administration ante partum. Am J Dis Child 1955;90:286–9.
5. Towell ME, Hyman AI. Catecholamine depletion in pregnancy. J Obstet Gynaecol Br Commonw 1966;73:431–8.
6. Product information. Smith Kline & French Laboratories, 1980.

Name: **RIFAMPIN**

Class: **Antituberculosis Agent**   Risk Factor: **C**

Fetal Risk Summary

No controlled studies have linked the use of rifampin with congenital defects (1, 2). One report described 9 malformations in 204 pregnancies that went to term (3). This incidence, 4.4%, is similar to the expected frequency of defects in a healthy non-exposed population but higher than the 1.8% rate noted in other tuberculosis patients (3). Rifampin may interfere with oral contraceptives resulting in unplanned pregnancies (see Oral Contraceptives) (4).

Author (ref)	No. Pts.	Indication	Gestational Age	Dose	Other Drugs	Fetal Effects	Comment
Steen (3)	226	Tuberculosis	Throughout	400–600 mg/day	Ethambutol Isoniazid	22 abortions (17 induced) 1 anencephaly 2 hydrocephalus 4 limb malformations 1 renal tract abnormalities 1 congenital hip dislocation	In animals, CNS and skeletal defects are the most common malformations seen.

Breast Feeding Summary

Rifampin is excreted into breast milk in concentrations of 1 to 3 μg/ml (5). No reports describing adverse effects in nursing infants have been located.

References

1. Reimers D. Missbildungen durch Rifampicin. Bericht ueber 2 faelle von normaler fetaler entwicklung nach rifampicin-therapie in der fruehsch wangerschaft. Munchen Med Wochenschr 1971;113:1690.
2. Warkany J. Antituberculous drugs. Teratology 1979;20:133–8.
3. Steen JSM, Stainton-Ellis DM. Rifampicin in pregnancy. Lancet 1977;2:604–5.
4. Gupta KC, Ali MY. Failure of oral contraceptives with rifampicin. Med J Zambia 1980; 15:23.
5. Vorherr H. Drug excretion in breast milk. Postgrad Med J 1974;56:97–104.

Name: **RITODRINE**

Class: **Sympathomimetic (Adrenergic)**   Risk Factor: **B**

Fetal Risk Summary

Ritodrine is a β-sympathomimetic used to prevent premature labor. Its effects on the mother, fetus and newborn have been reviewed in several publications (1–3). Ritodrine crosses the placenta, appearing in cord blood in amounts ranging from 20 to 100% of the maternal level (4). Although no congenital malformations have been observed, use of ritodrine prior to the 20th week of gestation has not been reported. The manufacturer considers ritodrine to be contraindicated before this time (5). Ritodrine increases fetal and maternal heart rates (6). Fetal rates up to 200 beats per minute have been recorded (1–3, 5). Use of ritodrine may result in transient maternal and fetal hyperglycemia followed by increases in levels of serum insulin. If delivery occurs before these effects have terminated (usually 48 to 72 hours), low neonatal blood glucose levels may be observed (6). Ketoacidosis with fetal death has been reported (7). An insulin-dependent diabetic was treated with ritodrine for preterm labor at 28 weeks of gestation. Fetal heart patterns were normal prior to therapy. Maternal hyperglycemia with ketoacidosis developed, and 6 hours later fetal heart activity was undetectable. She was subsequently delivered of a stillborn fetus weighing 970 g.

Ritodrine decreases the incidence of neonatal death and respiratory distress syndrome (8–10). Two-year follow-up studies of infants exposed to *in utero* ritodrine have failed to detect harmful effects on growth, incidence of disease, development or functional maturation (5, 11).

Breast Feeding Summary

No data available.

References

1. Barden TP, Peter JB, Merkatz IR. Ritodrine hydrochloride: a betamimetic agent for use in preterm labor. I. Pharmacology, clinical history, administration, side effects, and safety. Obstet Gynecol 1980;56:1–6.
2. Anonymous. Ritodrine for inhibition of preterm labor. Med Lett Drugs Ther 1980;22:89–90.
3. Finkelstein BW. Ritodrine (Yutopar, Merrell Dow Pharmaceuticals Inc.). Drug Intell Clin Pharm 1981;15:425–33.
4. Gandar R, De Zoeten LW, van der Schoot JB. Serum Levels of ritodrine in man. Eur J Clin Pharmacol 1980;17:117–22.
5. Product information and clinical summary of Yutopar, Merrell-National Laboratories, Inc., Cincinnati, 1980.
6. Leake RD, Hobel CJ, Oh W, Thiebeault DW, Okada DM, Williams PR. A controlled, prospective study of the effects of ritodrine hydrochloride for premature labor (abstract). Clin Res 1980;28:90A.
7. Schilthius MS, Aarnoudse JG. Fetal death associated with severe ritodrine induced ketoacidosis. Lancet 1980;1:1145.
8. Boog G, Ben Brahim M, Gandar R. Beta-mimetic drugs and possible prevention of respiratory distress syndrome. Br J Obstet Gynaecol 1975;82:285–8.
9. Merkatz IR, Peter JB, Barden TP. Ritodrine hydrochloride: a betamimetic agent for use in preterm labor. II. Evidence of efficacy. Obstet Gynecol 1980;56:7–12.
10. Lauersen NH, Merkatz IR, Tejani N, et al. Inhibition of premature labor: a multicenter comparison of ritodrine and ethanol. Am J Obstet Gynecol 1977;127:837–45.
11. Freysz H, Willard D, Lehr A, Messer J, Boog G. A long term evaluation of infants who received a beta-mimetic drug while in utero. J Perinat Med 1977;5:94–9.

S

Name: SALSALATE

Class: **Analgesic/Antipyretic** Risk Factor: **C***

Fetal Risk Summary

See Aspirin.

[*Risk Factor D if used in the 3rd trimester.]

Breast Feeding Summary

See Aspirin.

Name: SCOPOLAMINE

Class: **Parasympatholytic (Anticholinergic)** Risk Factor: **C**

Fetal Risk Summary

Scopolamine is an anticholinergic agent. The Collaborative Perinatal Project monitored 50,282 mother-child pairs, 309 of which used scopolamine in the 1st trimester (1). For anytime use, 881 exposures were recorded (2). In neither case was evidence found for an association with malformations. However, when the group of parasympatholytics were taken as a whole (2,323 exposures), a possible association with minor malformations was found (1). Scopolamine readily crosses the placenta (3). When administered to the mother at term, fetal effects include tachycardia, decreased heart rate variability and decreased heart rate deceleration (4–6). Maternal tachycardia is comparable to that with other anticholinergic agents, such as atropine or glycopyrrolate (7). Scopolamine toxicity in a newborn has been described (8). The mother had received six doses of scopolamine (1.8 mg total) with several other drugs during labor. Symptoms in the female infant consisted of fever, tachycardia and lethargy; she was also "barrel chested" without respiratory depression. Therapy with physostigmine reversed the condition.

Breast Feeding Summary

See Atropine.

References

1. Heinonen OP, Slone D, Shapiro S. *Birth Defects and Drugs in Pregnancy*. Littleton: Publishing Sciences Group, 1977:346–53.

2. *Ibid*, 439.
3. Moya F, Thorndike V. The effects of drugs used in labor on the fetus and newborn. Clin Pharmacol Ther 1963;4:628–53.
4. Shenker L. Clinical experiences with fetal heart rate monitoring of one thousand patients in labor. Am J Obstet Gynecol 1973;115:1111–6.
5. Boehm FH, Growdon JH Jr. The effect of scopolamine on fetal heart rate baseline variability. Am J Obstet Gynecol 1974;120:1099–1104.
6. Ayromlooi J, Tobias M, Berg P. The effects of scopolamine and ancillary analgesics upon the fetal heart rate recording. J Reprod Med 1980;25:323–6.
7. Diaz DM, Diaz SF, Marx GF. Cardiovascular effects of glycopyrrolate and belladonna derivatives in obstetric patients. Bull NY Acad Med 1980;56:245–8.
8. Evens RP, Leopold JC. Scopolamine toxicity in a newborn. Pediatrics 1980;329–30.

Name: **SECOBARBITAL**

Class: **Sedative/Hypnotic**   Risk Factor: **C**

Fetal Risk Summary

No reports linking the use of secobarbital with congenital defects have been located. The Collaborative Perinatal Project monitored 50,282 mother-child pairs, 378 of which had 1st trimester exposure to secobarbital (1). No evidence was found to suggest a relationship to large categories of major or minor malformations or to individual defects. Hemorrhagic disease of the newborn and barbiturate withdrawal are theoretical possibilities (see also Phenobarbital).

Breast Feeding Summary

Secobarbital is excreted into breast milk (2). The amount and effects on the nursing infant are not known.

References

1. Heinonen OP, Slone D, Shapiro S. *Birth Defects and Drugs in Pregnancy*. Littleton: Publishing Sciences Group, 1977:336–7.
2. Wilson JT, Brown RD, Cherek DR, et al. Drug excretion in human breast milk: principles, pharmacokinetics and projected consequences. Clin Pharmacokinet 1980;5:1–66.

Name: **SIMETHICONE**

Class: **Antiflatulent/Defoaming Agent**   Risk Factor: **C**

Fetal Risk Summary

Simethicone is a silicone product that is used as an antiflatulent. No reports linking the use of this agent with congenital defects have been located.

Breast Feeding Summary

No data available.

Name: **SODIUM SALICYLATE**

Class: **Analgesic/Antipyretic**   Risk Factor: **C***

Fetal Risk Summary

See Aspirin.

[*Risk Factor D if used in the 3rd trimester.]

Breast Feeding Summary

See Aspirin.

Name: **SODIUM THIOSALICYLATE**

Class: **Analgesic/Antipyretic**   Risk Factor: **C***

Fetal Risk Summary

See Aspirin.

[*Risk Factor D if used in the 3rd trimester.]

Breast Feeding Summary

See Aspirin.

Name: **SOMATOSTATIN**

Class: **Pituitary Hormone**   Risk Factor: **B**

Fetal Risk Summary

No data available.

Breast Feeding Summary

No data available.

Name: **SPECTINOMYCIN**

Class: **Antibiotic** Risk Factor: **B**

Fetal Risk Summary

No reports linking the use of spectinomycin with congenital defects have been located. The drug has been used to treat gonorrhea in pregnant patients allergic to penicillin. Available data do not suggest a threat to mother or fetus (1, 2).

Breast Feeding Summary

No data available.

References

1. McCormack WM, Finland M. Spectinomycin. Ann Intern Med 1976;84:712–6.
2. Anonymous. Treatment of syphilis and gonorrhea. Med Lett Drugs Ther 1977;19:105–7.

Name: **SPIRONOLACTONE**

Class: **Diuretic** Risk Factor: **D**

Fetal Risk Summary

Spironolactone is a potassium-conserving diuretic. No reports linking it with congenital defects have been located. Messina has commented, however, that spironolactone may be contraindicated during pregnancy based on the known antiandrogenic effects in humans and the feminization observed in male rat fetuses (1). Other investigators consider diuretics in general contraindicated in pregnancy, except for patients with cardiovascular disorders, since they do not prevent or alter the course of toxemia and they may decrease placental perfusion (2–4).

Breast Feeding Summary

No data available.

References

1. Messina M, Biffignandi P, Ghiga E, Jeantet MG, Molinatti GM. Possible contraindication of spironolactone during pregnancy. J Endocrinol Invest 1979;2:222.
2. Pitkin RM, Kaminetzky HA, Newton M, Pritchard JA. Maternal nutrition: a selective review of clinical topics. Obstet Gynecol 1972;40:773–85.
3. Lindheimer MD, Katz AI. Sodium and diuretics in pregnancy. N Engl J Med 1973;288:891–4.
4. Christianson R, Page EW. Diuretic drugs and pregnancy. Obstet Gynecol 1976;48:647–52.

Name: **STREPTOKINASE**

Class: **Thrombolytic**   Risk Factor: **C**

Fetal Risk Summary

No reports linking the use of streptokinase with congenital defects have been located. Only minimal amounts cross the placenta and are not sufficient to cause fibrinolytic effects in the fetus (1–7). Although the passage of streptokinase is blocked by the placenta, streptokinase antibodies do cross to the fetus (5). This passive sensitization would have clinical importance only if the neonate required streptokinase therapy. Ludwig has treated 24 patients in the 2nd and 3rd trimesters without fetal complications (5). Use in the 1st trimester for maternal thrombophlebitis has also been reported (6). No adverse effects were observed in the infant born at term.

Breast Feeding Summary

No data available.

References

1. Pfeifer GW. Distribution and placental transfer of 131-I streptokinase. Aust Ann Med 1970;19(Suppl):17–8.
2. Hall RJC, Young C, Sutton GC, Campbell S. Treatment of acute massive pulmonary embolism by streptokinase during labour and delivery. Br Med J 1972;4:647–9.
3. McTaggart DR, Ingram TG. Massive pulmonary embolism during pregnancy treated with streptokinase. Med J Aust 1977;1:18–20.
4. Benz JJ, Wick A. The problem of fibrinolytic therapy in pregnancy. Schweiz Med Wochenschr 1973;103:1359–63.
5. Ludwig H. Results of streptokinase therapy in deep venous thrombosis during pregnancy. Postgrad Med J 1973;49(Suppl 5):65–7.
6. Walter C, Koestering H. Therapeutische thrombolyse in der neunten schwangerschalftswoche. Dtsch Med Wochenschr 1969;94:32–4.
7. Witchitz S, Veyrat C, Moisson P, Scheinman N, Rozenstajn. Fibrinolytic treatment of thrombus on prosthetic heart valves. Br Heart J 1980;44:545–54.

Name: **STREPTOMYCIN**

Class: **Antibiotic**   Risk Factor: **D**

Fetal Risk Summary

Streptomycin is an aminoglycoside antibiotic. The drug rapidly crosses the placenta into the fetal circulation and amniotic fluid, obtaining concentrations usually less than 50% of the maternal serum level (1, 2). Early investigators, well aware of streptomycin-induced ototoxicity, were unable to observe this defect in infants exposed *in utero* to the agent (3–5). Eventually, ototoxicity was described in a 2-½-month-old infant whose mother had been treated for tuberculosis with 30 g of streptomycin during the last month of pregnancy (6).

The infant was deaf with a negative cochleopalpebral reflex. Several other case reports and small surveys describing similar toxicity followed this initial report (7, 8). In general, however, the incidence of congenital ototoxicity, cochlear or vestibular, from streptomycin is low, especially with careful dosage calculations and if the duration of fetal exposure is limited (9).

Except for eighth cranial nerve damage, no reports of congenital defects due to streptomycin have been located. The Collaborative Perinatal Project monitored 50,282 mother-child pairs, 135 of which had 1st trimester exposure to streptomycin (10). For use anytime during pregnancy, 355 exposures were recorded (11). In neither case was evidence found to suggest a relationship to large categories of major or minor malformations or to individual defects.

In a group of 1,619 newborns whose mothers were treated for tuberculosis during pregnancy with multiple drugs, including streptomycin, the incidence of congenital defects was the same as a healthy control group (2.34% vs 2.56%) (12). Other investigators had previously concluded that the use of streptomycin in pregnant tuberculosis patients was not teratogenic (13).

Breast Feeding Summary

Streptomycin is excreted into breast milk. Milk:plasma ratios of 0.5 to 1.0 have been reported (14). Since the oral absorption of this antibiotic is poor, ototoxicity in the infant would not be expected. However, three potential problems exist for the nursing infant: modification of bowel flora, direct effects on the infant and interference with the interpretation of culture results if a fever work-up is required.

References

1. Woltz J, Wiley M. Transmission of streptomycin from maternal blood to the fetal circulation and the amniotic fluid. Proc Soc Exp Biol Med 1945;60:106–7.
2. Heilman D, Heilman F, Hinshaw H, Nichols D, Herrell W. Streptomycin: absorption, diffusion, excretion and toxicity. Am J Med Sci 1945;210:576–84.
3. Watson E, Stow R. Streptomycin therapy: effects on fetus. JAMA 1948;137:1599–1600.
4. Rubin A, Winston J, Rutledge M. Effects of streptomycin upon the human fetus. Am J Dis Child 1951;82:14–6.
5. Kistner R. The use of streptomycin during pregnancy. Am J Obstet Gynecol 1950;60:422–6.
6. Lerox M. Existe-t-il une surdite congenitale acquise due a la streptomycine? Am Otolaryngol 1950;67:194–6.
7. Nishimura H, Tanimura T. Clinical Aspects of the Teratogenicity of Drugs. Amsterdam: Excerpta Medica, 1976:130.
8. Donald PR, Sellars SL. Streptomycin ototoxicity in the unborn child. S Afr Med J 1981;60:316–8.
9. Mann J, Moskowitz R. Plaque and pregnancy. A case report. JAMA 1977;237:1854–5.
10. Heinonen OP, Slone D, Shapiro S. Birth Defects and Drugs in Pregnancy. Littleton: Publishing Sciences Group, 1977:297–301.
11. Ibid, 435.
12. Marynowski A, Sianozecka E. Comparison of the incidence of congenital malformations in neonates from healthy mothers and from patients treated because of tuberculosis. Ginekol Pol 1972;43:713–5.
13. Lowe C. Congenital defects among children born under supervision or treatment for pulmonary tuberculosis. Br J Prev Soc Med 1964;18:14–6.
14. Wilson JT. Milk/plasma ratios and contraindicated drugs. In Wilson JT, ed. Drugs in Breast Milk. Australia: ADIS Press, 1981:79.

Name: **SUCCINYLSULFATHIAZOLE**

Class: **Anti-infective**   Risk Factor: **B***

Fetal Risk Summary

See Sulfonamides.

[* Risk Factor D if administered near term.]

Breast Feeding Summary

See Sulfonamides.

Name: **SULFACETAMIDE**

Class: **Anti-infective**   Risk Factor: **B***

Fetal Risk Summary

See Sulfonamides.

[* Risk Factor D if administered near term.]

Breast Feeding Summary

See Sulfonamides.

Name: **SULFACHLORPYRIDAZINE**

Class: **Anti-infective**   Risk Factor: **B***

Fetal Risk Summary

See Sulfonamides.

[* Risk Factor D if administered near term.]

Breast Feeding Summary

See Sulfonamides.

Name: **SULFACYTINE**

Class: **Anti-infective**   Risk Factor: **B***

Fetal Risk Summary

See Sulfonamides.

[* Risk Factor D if administered near term.]

Breast Feeding Summary

See Sulfonamides.

Name: **SULFADIAZINE**

Class: **Anti-infective**   Risk Factor: **B***

Fetal Risk Summary

See Sulfonamides.

[* Risk Factor D if administered near term.]

Breast Feeding Summary

See Sulfonamides.

Name: **SULFADIMETHOXINE**

Class: **Anti-infective**   Risk Factor: **B***

Fetal Risk Summary

See Sulfonamides.

[* Risk Factor D if administered near term.]

Breast Feeding Summary

See Sulfonamides.

Name: **SULFADOXINE**
Class: **Anti-infective**   Risk Factor: **B***

Fetal Risk Summary
See Sulfonamides.

[* Risk Factor D if administered near term.]

Breast Feeding Summary
See Sulfonamides.

Name: **SULFAETHIDOLE**
Class: **Anti-infective**   Risk Factor: **B***

Fetal Risk Summary
See Sulfonamides.

[* Risk Factor D if administered near term.]

Breast Feeding Summary
See Sulfonamides.

Name: **SULFAGUANIDINE**
Class: **Anti-infective**   Risk Factor: **B***

Fetal Risk Summary
See Sulfonamides.

[* Risk Factor D if administered near term.]

Breast Feeding Summary
See Sulfonamides.

Name: **SULFAMERAZINE**

Class: **Anti-infective**   Risk Factor: **B***

Fetal Risk Summary

See Sulfonamides.

[* Risk Factor D if administered near term.]

Breast Feeding Summary

See Sulfonamides.

Name: **SULFAMETHAZINE**

Class: **Anti-infective**   Risk Factor: **B***

Fetal Risk Summary

See Sulfonamides.

[* Risk Factor D if administered near term.]

Breast Feeding Summary

See Sulfonamides.

Name: **SULFAMETHIZOLE**

Class: **Anti-infective**   Risk Factor: **B***

Fetal Risk Summary

See Sulfonamides.

[* Risk Factor D if administered near term.]

Breast Feeding Summary

See Sulfonamides.

Name: **SULFAMETHOXAZOLE**

Class: **Anti-infective**   Risk Factor: **B***

Fetal Risk Summary

See Sulfonamides.

[* Risk Factor D if administered near term.]

Breast Feeding Summary

See Sulfonamides.

Name: **SULFAMETHOXYDIAZINE**

Class: **Anti-infective**   Risk Factor: **B***

Fetal Risk Summary

See Sulfonamides.

[* Risk Factor D if administered near term.]

Breast Feeding Summary

See Sulfonamides.

Name: **SULFAMETHOXYPYRIDAZINE**

Class: **Anti-infective**   Risk Factor: **B***

Fetal Risk Summary

See Sulfonamides.

[* Risk Factor D if administered near term.]

Breast Feeding Summary

See Sulfonamides.

Name: **SULFAMETOPYRAZINE**

Class: **Anti-infective**   Risk Factor: **B***

Fetal Risk Summary

See Sulfonamides.

[* Risk Factor D if administered near term.]

Breast Feeding Summary

See Sulfonamides.

Name: **SULFANILAMIDE**

Class: **Anti-infective**   Risk Factor: **B***

Fetal Risk Summary

See Sulfonamides.

[* Risk Factor D if administered near term.]

Breast Feeding Summary

See Sulfonamides.

Name: **SULFANILCARBAMIDE**

Class: **Anti-infective**   Risk Factor: **B***

Fetal Risk Summary

See Sulfonamides.

[* Risk Factor D if administered near term.]

Breast Feeding Summary

See Sulfonamides.

Name: SULFAPHENAZOLE

Class: **Anti-infective**   Risk Factor: **B***

Fetal Risk Summary

See Sulfonamides.

[* Risk Factor D if administered near term.]

Breast Feeding Summary

See Sulfonamides.

Name: SULFAPYRIDINE

Class: **Anti-infective**   Risk Factor: **B***

Fetal Risk Summary

See Sulfonamides.

[* Risk Factor D if administered near term.]

Breast Feeding Summary

See Sulfonamides.

Name: SULFASALAZINE

Class: **Anti-infective**   Risk Factor: **B***

Fetal Risk Summary

Sulfasalazine is a compound composed of 5-aminosalicylic acid (5-ASA) joined to sulfapyridine by an azo- linkage (refer to Sulfonamides for a complete review of this class of agents). Sulfasalazine is used for the treatment of ulcerative colitis and Crohn's disease. No increase in congenital defects or newborn toxicity has been observed from its use in pregnancy (1–7). Only one report has associated sulfasalazine with congenital deformities (see table below) (8). Sulfasalazine and its metabolite, sulfapyridine, readily cross the placenta to the fetal circulation (5, 6). Fetal concentrations are approximately the same as maternal concentrations. Placental transfer of 5-ASA is limited since only negligible amounts are absorbed from the cecum and colon, and this is rapidly excreted in the urine (9).

At birth, concentrations of sulfasalazine and sulfapyridine in 11 infants were 4.6 and 18.2 µg/ml, respectively (6). Neither of these levels were sufficient to cause significant displacement of bilirubin from albumin (6). Kernicterus and severe neonatal jaundice have not been reported following maternal use of sulfasalazine, even when the drug was given up to the time of delivery (6, 7). Caution is advised, however, since other sulfonamides have caused jaundice in the newborn when given near term (see Sulfonamides).

Sulfasalazine may adversely affect spermatogenesis in male patients with inflammatory bowel disease (10, 11). Sperm counts and motility are both reduced and require two months or longer after stopping the drug to return to normal levels (10).

Author (ref)	No. Pts.	Indica- tion	Gestational Age	Dose	Other Drugs	Fetal Effects	Comment
Craxi (8)	1	Ulcerative colitis	Throughout	3 g/day	Not stated	Full term female infant—ex- pired Bilateral cleft lip/palate Severe hydrocephalus	

[* Risk Factor D if administered near term.]

Breast Feeding Summary

Sulfapyridine (SP) is excreted into breast milk (see also Sulfonamides) (5, 9). Unmetabolized sulfasalazine (SASP) was detected in one study but not in another (see table below). Levels of 5-aminosalicyclic acid were undetectable. No adverse effects were observed in the four infants exposed to the drug in milk (5, 9).

Author (ref)	No. Pts.	Dose	Concentration (μg/ml)		M:P Ratio	Effect on Infant
			Serum	Milk		
Azad Khan (5)	3	2 g/day	8.8 (SASP) 19.0 (SP)	2.7 (SASP) 10.3 (SP)	0.3 (SASP) 0.5 (SP)	None mentioned
Berlin (9)	1	2 g/day	0 (SASP) 12.0 (SP) 17.9 (SP)	0 (SASP) 7.5 (SP) 10.7 (SP)	— 0.63 0.60 (repeat test 1 month after 1st sample)	Infant urine contained 3–4 μg/ml (1.2–1.6 mg/24 hr or 30–40% of total dose in milk)

References

1. McEwan HP. Anorectal conditions in obstetric practice. Proc R Soc Med 1972;65:279–81.
2. Willoughby CP, Truelove SC. Ulcerative colitis and pregnancy. Gut 1980;21:469–74.
3. Levy N, Roisman I, Teodor I. Ulcerative colitis in pregnancy in Israel. Dis Colon Rectum 1981;24:351–4.
4. Mogadam M, Dobbins WO III, Korelitz BI, Ahmed SW. Pregnancy in inflammatory bowel disease: effect of sulfasalazine and corticosteroids on fetal outcome. Gastroenterology 1981;80:72–6.
5. Azad Khan AK, Truelove SC. Placental and mammary transfer of sulphasalazine. Br Med J 1979;2:1553.
6. Jarnerot G, Into-Malmberg MB, Esbjorner E. Placental transfer of sulphasalazine and sulpha- pyridine and some of its metabolites. Scand J Gastroenterol 1981;16:693–7.
7. Modadam M. Sulfasalazine, IBD, and pregnancy: reply. Gastroenterology 1981;81:194.
8. Craxi A, Pagliarello F. Possible embryotoxicity of sulfasalazine. Arch Intern Med 1980;140:1674.
9. Berlin CM Jr, Yaffe SJ. Disposition of salicylazosulfapyridine (Azulfidine) and metabolites in human breast milk. Dev Pharmacol Ther 1980;1:31–9.

10. Toovey S, Hudson E, Hendry WF, Levi AJ. Sulphasalazine and male infertility: reversibility and possible mechanism. Gut 1981;22:445–51.
11. Freeman JG, Reece VAC, Venables CW. Sulphasalazine and spermatogenesis. Digestion 1982;23:68–71.

Name: **SULFASYMAZINE**

Class: **Anti-infective**   Risk Factor: **B***

Fetal Risk Summary

See Sulfonamides.

[* Risk Factor D if administered near term.]

Breast Feeding Summary

See Sulfonamides.

Name: **SULFATHIAZOLE**

Class: **Anti-infective**   Risk Factor: **B***

Fetal Risk Summary

See Sulfonamides.

[* Risk Factor D if administered near term.]

Breast Feeding Summary

See Sulfonamides.

Name: **SULFISOXAZOLE**

Class: **Anti-infective**   Risk Factor: **B***

Fetal Risk Summary

See Sulfonamides.

[* Risk Factor D if administered near term.]

Breast Feeding Summary

See Sulfonamides.

Name: **SULFONAMIDES**
Class: **Anti-infective**   Risk Factor: **B***

Fetal Risk Summary

Sulfonamides are a large class of antibacterial agents. While there are differences in their bioavailability, all share similar actions in the fetal and newborn periods, and they will be considered as a single group. The sulfonamides readily cross the placenta to the fetus during all stages of gestation (1–9). Equilibrium with maternal blood is usually established after 2 to 3 hours, with fetal levels averaging 70 to 90% of maternal. Significant levels may persist in the newborn for several days after birth when given near term. The primary danger of sulfonamide administration during pregnancy is manifested when these agents are given close to delivery. Toxicities that may be observed in the newborn include jaundice, hemolytic anemia and, theoretically, kernicterus. Severe jaundice in the newborn has been related to maternal sulfonamide ingestion at term by several authors (10–15). Premature infants seem especially prone to development of hyperbilirubinemia (14). However, a study of 94 infants exposed to sulfadiazine *in utero* for maternal prophylaxis of rheumatic fever failed to show an increase in prematurity, hyperbilirubinemia or kernicterus (16). Hemolytic anemia has been reported in two newborns and in a fetus following *in utero* exposure to sulfonamides (10, 11, 15). Both newborns survived. In the case involving the fetus, the mother had homozygous glucose-6-phosphate dehydrogenase (G-6-PD) deficiency (15). She was treated with sulfisoxazole for a urinary tract infection 2 weeks prior to delivery of a stillborn male infant. Autopsy revealed a 36-week infant with maceration, severe anemia and hydrops fetalis.

Sulfonamides compete with bilirubin for binding to plasma albumin. *In utero*, the fetus clears free bilirubin by the placental circulation, but after birth, this mechanism is no longer available. Unbound bilirubin is free to cross the blood-brain barrier and may result in kernicterus. While this toxicity is well known when sulfonamides are administered directly to the neonate, kernicterus in the newborn following *in utero* exposure has not been reported.

Most reports of sulfonamide exposure during gestation have failed to demonstrate an association with congenital malformations (9, 10, 17–23). Offspring of patients treated throughout pregnancy with sulfasalazine (sulfapyridine plus 5-aminosalicylic acid) for ulcerative colitis or Crohn's disease have not shown an increase in adverse effects (see also Sulfasalazine) (9, 20, 22). In contrast, a retrospective study of 1,369 patients found that significantly more mothers of 458 infants with congenital malformations took sulfonamides than did mothers in the control group (24). A 1975 study examined the *in utero* drug exposures of 599 children born with oral clefts (25). A significant difference ($p < 0.05$), as compared with matched controls, was found with 1st and 2nd trimester sulfonamide use only when other defects, in addition to the clefts, were present.

Sulfonamides are teratogenic in some species of animals, a finding which has prompted warnings of human teratogenicity (26, 27). In 2 reports, inves-tigators associated *in utero* sulfonamide exposure with tracheoeosophageal fistula and cataracts, but additional descriptions of these effects have not appeared (28, 29). A mother treated for food poisoning with sulfaguanidine in early pregnancy delivered a child with multiple anomalies (30). The author attributed the defects to use of the drug.

The Collaborative Perinatal Project monitored 50,282 mother-child pairs, 1,455 of which had 1st trimester exposure to sulfonamides (31). For use anytime during pregnancy, 5,689 exposures were reported (32). In neither case was evidence found to suggest a relationship to large categories of major or minor malformations. Several possible associations were found with individ-ual defects after anytime use but the statistical significance of these are not known (33). Independent confirmation is required.

Ductus arteriosus persistens (8 cases)
Coloboma (4 cases)
Hypoplasia of limb or part thereof (7 cases)
Miscellaneous foot defects (4 cases)
Urethral obstruction (13 cases)
Hypoplasia/atrophy of adrenals (6 cases)
Benign tumors (12 cases)

Taken in sum, sulfonamides do not appear to pose a significant teratogenic risk. Due to the potential toxicity to the newborn, these agents should be avoided near term.

[* Risk Factor D if used in the 3rd trimester.]

Breast Feeding Summary

Sulfonamides are excreted into breast milk in low concentrations. Milk levels of sulfanilamide (free and conjugated) are reported to range from 6 to 94 μg/ml (3, 34–39). Up to 1.6% of the total dose could be recovered from the milk (34, 37). Milk levels often exceeded serum levels and persisted for several days after maternal consumption of the drug was stopped. Milk:plasma ratios during therapy with sulfanilamide were 0.5 to 0.6 (38). Reports of adverse effects in nursing infants are rare. Von Friesen found reports of diarrhea and rash in breast-fed infants whose mothers were receiving sulfapyridine or sulfathiazole (6). Milk levels of sulfapyridine, the active metabolite of sulfa-salazine, were 10.3 μg/ml, a M:P ratio of 0.5 (9). Based on this data, the nursing infant would receive approximately 3 to 4 mg/kg of sulfapyridine per day, an apparently non-toxic amount for a healthy neonate (16). Sulfisoxazole, a very water-soluble drug, was reported to produce a low M:P ratio of 0.06 (40). The conjugated form achieved a ratio of 0.22. The total amount of sulfisoxazole recovered in milk over 48 hours after a 4-g divided dose was only 0.45%. Although controversial, breast feeding during maternal adminis-tration of sulfisoxazole seems to present a very low risk for the healthy neonate (41, 42).

In summary, sulfonamide excretion into breast milk apparently does not pose a significant risk for the healthy, full term neonate. Exposure to sulfonamides *via* breast milk should be avoided in premature infants and in infants with hyperbilirubinemia or G-6-PD deficiency.

References

1. Barker RH. The placental transfer of sulfanilamide. N Engl J Med 1938;219:41.
2. Speert H. The passage of sulfanilamide through the human placenta. Bull Johns Hopkins Hosp 1938;63:337-9.
3. Stewart HL Jr, Pratt JP. Sulfanilamide excretion in human breast milk and effect on breast-fed babies. JAMA 1938;111:1456-8.
4. Speert H. The placental transmission of sulfanilamide and its effects upon the fetus and newborn. Bull Johns Hopkins Hosp 1940;66:139-55.
5. Speert H. Placental transmission of sulfathiazole and sulfadiazine and its significance for fetal chemotherapy. Am J Obstet Gynecol 1943;45:200-7.
6. von Freisen B. A study of small dose sulphamerazine prophylaxis in obstetrics. Acta Obstet Gynecol Scand 1951;31(Suppl):75-116.
7. Sparr RA, Pritchard JA. Maternal and newborn distribution and excretion of sulfamethoxy-pyridazine (Kynex). Obstet Gynecol 1958;12:131-4.
8. Nishimura H, Tanimura T. *Clinical Aspects of the Teratogenicity of Drugs.* Amsterdam: Excerpta Medica, 1976:88.
9. Azad Khan AK, Truelove SC. Placental and mammary transfer of sulphasalazine. Br Med J 1979;2:1553.
10. Heckel GP. Chemotherapy during pregnancy. Danger of fetal injury from sulfanilamide and its derivatives. JAMA 1941;117:1314-6.
11. Ginzler AM, Cherner C. Toxic manifestations in the newborn infant following placental transmission of sulfanilamide. With a report of 2 cases simulating erythroblastosis fetalis. Am J Obstet Gynecol 1942;44:46-55.
12. Lucey JF, Driscoll TJ Jr. Hazard to newborn infants of administration of long-acting sulfona-mides to pregnant women. Pediatrics 1959;24:498-9.
13. Kantor HI, Sutherland DA, Leonard JT, Kamholz FH, Fry ND, White WL. Effect on bilirubin metabolism in the newborn of sulfisoxazole administration to the mother. Obstet Gynecol 1961;17:494-500.
14. Dunn PM. The possible relationship between the maternal administration of sulphamethoxy-pyridazine and hyperbilirubinaemia in the newborn. J Obstet Gynaecol Br Commonw 1964;71:128-31.
15. Perkins RP. Hydrops fetalis and stillbirth in a male glucose-6-phosphate dehydrogenase-deficient fetus possibly due to maternal ingestion of sulfisoxazole. Am J Obstet Gynecol 1971;111:379-81.
16. Baskin CG, Law S, Wenger NK. Sulfadiazine rheumatic fever prophylaxis during pregnancy: does it increase the risk of kernicterus in the newborn? Cardiology 1980;65:222-5.
17. Bonze EJ, Fuerstner PG, Falls FH. Use of sulfanilamide derivative in treatment of gonorrhea in pregnant and nonpregnant women. Am J Obstet Gynecol 1939;38:73-9.
18. Carter MP, Wilson F. Antibiotics and congenital malformations. Lancet 1963;1:1267-8.
19. Little PJ. The incidence of urinary infection in 5000 pregnant women. Lancet 1966;2:925-8.
20. McEwan HP. Anorectal conditions in obstetric patients. Proc R Soc Med 1972;65:279-81.
21. Williams JD, Smith EK. Single-dose therapy with streptomycin and sulfametopyrazine for bacteriuria during pregnancy. Br Med J 1970;4:651-3.
22. Mogadam M, Dobbins WO III, Korelitz BI, Ahmed SW. Pregnancy in inflammatory bowel disease: effect of sulfasalazine and corticosteroids on fetal outcome. Gastroenterology 1981;80:72-6.
23. Richards IDG. A retrospective inquiry into possible teratogenic effects of drugs in pregnancy. Adv Exp Med Biol 1972;27:441-55.
24. Nelson MM, Forfar JO. Association between drugs administered during pregnancy and congenital abnormalities of the fetus. Br Med J 1971;1:523-7.
25. Saxen I. Associations between oral clefts and drugs taken during pregnancy. Int J Epidemiol 1975;4:37-44.
26. Anonymous. Teratogenic effects of sulphonamides. Br Med J 1965;1:142.
27. Green KG. "Bimez" and teratogenic action. Br Med J 1963;2:56.

28. Ingalls TH, Prindle RA. Esophageal atresia with tracheoeosophageal fistula. Epidemiologic and teratologic implications. N Engl J Med 1949;240:987–95.
29. Harly JD, Farrar JF, Gray JB, Dunlop IC. Aromatic drugs and congenital cataracts. Lancet 1964;1:472–3.
30. Pogorzelska E. A case of multiple congenital anomalies in a child of a mother treated with sulfaguanidine. Patol Pol 1966;17:383–6.
31. Heinonen OP, Slone D, Shapiro S. Birth Defects and Drugs in Pregnancy. Littleton: Publishing Sciences Group, 1977:296–313.
32. Ibid, 435.
33. Ibid, 485–6.
34. Adair FL, Hesseltine HC, Hac LR. Experimental study of the behavior of sulfanilamide. JAMA 1938;111:766–70.
35. Hepburn JS, Paxson NF, Rogers AN. Secretion of ingested sulfanilamide in breast milk and in the urine of the infant. J Biol Chem 1938;123:LIV–LV.
36. Pinto SS. Excretion of sulfanilamide and acetylsulfanilamide in human milk. JAMA 1938;111:1914–6.
37. Hac LR, Adair FL, Hesseltine HC. Excretion of sulfanilamide and acetylsulfanilamide in human breast milk. Am J Obstet Gynecol 1939;38:57–66.
38. Foster FP. Sulfanilamide excretion in breast milk: report of a case. Proc Staff Meet Mayo Clin 1939;14:153–5.
39. Hepburn JS, Paxson NF, Rogers AN. Secretion of ingested sulfanilamide in human milk and in the urine of the nursing infant. Arch Pediatr 1942;59:413–8.
40. Kauffman RE, O'Brien C, Gilford P. Sulfisoxazole secretion into human milk. J Pediatr 1980;97:839–41.
41. Elliott GT, Quinn SI. Sulfisoxazole in human milk. J Pediatr 1981;99:171–2.
42. Kauffman RE. Reply. J Pediatr 1981;99:172.

Name: **SULINDAC**

Class: **Nonsteroidal Anti-inflammatory**   Risk Factor: **B***

Fetal Risk Summary

No reports linking the use of sulindac with congenital defects have been located. Theoretically, sulindac, a prostaglandin synthetase inhibitor, could cause constriction of the ductus arteriosus in utero (1). Persistent pulmonary hypertension of the newborn should also be considered (2). Drugs in this class have been shown to inhibit labor and prolong pregnancy (2). The manufacturer recommends that the drug not be used during pregnancy (3).

[* Risk Factor D if used in the 3rd trimester or near delivery.]

Breast Feeding Summary

No data available (4). The manufacturer recommends that the drug not be used when breast feeding (3).

References

1. Levin DL. Effects of inhibition of prostaglandin synthesis on fetal development, oxygenation, and the fetal circulation. Semin Perinatol 1980;4:35–44.
2. Fuchs F. Prevention of prematurity. Am J Obstet Gynecol 1976;126:809–20.
3. Product information. Clinoril. Merck Sharp & Dohme, 1982.
4. Personal communication. Whalen JJ, Merck Sharp & Dohme, 1981.

Name: **TENIPOSIDE**

Class: **Antineoplastic**   Risk Factor: **D**

Fetal Risk Summary

Teniposide, a podophyllin derivative, has been used in the 2nd and 3rd trimesters of one pregnancy (1). An apparently normal infant was delivered at 37 weeks of gestation. Long term studies of growth and mental development in offspring exposed to antineoplastic agents during the 2nd trimester, the period of neuroblast multiplication, have not been conducted (2).

Breast Feeding Summary

No data available.

References

1. Lowenthal RM, Funnell CF, Hope DM, Stewart IG, Humphrey DC. Normal infant after combination chemotherapy including teniposide for Burkitt's lymphoma in pregnancy. Med Pediatr Oncol 1982;10:165–9.
2. Dobbing J. Pregnancy and leukaemia. Lancet 1977;1:1155.

Name: **TERBUTALINE**

Class: **Sympathomimetic (Adrenergic)**   Risk Factor: **B**

Fetal Risk Summary

No reports linking the use of terbutaline with congenital defects have been located. Terbutaline, a β-sympathomimetic, has been used to prevent premature labor (see also parent compound Metaproterenol). Haller has recently reviewed the use of this drug as a tocolytic agent (1). Terbutaline may cause fetal and maternal tachycardia (1–4). Fetal rates are usually less than 175 beats per minute (3). Drops in maternal blood pressure may occur, but fetal distress as a consequence has not been observed (4, 5). Like all β-mimetics, terbutaline may cause transient maternal hyperglycemia followed by an increase in serum insulin levels (1, 6). Sustained neonatal hypoglycemia may be observed if maternal effects have not terminated prior to delivery (6). Terbutaline decreases the incidence of neonatal respiratory distress syndrome similar to other β-mimetics (7). Long term evaluation of infants exposed to *in utero* terbutaline has been reported (8). No harmful effects in the infants (2 to 12 months) were found.

Breast Feeding Summary

No data available.

References

1. Haller DL. The use of terbutaline for premature labor. Drug Intell Clin Pharm 1980;14:757–64.
2. Andersson KE, Bengtsson LP, Gustafson I, Ingermarsson I. The relaxing effect of terbutaline on the human uterus during term labor. Am J Obstet Gynecol 1975;121:602–9.
3. Ingermarrson I. Effect of terbutaline on premature labor. A double-blind placebo-controlled study. Am J Obstet Gynecol 1976;125:520–4.
4. Ravindran R, Viegas OJ, Padilla LM, LaBlonde P. Anesthetic considerations in pregnant patients receiving terbutaline therapy. Anesth Analg (Clev) 1980;59:391–2.
5. Vargas GC, Macedo GJ, Amved AR, Lowenberg FE. Terbutaline, a new uterine inhibitor. Ginecol Obstet Mex 1974;36:75–88.
6. Epstein MF, Nicholls RN, Stubblefield PG. Neonatal hypoglycemia after beta-sympathomimetic tocolytic therapy. J Pediatr 1979;94:449–53.
7. Bergman B, Hedner T. Antepartum administration of terbutaline and the incidence of hyaline membrane disease in preterm infants. Acta Obstet Gynecol Scand 1978;57:217–21.
8. Wallace R, Caldwell D, Ansbacher R, Otterson W. Inhibition of premature labor by terbutaline. Obstet Gynecol 1978;51:387–93.

Name: **TETRACYCLINE**

Class: **Antibiotic**   Risk Factor: **D**

Fetal Risk Summary

Tetracyclines are a class of antibiotics that should be used with extreme caution, if at all, in pregnancy. The following discussion, unless otherwise noted, applies to all members of this class. Problems attributable to the use of the tetracyclines during or around the gestational period can be classified into four areas:

  Adverse effects on fetal teeth and bones

  Maternal liver toxicity

  Congenital defects

  Miscellaneous effects

  Placental transfer of a tetracycline was first demonstrated by Guilbeau in 1950 (1). The tetracyclines were considered safe for the mother and fetus and were routinely used for maternal infections during the following decade (2–5). It was not until 1961 that Cohlan observed an intense yellow-gold fluorescence in the mineralized structures of a fetal skeleton whose mother had taken tetracycline just prior to delivery (6). Harcourt followed this report with the description of a 2-year-old child whose erupted deciduous teeth formed normally but were stained a bright yellow due to tetracycline exposure *in utero* (7). Fluorescence under ultraviolet light and yellow-colored deciduous teeth which eventually changed to yellow-brown were associated with maternal tetracycline ingestion during pregnancy by several other investigators (8-22). An increase in enamel hypoplasia and caries was initially suspected but later shown not to be related to *in utero* tetracycline exposure (14, 15, 22). Newborn growth and development were normal in all of these reports, although tetracycline has been shown to cause inhibition of fibula growth in premature infants (6). The mechanism for the characteristic dental defect produced by tetracycline is due to the potent chelating ability of the drug (13). Tetracycline forms a complex with calcium orthophosphate and becomes incorporated into bones and teeth undergoing calcification. In the latter structure, this complex causes a permanent discoloration, as remodeling and calcium exchange do not occur after calcification is completed. Since the deciduous teeth begin to calcify at around 5 or 6 months *in utero*, use of tetracycline after this time will result in staining.

The first case linking tetracycline with acute fatty liver of pregnancy was described by Schultz in 1963, although two earlier papers reported the disease without associating it with the drug (23-25). This rare but often fatal syndrome usually follows intravenous dosing of more than 2 g per day. Many of the pregnant patients were being treated for pyelonephritis (24-37). The disease may also be due to non-drug causes. The symptoms include jaundice, azotemia, acidosis and terminal, irreversible shock. Pancreatitis and nonoliguric renal failure are often related findings. The fetus may not be affected directly, but as a result of the maternal pathology, stillborns and premature births are common. In an experimental study, Allen demonstrated that increasing doses of tetracycline caused increasing fatty metamorphosis of the liver (38). The possibility that chronic maternal use of tetracycline before conception could result in fatal hepatotoxicity of pregnancy was recently raised (36). The authors speculated that tetracycline deposited in the bone of a 21-year-old patient was released during pregnancy, resulting in liver damage.

The Collaborative Perinatal Project monitored 50,282 mother-child pairs, 341 of which had 1st trimester exposure to tetracycline, 14 to chlortetracycline, 90 to demeclocycline and 119 to oxytetracycline (39). For use anytime in pregnancy, 1,336 exposures were recorded for tetracycline, 0 for chlortetracycline, 280 for demeclocycline and 328 for oxytetracycline (40). The findings of this study were:

Tetracycline: Evidence was found to suggest a relationship to minor, but not major, malformations. Three possible associations were found with individual defects, but the statistical significance of these are unknown (41). Independent confirmation is required to determine the actual risk.

Hypospadias (1st trimester only) (5 cases)

Inguinal hernia (25 cases)

Hypoplasia of limb or part thereof (6 cases)

Chlortetracycline: No evidence was found to suggest a relationship to large categories of major or minor malformations or to individual defects. However, the sample size is extremely small and safety should not be inferred from these negative results.

Demeclocycline: Evidence was found to suggest a relationship to major or minor malformations but the sample size is small (39). Two possible associations were found with individual defects, but the statistical significance of these are unknown (41). Independent confirmation is required to determine the actual risk.

Clubfoot (1st trimester only) (3 cases)

Inguinal hernia (8 cases)

Oxytetracycline: Evidence was found to suggest a relationship to major and minor malformations (39). One possible association was found with individual defects, but the statistical significance of this is unknown (41). Independent confirmation is required to determine the actual risk.

Inguinal hernia (14 cases)

In 1962, a woman treated with tetracycline in the 1st trimester for acute bronchitis delivered an infant with congenital defects of both hands (42, 43). The mother had a history of minor congenital defects on her side of the family and doubt was cast on the role of the drug in this anomaly (44).

A possible association between the use of tetracyclines in pregnancy or during lactation and congenital cataracts has been reported in 4 patients (45). The effects of other drugs, including several antibiotics and maternal infection, could not be determined and a causal relationship to the tetracyclines seems remote.

An infant with multiple anomalies whose mother had been treated with clomocycline for acne daily during the first 8 weeks of pregnancy has been described (46). Some of the defects, particularly the incomplete fibrous ankylosis and bone changes, made the authors suspect this tetracycline as the likely cause.

Under miscellaneous effects, two reports have appeared which, although they do not directly relate to effects on the fetus, do directly affect pregnancy. In 1974, Briggs observed that a one-week administration of 500 mg of chlortetracycline per day to male subjects was sufficient to produce sperm levels of the drug averaging 4.5 $\mu g/ml$ (47). He theorized that tetracycline overdose could modify the fertilizing capacity of human sperm by inhibiting capacitation. Finally, a possible interaction between oral contraceptives and tetracycline resulting in pregnancy has been reported (48). The mechanism for this interaction may involve the interruption of enterohepatic circulation of contraceptive steroids by inhibiting gut bacterial hydrolysis of steroid conjugates resulting in a lower concentration of circulating steroids.

Breast Feeding Summary

Tetracycline is excreted into breast milk in low concentrations. Milk:plasma ratios vary between 0.25 and 1.5 (4, 49, 50). Theoretically, dental staining and inhibition of bone growth could occur in breast-fed infants whose mothers were consuming tetracycline. However, this theoretical possibility seems remote, since tetracycline serum levels in infants exposed in such a manner were undectable (less than 0.05 $\mu g/ml$) (4). Three potential problems may exist for the nursing infant even though there are no reports in this regard:

modification of bowel flora, direct effects on the infant and interference with the interpretation of culture results if a fever work-up is required.

Author (ref)	No. Pts.	Dose	Concentration (μg/ml)		M:P Ratio	Effect on Infant
			Serum	Milk		
Posner (4)	5	2 g/day for 3 days	1.92	1.14	0.59	Drug not detectable in serum of infants (less than 0.05 μg/ml)
Knowles (49)	2	1.5–2.0 g/day	8.0	1–2.5	0.25–1.5	—
	Not stated	2.5 g once	—	4 (at 8 hr)	—	—
Graf (50)	1	275 mg/day intravenous (pyrrolidino-methyl form)	—	—	1.5	—

References

1. Guilbeau JA, Schoenbach EG, Schaub IG, Latham DV. Aureomycin in obstetrics: therapy and prophylaxis. JAMA 1950;143:520–6.
2. Charles D. Placental transmission of antibiotics. J Obstet Gynaecol Br Emp 1954;61:750–7.
3. Gibbons RJ, Reichelderfer TE. Transplacental transmission of demethychlortetracycline and toxicity studies in premature and full term newly born infants. Antibiot Med Clin Ther 1960;7:618–22.
4. Posner AC, Prigot A, Konicoff NG. Further observations on the use of tetracycline hydrochloride in prophylaxis and treatment of obstetric infections. In Antibiotics Annual, 1954–55, New York: Medical Encyclopedia, 594–8.
5. Posner AC, Konicoff NG, Prigot A. Tetracycline in obstetric infections. In Antibiotics Annual, 1955–56. New York: Medical Encyclopedia, 345–8.
6. Cohlan SQ, Bevelander G, Bross S. Effect of tetracycline on bone growth in the premature infant. Antimicrob Agents Chemother 1961:340–7.
7. Harcourt JK, Johnson NW, Storey E. In vivo incorporation of tetracycline in the teeth of man. Arch Oral Biol 1962;7:431–7.
8. Rendle-Short TJ. Tetracycline in teeth and bone. Lancet 1962;1:1188.
9. Douglas AC. The deposition of tetracycline in human nails and teeth: a complication of long term treatment. Br J Dis Chest 1963;57:44–7.
10. Kutscher AH, Zegarelli EV, Tovell HM, Hochberg B. Discoloration of teeth induced by tetracycline. JAMA 1963;184:586–7.
11. Kline AH, Blattner RJ, Lunin M. Transplacental effect of tetracyclines on teeth. JAMA 1964;188:178–80.
12. Macaulay JC, Leistyna JA. Preliminary observations on the prenatal administration of demethylchlortetracycline HCl. Pediatrics 1964;34:423–4.
13. Stewart DJ. The effects of tetracyclines upon the dentition. Br J Dermatol 1964;76:374–8.
14. Swallow JN. Discoloration of primary dentition after maternal tetracycline ingestion in pregnancy. Lancet 1964;2:611–2.
15. Porter PJ, Sweeney EA, Golan H, Kass EH. Controlled study of the effect of prenatal tetracycline on primary dentition. Antimicrob Agents Chemother 1965:668–71.
16. Toaff R, Ravid R. Tetracyclines and the teeth. Lancet 1966;2:281–2.
17. Kutscher AH, Zegarelli EV, Tovell HM, Hochberg B, Hauptman J. Discoloration of deciduous teeth induced by administrations of tetracycline antepartum. Am J Obstet Gynecol 1966;96:291–2.
18. Brearley LJ, Stragis AA, Storey E. Tetracycline-induced tooth changes. Part 1. Prevalence in pre-school children. Med J Aust 1968;2:653–8.
19. Brearley LJ, Storey E. Tetracycline-induced tooth changes. Part 2. Prevalence, localization and nature of staining in extracted deciduous teeth. Med J Aust 1968;2:714–9.

20. Baker KL, Storey E. Tetracycline-induced tooth changes. Part 3. Incidence in extracted first permanent molar teeth. Med J Aust 1970;1:109-13.

21. Anthony JR. Effect on deciduous and permanent teeth of tetracycline deposition in utero. Postgrad Med 1970;48:165-8.

22. Genot MT, Golan HP, Porter PJ, Kass EH. Effect of administration of tetracycline in pregnancy on the primary dentition of the offspring. J Oral Med 1970;25:75-9.

23. Bruno M, Ober WB. Clinicopathologic conference: jaundice at the end of pregnancy. NY State J Med 1962;62:3792-800.

24. Lewis PL, Takeda M, Warren MJ. Obstetric acute yellow atrophy. Report of a case. Obstet Gynecol 1963;22:121-7.

25. Schultz JC, Adamson JS Jr, Workman WW, Normal TD. Fatal liver disease after intravenous administration of tetracycline in high dosage. N Engl J Med 1963;269:999-1004.

26. Briggs RC. Tetracycline and liver disease. N Engl J Med 1963;269:1386.

27. Leonard GL. Tetracycline and liver disease. N Engl J Med 1963;269:1386.

28. Gough GS, Searcy RL. Additional case of fatal liver disease with tetracycline therapy. N Engl J Med 1964;270:157-8.

29. Whalley PJ, Adams RH, Combes B. Tetracycline toxicity in pregnancy. JAMA 1964;189:357-62.

30. Kunelis CT, Peters JL, Edmondson HA. Fatty liver of pregnancy and its relationship to tetracycline therapy. Am J Med 1965;38:359-77.

31. Lew HT, French SW. Tetracycline nephrotoxicity and nonoliguric acute renal failure. Arch Intern Med 1966;118:123-8.

32. Meihoff WE, Pasquale DN, Jacoby WJ Jr. Tetracycline-induced hepatic coma, with recovery. A report of a case. Obstet Gynecol 1967;29:260-5.

33. Aach R, Kissane J. Clinicopathologic conference: a seventeen year old girl with fatty liver of pregnancy following tetracycline therapy. Am J Med 1967;43:274-83.

34. Whalley PJ, Martin FG, Adams RH, Combes B. Disposition of tetracycline by pregnant women with acute pyelonephritis. Obstet Gynecol 1970;36:821-6.

35. Pride GL, Cleary RE, Hamburger RJ. Disseminated intravascular coagulation associated with tetracycline-induced hepatorenal failure during pregnancy. Am J Obstet Gynecol 1973;115:585-6.

36. Wenk RE, Gebhardt FC, Behagavan BS, Lustgarten JA, McCarthy EF. Tetracycline-associated fatty liver of pregnancy, including possible pregnancy risk after chronic dermatologic use of tetracycline. J Reprod Med 1981;26:135-41.

37. King TM, Bowe ET, D'Esopo DA. Toxic effects of the tetracyclines. Bull Sloane Hosp Women 1964;10:35-41.

38. Allen ES, Brown WE. Hepatic toxicity of tetracycline in pregnancy. Am J Obstet Gynecol 1966;95:12-8.

39. Heinonen O, Slone D, Shaprio S. Birth Defects and Drugs in Pregnancy. Littleton: Publishing Sciences Group, 1977:297-313.

40. Ibid, 435.

41. Ibid, 472, 485.

42. Wilson F. Congenital defects in the newborn. Br Med J 1962;2:255.

43. Carter MP, Wilson F. Tetracycline and congenital limb abnormalities. Br Med J 1962;2:407-8.

44. Mennie AT. Tetracycline and congenital limb abnormalities. Br Med J 1962;2:480.

45. Harley JD, Farrar JF, Gray JB, Dunlop IC. Aromatic drugs and congenital cataracts. Lancet 1964;1:472.

46. Corcoran R, Castles JM. Tetracycline for acne vulgaris and possible teratogenesis. Br Med J 1977;2:807-8.

47. Briggs M. Tetracycline and steroid hormone binding to human spermatozoa. Acta Endocrinol 1974;75:785-92.

48. Bacon JF, Shenfield GM. Pregnancy attributable to interaction between tetracycline and oral contraceptives. Br Med J 1980;1:283.

49. Knowles JA. Drugs in milk. Pediatr Curr 1972;21:28-32.

50. Graf VH, Reimann S. Untersuchungen uber die konzentration von pyrrolidino-methyl-tetra-cycline in der muttermilch. Dtsch Med Wochenschr 1959;84:1694.

Name: **THEOPHYLLINE**

Class: **Spasmolytic/Vasodilator**   Risk Factor: **C**

Fetal Risk Summary

Theophylline is the bronchodilator of choice for asthma and chronic obstructive pulmonary disease in the pregnant patient (1-6). No reports linking the use of theophylline with congenital defects have been located. Theophylline crosses the placenta and newborns may have therapeutic serum levels (7-9). Transient tachycardia, irritability and vomiting were reported in 3 infants from *in utero*-acquired theophylline (7, 8). These effects are more likely to occur when maternal serum levels at term are in the high therapeutic range or above (therapeutic range 8-20 μg/ml) (9). In 67 asthmatic pregnant patients at risk for premature delivery, aminophylline (theophylline ethylenediamine) was found to exert a beneficial effect by reducing the perinatal death rate and the frequency of respiratory distress syndrome (10). No complications or adverse effects due to drug administration were observed.

The Collaborative Perinatal Project monitored 193 mother-child pairs with 1st trimester exposure to theophylline or aminophylline (11). No evidence was found for an association with malformations. Concern over the depressant effects of methylxanthines on lipid synthesis in developing neural systems has been reported (12). Recent observations that infants treated with theophylline for apnea exhibit no overt neurologic deficits at 9 to 27 months of age are encouraging (13, 14). However, the long term effects of these drugs on human brain development are not known (12). Little is known about the pharmacokinetics of theophylline during pregnancy. A recent report suggests that plasma concentrations of theophylline fall during the 3rd trimester due to an increased maternal volume of distribution (15). Those patients that require theophylline during pregnancy should be monitored accordingly.

Breast Feeding Summary

Theophylline is excreted into breast milk (16, 17). A milk:plasma ratio of 0.7 has been measured (17). Estimates indicate that less than 1% of the maternal dose is excreted into breast milk (16, 17). However, one infant became irritable secondary to a rapidly absorbed oral solution of aminophylline taken by the mother (16). Because very young infants may be more sensitive to levels which would be non-toxic in older infants, less rapidly absorbed theophylline preparations may be advisable for nursing mothers (8, 18).

References

1. Greenberger P, Patterson R. Safety of therapy for allergic symptoms during pregnancy. Ann Intern Med 1978;89:234-7.
2. Weinstein AM, Dubin BD, Podleski WK, Spector SL, Farr RS. Asthma and pregnancy. JAMA 1979;241:1161-5.
3. Hernandez E, Angell CS, Johnson JWC. Asthma in pregnancy: current concepts. Obstet Gynecol 1980;55:739-43.
4. Turner ES, Greenberger PA, Patterson R. Management of the pregnant asthmatic patient. Ann Intern Med 1980;93:905-18.

Theophylline–Thioguanine

5. Pratt WR. Allergic diseases in pregnancy and breast feeding. Ann Allergy 1981;47:355–60.
6. Lalli CM, Raju L. Pregnancy and chronic obstructive pulmonary disease. Chest 1981;80:759–61.
7. Arwood LL, Dasta JF, Friedman C. Placental transfer of theophylline: two case reports. Pediatrics 1979;63:844–6.
8. Yeh TF, Pildes RS. Transplacental aminophylline toxicity in a neonate. Lancet 1977;1:910.
9. Labovitz E, Spector S. Placental theophylline transfer in pregnant asthmatics. JAMA 1982;247:786–8.
10. Hadjigeorgiou E, Kitsiou S, Psaroudakis A, Segos C, Nicolopoulos D, Kaskarelis D. Antepartum aminophylline treatment for prevention of the respiratory distress syndrome in premature infants. Am J Obstet Gynecol 1979;135:257–60.
11. Heinonen OP, Slone D, Shapiro S. Birth Defects and Drugs in Pregnancy. Littleton: Publishing Sciences Group, 1977:367,370.
12. Volpe JJ. Effects of methylxanthines on lipid synthesis in developing neural systems. Semin Perinatol 1981;5:395–405.
13. Aranda JV, Dupont C. Metabolic effects of methylxanthines in premature infants. J Pediatr 1976;89:833–4.
14. Nelson RM, Resnick MB, Holstrum WJ, Eitzman DV. Development outcome of premature infants treated with theophylline. Dev Pharmacol Ther 1980;1:274–80.
15. Sutton PL, Koup JR, Rose JQ, Middleton E. The pharmacokinetics of theophylline in pregnancy. J Allergy Clin Immunol 1978;61:174.
16. Yurchak AM, Jusko WJ. Theophylline secretion into breast milk. Pediatrics 1976;57:518–25.
17. Stec GP, Greenberger P, Ruo TI, et al. Kinetics of theophylline transfer to breast milk. Clin Pharmacol Ther 1980;28:404–8.
18. Berlin CM. Excretion of methylxanthines in human milk. Semin Perinatol 1981;5:389–94.

Name: THIOGUANINE

Class: **Antineoplastic**   Risk Factor: **D**

Fetal Risk Summary

The use of thioguanine in pregnancy has been reported in 16 patients, 4 during the 1st trimester (1–12). Use in the 1st and 2nd trimesters has been associated with congenital malformations and chromosomal abnormalities (see table below) (1, 11). Data from one review indicated that 40% of the infants exposed to anticancer drugs were of low birth weight (13). This finding was not related to the timing of exposure. Long term studies of growth and mental development in offspring exposed to thioguanine during the 2nd trimester, the period of neuroblast multiplication, have not been conducted (14).

Although abnormal chromosomal changes were observed in one aborted fetus, karyotyping of cultured cells in two other newborns did not show anomalies (1, 4). Paternal use of thioguanine with other antineoplastic agents prior to conception may have been associated with congenital defects observed in two infants: an anencephalic stillborn and one with tetralogy of Fallot with syndactyly of the 1st and 2nd toes (15). Congenital defects were not observed in the offspring of a third male exposed to thioguanine before fertilization (16).

Author (ref)	No. Pts.	Indication	Gestational Age	Dose	Other Drugs	Fetal Effects	Comments
Maurer (1)	1	Myelogenous leukemia	2nd trimester	100 mg/m² intravenously	Cytarabine	Elective abortion at 24 weeks of gestation Trisomy for group C autosomes without mosaicism	Relationship to drug unknown
Schafer (11)	1	Myeloblastic leukemia	Throughout	120 mg/day for 5 days each month	Cytarabine	Two medial digits of both feet missing Distal phalanges of both thumbs missing with hypoplastic remnant of right thumb	Normal infants before and after case infant

Breast Feeding Summary

No data available.

References

1. Maurer LH, Forcier RJ, McIntyre OR, Benirschke K. Fetal group C trisomy after cytosine arabinoside and thioguanine. Ann Intern Med 1971;75:809–10.
2. Pawliger DF, McLean FW, Noyes WD. Normal fetus after cytosine arabinoside therapy. Ann Intern Med 1971;74:1012.
3. Au-Yong R, Collins P, Young JA. Acute myeloblastic leukaemia during pregnancy. Br Med J 1972;4:493–4.
4. Raich PC, Curet LB. Treatment of acute leukemia during pregnancy. Cancer 1975;36:861–2.
5. Gokal R, Durrant J, Baum JD, Bennett MJ. Successful pregnancy in acute monocytic leukaemia. Br J Cancer 1976;34:299–302.
6. Lilleyman JS, Hill AS, Anderton KJ. Consequences of acute myelogenous leukemia in early pregnancy. Cancer 1977;40:1300–3.
7. Moreno H, Castleberry RP, McCann WP. Cytosine arabinoside and 6-thioguanine in the treatment of childhood acute myeloblastic leukemia. Cancer 1977;40:998–1004.
8. Manoharan A, Leyden MJ. Acute non-lymphocytic leukaemia in the third trimester of pregnancy. Aust NZ J Med 1979;9:71–4.
9. Taylor G, Blom J. Acute leukemia during pregnancy. South Med J 1980;73:1314–5.
10. Tobias JS, Bloom HJG. Doxorubicin in pregnancy. Lancet 1980;1:776.
11. Schafer AI. Teratogenic effects of antileukemic chemotherapy. Arch Intern Med 1981;141:514–5.
12. Plows CW. Acute myelomonocytic leukemia in pregnancy: report of a case. Am J Obstet Gynecol 1982;143:41–3.
13. Nicholson HO. Cytotoxic drugs in pregnancy: review of reported cases. J Obstet Gynaecol Br Commonw 1968;75:307–12.
14. Dobbing J. Pregnancy and leukaemia. Lancet 1977;1:1155.
15. Russell JA, Powles RL, Oliver RTD. Conception and congenital abnormalities after chemotherapy of acute myelogenous leukaemia in two men. Br Med J 1976;1:1508.
16. Matthews JH, Wood JK. Male fertility during chemotherapy for acute leukemia. N Engl J Med 1980;303:1235.

Name: **THIOPROPAZATE**

Class: **Tranquilizer**   Risk Factor: **C**

Fetal Risk Summary

Thiopropazate is a piperazine phenothiazine in the same group as prochlor-perazine (see Prochlorperazine). Phenothiazines readily cross the placenta (1). No specific information on the use of thiopropazate in pregnancy has been located. Although occasional reports have attempted to link various phenothi-azine compounds with congenital malformations, the bulk of the evidence indicates that these drugs are safe for the mother and fetus (see also Chlor-promazine).

Breast Feeding Summary

No data available.

Reference

1. Moya F, Thorndike V. Passage of drugs across the placenta. Am J Obstet Gynecol 1962;84:1778–98.

Name: **THIORIDAZINE**

Class: **Tranquilizer**   Risk Factor: **C**

Fetal Risk Summary

Thioridazine is a piperidyl phenothiazine. The phenothiazines readily cross the placenta (1). Extrapyramidal symptoms were seen in a newborn exposed to thioridazine *in utero*, but the reaction was probably due to chlorpromazine (2). A case of a congenital heart defect was described in 1969 (3). However, Scanlan found no anomalies in the offspring of 23 patients exposed throughout gestation to thioridazine (4). Twenty of the infants were evaluated for up to 13 years. Although occasional reports have attempted to link various phenothi-azine compounds with congenital malformations, the bulk of the evidence indicates that these drugs are safe for the mother and fetus (see Chlorpro-mazine).

Breast Feeding Summary

No data available.

References

1. Moya F, Thorndike V. Passage of drugs across the placenta. Am J Obstet Gynecol 1962;84:1778–98.
2. Hill RM, Desmond MM, Kay JL. Extrapyramidal dysfunction in an infant of a schizophrenic mother. J Pediatr 1966;69:589–95.

3. Vince DJ. Congenital malformations following phenothiazine administration during pregnancy. Can Med Assoc J 1969;100:223.
4. Scanlan FJ. The use of thioridazine (Mellaril) during the first trimester. Med J Aust 1972;1:1271–2.

Name: THIOTEPA

Class: **Antineoplastic**   Risk Factor: **D**

Fetal Risk Summary

No data available.

Breast Feeding Summary

No data available.

Name: THIOTHIXENE

Class: **Tranquilizer**   Risk Factor: **C**

Fetal Risk Summary

Thiothixene is structurally and pharmacologically related to trifluoperazine and chlorprothixene. No specific data on its use in pregnancy has been located (see also Trifluoperazine).

Breast Feeding Summary

No data available.

Name: THIPHENAMIL

Class: **Parasympatholytic (Anticholinergic)**   Risk Factor: **C**

Fetal Risk Summary

Thiphenamil is an anticholinergic agent used in the treatment of parkinsonism. No reports of its use in pregnancy have been located (see also Atropine).

Breast Feeding Summary

No data available (see also Atropine).

Name: **TICARCILLIN**

Class: **Antibiotic**   Risk Factor: **B**

Fetal Risk Summary

Ticarcillin is a penicillin antibiotic. The drug rapidly crosses the placenta into the fetal circulation and amniotic fluid (1). Following a 1-g intravenous (IV) dose, single determinations of the amniotic fluid from 6 patients, 15 to 76 minutes after injection, yielded levels ranging from 1.0 to 3.3 µg/ml. Similar measurements of ticarcillin in cord serum ranged from 12.6 to 19.2 µg/ml.

No reports linking the use of ticarcillin with congenital defects have been located. The Collaborative Perinatal Project monitored 50,282 mother-child pairs, 3,546 of which had 1st trimester exposure to penicillin derivatives (2). For use anytime during pregnancy, 7,171 exposures were recorded (3). In neither case was evidence found to suggest a relationship to large categories of major or minor malformations or to individual defects.

Breast Feeding Summary

Ticarcillin is excreted into breast milk in low concentrations. After a 1-g IV dose given to 5 patients, only trace amounts of drug were measured at intervals up to 6 hours (1). Although these amounts are probably not significant, three potential problems exist for the nursing infant: modification of bowel flora, direct effects on the infant (e.g., allergic response) and interference with the interpretation of culture results if a fever work-up is required.

References

1. Cho N, Nakayama T, Vehara K, Kunii K. Laboratory and clinical evaluation of ticarcillin in the field of obstetrics and gynecology. Chemotherapy (Tokyo) 1977;25:2911–23.
2. Heinonen OP, Slone, D, Shapiro S. *Birth Defects and Drugs in Pregnancy.* Littleton: Publishing Sciences Group, 1977:297–313.
3. *Ibid*, 435.

Name: **TOBRAMYCIN**

Class: **Antibiotic**   Risk Factor: **C**

Fetal Risk Summary

Tobramycin is an aminoglycoside antibiotic. The drug crosses the placenta into the fetal circulation and amniotic fluid (1). Studies in patients undergoing elective abortions in the 1st and 2nd trimesters indicate that tobramycin distributes to most fetal tissues except the brain and cerebrospinal fluid. Aminotic fluid levels generally did not occur until the 2nd trimester. The highest fetal concentrations were found in the kidneys and urine. Reports measuring the passage of tobramycin in the 3rd trimester and at term are lacking.

No reports linking the use of tobramycin with congenital defects have been located. Ototoxicity, which is known to occur after tobramycin therapy, has not been reported as an effect of *in utero* exposure. However, eighth cranial nerve toxicity in the fetus is well known following exposure to other aminoglycosides (see Kanamycin and Streptomycin) and may potentially occur with tobramycin.

Breast Feeding Summary

Tobramycin is excreted into breast milk. Following an 80-mg intramuscular dose given to 5 patients, milk levels varied from trace to 0.52 μg/ml over 8 hours (2). Peak levels occurred at 4 hours post-injection. Since oral absorption of this antibiotic is poor, ototoxicity in the infant would not be expected. However, three potential problems exist for the nursing infant: modification of bowel flora, direct effects on the infant and interference with the interpretation of culture results if a fever work-up is required.

References

1. Bernard B, Garcia-Cazares S, Ballard C, Thrupp L, Mathies A, Wehrle P. Tobramycin: maternal-fetal pharmacology. Antimicrob Agents Chemother 1977;11:688–94.
2. Takase Z. Laboratory and clinical studies on tobramycin in the field of obstetrics and gynecology. Chemotherapy (Tokyo) 1975;23:1402.

Name: **TOLAZAMIDE**

Class: **Oral Hypoglycemic**   Risk Factor: **D**

Fetal Risk Summary

Tolazamide is a sulfonylurea used for the treatment of adult-onset diabetes mellitus. It is not indicated for the pregnant diabetic since tolazamide will not provide good control in patients who cannot be controlled by diet alone. Oral hypoglycemics may cause prolonged symptomatic hypoglycemia in newborns if exposed near term (see Chlorpropamide).

Breast Feeding Summary

No data available.

Name: **TOLAZOLINE**

Class: **Vasodilator**   Risk Factor: **C**

Fetal Risk Summary

Tolazoline is structurally and pharmacologically related to phentolamine (see also Phentolamine). Experience with tolazoline in pregnancy is limited. The Collaborative Perinatal Project monitored 2 1st trimester exposures to tolazoline plus 13 other patients exposed to other vasodilators (1). From this small group of 15 patients, 4 malformed children were produced, a statisically significant incidence ($p < 0.02$). It was not stated if tolazoline was taken by any of the mothers of the affected infants. Although the data serves as a warning, the number of patients is so small that conclusions as to the relative safety of this drug in pregnancy cannot be made.

Breast Feeding Summary

No data available.

Reference

1. Heinonen OP, Slone D, Shapiro S. *Birth Defects and Drugs in Pregnancy.* Littleton: Publishing Sciences Group, 1977:371–3.

Name: **TOLBUTAMIDE**

Class: **Oral Hypoglycemic**   Risk Factor: **D**

Fetal Risk Summary

Tolbutamide is a sulfonylurea used for the treatment of adult-onset diabetes mellitus. It is not indicated for the pregnant diabetic. When administered near term, the drug crosses the placenta (1, 2). Neonatal serum levels are higher than corresponding maternal concentrations. In one infant whose mother took 500 mg per day, serum levels at 27 hours were 7.2 mg/100 ml (maternal 2.7 mg/100 ml) (2). Prolonged symptomatic hypoglycemia has not been reported with tolbutamide but has been observed with other oral hypoglycemics (see also Acetohexamide and Chlorpropamide). However, tolbutamide should be stopped at least 48 hours before delivery to avoid this potential complication (3). Although teratogenic in animals, an increased incidence of congenital defects, other than that expected in diabetes mellitus, has not been found with tolbutamide (4–14). Four malformed infants have been attributed to tolbutamide but the relationship is unclear (2, 15–17). Maternal diabetes is known to increase the rate of malformations by two to four fold, but the mechanism(s) are not understood (see also Insulin). Neonatal thrombocytopenia, persisting for about two weeks, may have been induced by tolbutamide (2). In spite of this relative lack of teratogenicity, tolbutamide should be avoided in pregnancy since the drug will not provide good control in patients who cannot be controlled by diet alone (3). The manufacturer recommends that it not be used in pregnancy (18).

Author (ref)	No. Pts.	Indica-tion	Gestational Age	Dose	Other Drugs	Fetal Effects	Comment
Larson (15)	1	Diabetes mellitus	Throughout	500 mg/day	Not stated	Hands/feet anomalies; finger/toe syndactyly; external ear defect; atresia of external auditory canal; gastrointestinal/ heart/renal anomalies	—
Campbell (16)	1	Diabetes mellitus	Throughought	Not stated	Not stated	Grossly malformed	Relationship unknown
Soler (17)	1	Diabetes mellitus	2nd and 3rd trimesters	1 g/day	Not stated	Severe talipes, absent left toe	Probably not related to drug
Schiff (2)	1	Diabetes mellitus	Throughout	500 mg/day	Not stated	Right-sided preauricular skin tag; accessory right thumb; thrombocytopenia (nadir 19,000 mm^3 on 4th day)	Infant serum level 7.2 mg/100 ml (27 hours)

Breast Feeding Summary

Tolbutamide is excreted into breast milk. Following long term dosing with 500 mg orally twice daily, milk levels 4 hours after a dose in two patients averaged 3 and 18 μg/ml, respectively (19). Milk:plasma ratios were 0.09 and 0.40, respectively. The effect on an infant from these levels is unknown.

References

1. Miller DI, Wishinsky H, Thompson G. Transfer of tolbutamide across the human placenta. Diabetes 1962;11(Suppl):93–7.
2. Schiff D, Aranda J, Stern L. Neonatal thrombocytopenia and congenital malformation associated with administration of tolbutamide to the mother. J Pediatr 1970; 77:457–8.
3. Friend JR. Diabetes. Clin Obstet Gynaecol 1981; 8:353–82.
4. Ghanem MH. Possible teratogenic effect of tolbutamide in the pregnant prediabetic. Lancet 1961; 1:1227.
5. Dolger H, Bookman JJ, Nechemias C. The diagnostic and therapeutic value of tolbutamide in pregnant diabetics. Diabetes 1962;11(Suppl):97–8.
6. Jackson WPU, Campbell GD, Notelovitz M, Blumsohn D. Tolbutamide and chlorpropamide during pregnancy in human diabetes. Diabetes 1962; 11(Suppl):98–101.
7. Campbell GD. Chlorpropamide and foetal damage. Br Med J 1963;1:59–60.
8. Macphail I. Chlorpropamide and foetal damage. Br Med J 1963; 1:192.
9. Jackson WPU, Campbell GD. Chlorpropamide and perinatal mortality. Br Med J 1963;2:1652.
10. Malins JM, Cooke AM, Pyke DA, Fitzgerald MG. Sulphonylurea drugs in pregnancy. Br Med J 1964;2:187.
11. Moss JM, Connor EJ. Pregnancy complicated by diabetes. Report of 102 pregnancies including eleven treated with oral hypoglycemic drugs. Med Ann Dist Columb 1965;34:253-60.
12. Adam PAJ, Schwartz R. Diagnosis and treatment: should oral hypoglycemic agents be used in pediatric and pregnant patients? Pediatrics 1968;42:819–23.
13. Dignan PSJ. Teratogenic risk and counseling in diabetes. Clin Obstet Gynecol 1981;24:149-59.
14. Burt RL. Reactivity to tolbutamide in normal pregnancy. Obstet Gynecol 1958; 12:447–53.

15. Larsson Y, Sterky G. Possible teratogenic effect of tolbutamide in a pregnant prediabetic. Lancet 1960; 2:1424–6.
16. Campbell GD. Possible teratogenic effect of tolbutamide in pregnancy. Lancet 1961; 1:891–2.
17. Soler NG, Walsh CH, Malins JM. Congenital malformations in infants of diabetic mothers. Q J Med 1976;45:303–13.
18. Product information. Orinase. The Upjohn Company, 1981.
19. Moiel RH, Ryan JR. Tolbutamide (Orinase) in human breast milk. Clin Pediatr 1967;6:480.

Name: **TOLMETIN**

Class: **Nonsteroidal Anti-inflammatory**   Risk Factor: **B***

Fetal Risk Summary

No reports linking the use of tolmetin with congenital defects have been located. Theoretically, tolmetin, a prostaglandin synthetase inhibitor, could cause constriction of the ductus arteriosus *in utero* (1). Persistent pulmonary hypertension of the newborn should also be considered (2). Drugs in this class have been shown to inhibit labor and prolong pregnancy (2). The manufacturer recommends that the drug not be used during pregnancy (3).

[*Risk Factor D if used in 3rd trimester or near delivery.]

Breast Feeding Summary

No data available. The manufacturer recommends that the drug not be used when breast feeding (4).

References

1. Levin DL. Effects of inhibition of prostaglandin synthesis on fetal development, oxygenation, and the fetal circulation. Semin Perinatol 1980;4:35–44.
2. Fuchs F. Prevention of prematurity. Am J Obstet Gynecol 1976;126:809–20.
3. Product information. Tolectin. McNeil Pharmaceutical, 1982.
4. Personal communication. Collier JM, McNeil Laboratories, 1979.

Name: **TRANYLCYPROMINE**

Class: **Antidepressant**   Risk Factor: **C**

Fetal Risk Summary

Tranylcypromine is a monoamine oxidase inhibitor. The Collaborative Perinatal Project monitored 21 mother-child pairs exposed to these drugs during the 1st trimester, 13 of which were exposed to tranylcypromine (1). An increased risk of malformations was found. Details of the 13 cases with exposure to tranylcypromine are not available.

Breast Feeding Summary

No data available.

Reference

1. Heinonen OP, Slone D, Shapiro S. *Birth Defects and Drugs in Pregnancy.* Littleton: Publishing Sciences Group, 1977:336–7.

Name: **TRIAMTERENE**

Class: **Diuretic**   Risk Factor: **D**

Fetal Risk Summary

Triamterene is a potassium-conserving diuretic. No reports linking it with congenital defects have been located. The drug crosses to the fetus in animals, but this has not been studied in humans (1). No defects were observed in 5 infants exposed to triamterene in the 1st trimester in one study (2). For use anytime during pregnancy, 271 exposures were recorded without an increase in malformations (3). Many investigators consider diuretics contraindicated in pregnancy, except for patients with heart disease, since they do not present or alter the course of toxemia and they may decrease placental perfusion (4–6).

Breast Feeding Summary

Triamterene is excreted into cow's milk (1). Human data is not available.

References

1. Product information. Dyrenium. Smith Kline & French Laboratories, 1982.
2. Heinonen OP, Slone D, Shapiro S. *Birth Defects and Drugs in Pregnancy.* Littleton: Publishing Sciences Group, 1977:372.
3. *Ibid*, 441.
4. Pitkin RM, Kaminetzky HA, Newton M, Pritchard JA. Maternal nutrition: a selective review of clinical topics. Obstet Gynecol 1972;40:773–85.
5. Lindheimer MD, Katz AI. Sodium and diuretics in pregnancy. N Engl J Med 1973;288:891–4.
6. Christianson R, Page EW. Diuretic drugs and pregnancy. Obstet Gynecol 1976;48:647–52.

Name: **TRICHLORMETHIAZIDE**

Class: **Diuretic**   Risk Factor: **D**

Fetal Risk Summary

See Chlorothiazide.

Breast Feeding Summary

See Chlorothiazide

Name: **TRIDIHEXETHYL**

Class: **Parasympatholytic (Anticholinergic)**   Risk Factor: **C**

Fetal Risk Summary

Tridihexethyl is an anticholinergic quaternary ammonium chloride. In a large prospective study, 2,323 patients were exposed to this class of drugs during the 1st trimester, 6 of whom took tridihexethyl (1). A possible association was found between the total group and minor malformations.

Breast Feeding Summary

No data available (see also Atropine).

Reference

1. Heinonen OP, Slone D, Shapiro S. *Birth Defects and Drugs in Pregnancy.* Littleton: Publishing Sciences Group, 1977:346–53.

Name: **TRIFLUOPERAZINE**

Class: **Tranquilizer**   Risk Factor: **C**

Fetal Risk Summary

Trifluoperazine is a piperazine phenothiazine. The drug readily crosses the placenta (1). Trifluoperazine has been used for the treatment of nausea and vomiting of pregnancy, but it is primarily used as a psychotropic agent. In 1962, the Canadian Food and Drug Directorate released a warning that 8 cases of congenital defects had been associated with trifluoperazine therapy (2). This correlation was refuted in a series of articles from the medical staff of the manufacturer of the drug (3–5). In 480 trifluoperazine-treated pregnant women, the incidence of liveborn infants with congenital malformations was 1.1%, as compared to 8,472 non-treated controls with an incidence of 1.5% (4). Two reports of phocomelia appeared in 1962–63, and a case of a congenital heart defect in 1969 (see table below) (6–8). In none of these cases is there a clear relationship between use of the drug and the defect. Extrapyramidal symptoms have been described in a newborn exposed to trifluoperazine *in utero*, but the reaction was probably due to chlorpromazine (see Chlorpromazine) (9).

The Collaborative Perinatal Project monitored 50,282 mother-child pairs, 42 of which had 1st trimester exposure to trifluoperazine (10). No evidence was found to suggest a relationship to malformations or an effect on perinatal mortality rate, birth weight or intelligence quotient scores at 4 years of age.

In summary, although some reports have attempted to link trifluoperazine with congenital defects, the bulk of the evidence indicates that the drug is safe for mother and fetus. Other reviewers have also concluded that the phenothiazines are not teratogenic (11, 12).

Author (ref)	No. Pts.	Indica- tion	Gestational Age	Dose	Other Drugs	Fetal Effects	Comment
Corner (6)	1	Not stated	1st and 2nd tri- mesters	4 mg/day	Not stated	Twins—both with phocomelia of all 4 limbs	
Hall (7)	1	Pruritus	1st tri- mester	3 mg/day for 2 days	Prochlorpro- mazine (2nd trimester)	Phocomelia of upper limbs	
Vince (8)	1	Psychia- tric	Through- out	4 mg/day	Thioridazine	Complete transposition of great vessels in heart	

Breast Feeding Summary

No data available.

References

1. Moya F, Thorndike V. Passage of drugs across the placenta. Am J Obstet Gynecol 1962;84:1778–98.
2. Canadian Department of National Health and Welfare, Food and Drug Directorate. Letter of notification to Canadian physicians. Ottawa, December 7, 1962.
3. Moriarity AJ. Trifluoperazine and congenital malformations. Can Med Assoc J 1963;88:97.
4. Moriarty AJ, Nance MR. Trifluoperazine and pregnancy. Can Med Assoc J 1963; 88:375–6.
5. Schrire I. Trifluoperazine and foetal abnormalities. Lancet 1963;1:174.
6. Corner BD. Congenital malformations. Clinical considerations. Med J Southwest 1962;77:46–52.
7. Hall G. A case of phocomelia of the upper limbs. Med J Aust 1963;1:449–50.
8. Vince DJ. Congenital malformations following phenothiazine administration during pregnancy. Can Med Assoc J 1969;100:223.
9. Hill RM, Desmond MM, Kay JL. Extrapyramidal dysfunction in an infant of a schizophrenic mother. J Pediatr 1966;69:589–95.
10. Slone D, Siskind V, Heinonen OP, Monson RR, Kaufman DW, Shapiro S. Antenatal exposure to the phenothiazines in relation to congenital malformations, perinatal mortality rate, birth weight, and intelligence quotient score. Am J Obstet Gynecol 1977;128:486–8.
11. Ayd FJ Jr. Children born of mothers treated with chlorpromazine during pregnancy. Clin Med 1964;71:1758–63.
12. Ananth J. Congenital malformations with psychopharmacologic agents. Compr Psychiatry 1975;16:437–45.

Name: **TRIFLUPROMAZINE**

Class: **Tranquilizer**   Risk Factor: **C**

Fetal Risk Summary

Triflupromazine is a propylamino phenothiazine in the same class as chlorpromazine. The phenothiazines readily cross the placenta (1). The Collaborative Perinatal Project monitored 50,282 mother-child pairs, 36 of which had 1st trimester exposure to triflupromazine (2). No evidence was found to suggest a relationship to malformations or an effect on perinatal mortality rates, birth weight or intelligence quotient scores at 4 years of age. Although occasional reports have attempted to link various phenothiazine compounds with congenital defects, the bulk of the evidence indicates that these drugs are safe for the mother and fetus (see also Chlorpromazine).

Breast Feeding Summary

No data available.

References

1. Moya F, Thorndike V. Passage of drugs across the placenta. Am J Obstet Gynecol 1962;84:1778–98.
2. Slone D, Siskind V, Heinonen OP, Monson RR, Kaufman DW, Shapiro S. Antenatal exposure to the phenothiazines in relation to congenital malformations, perinatal mortality rate, birth weight, and intelligence quotient score. Am J Obstet Gynecol 1977;128:486–8.

Name: **TRIHEXYPHENIDYL**

Class: **Parasympatholytic (Anticholinergic)**   Risk Factor: **C**

Fetal Risk Summary

Trihexyphenidyl is an anticholinergic agent used in the treatment of parkinsonism. In a large prospective study, 2,323 patients were exposed to this class of drugs during the 1st trimester, 9 of whom took trihexyphenidyl (1). A possible association was found between the total group and minor malformations.

Breast Feeding Summary

No data available (see also Atropine).

Reference

1. Heinonen OP, Slone D, Shapiro S. Birth Defects and Drugs in Pregnancy. Littleton: Publishing Sciences Group, 1977:346–53.

Name: **TRIMEPRAZINE**

Class: **Antihistamine**   Risk Factor: **C**

Fetal Risk Summary

Trimeprazine is a phenothiazine antihistamine that is primarily used as an antipruritic. The Collaborative Perinatal Project monitored 50,282 mother-child pairs, 14 of which had 1st trimester exposure to trimeprazine (1). From this small sample, no evidence was found to suggest a relationship to large categories of major or minor malformations or to individual malformations. For use anytime in pregnancy, 140 exposures were recorded (2). Based on defects in 5 children, a possible association with malformations was found, but the significance of this is unknown.

In a 1971 study, infants of mothers who had ingested antihistamines during the 1st trimester actually had significantly fewer abnormalities when compared to controls (3). Trimeprazine was the eighth most commonly used antihistamine.

Breast Feeding Summary

Trimeprazine is excreted into human milk but the levels are probably not sufficient to affect the infant (4).

References

1. Heinonen OP, Slone D, Shapiro S. *Birth Defects and Drugs in Pregnancy.* Littleton: Publishing Sciences Group, 1977:323.
2. *Ibid,* 437.
3. Nelson MM, Forfar JO. Associations between drugs administered during pregnancy and congenital abnormalities. Br Med J 1971;1:523–7.
4. O'Brien TE. Excretion of drugs in human milk. Am J Hosp Pharm 1974; 31:844–54.

Name: **TRIMETHADIONE**

Class: **Anticonvulsant**   Risk Factor: **X**

Fetal Risk Summary

Trimethadione is an oxazolidinedione anticonvulsant used in the treatment of petit mal epilepsy. Several case histories have suggested a phenotype for a fetal trimethadione syndrome of congenital malformations (1–7). The use of trimethadione in 9 families was associated with a 69% incidence of congenital defects—25 malformed children from 36 pregnancies. Three of these families reported 5 normal births after the anticonvulsant medication was stopped (1, 4). The incidence of fetal loss in these families was also increased over that seen in the general epileptic population. Because trimethadione has demonstrated both clinical and experimental fetal risk greater than other anticonvulsants, its use should be abandoned in favor of other medications used in the treatment of petit mal epilepsy (8–11).

Features of Fetal Trimethadione Syndrome (25 Cases)

	No. Cases*	%		No. Cases*	%
Growth:			Cardiac:		
prenatal deficiency	8	32	septal defect	5	20
postnatal deficiency	6	24	not stated	4	16
Performance (19 cases):			PDA	4	16
mental retardation	7	28	Limb:		
impaired vision (myopia)	5	20	simian crease	7	28
speech disorder	4	16	malformed hand	2	8
impaired hearing	2	8	clubfoot	1	4
Craniofacial:			Genitourinary:		
low set, cupped or	18	72	kidney and ureter	5	20
abnormal ears			abnormality		
high arched or cleft	16	64	inguinal hernia(s)	3	12
lip and/or palate			hypospadias	3	12
microcephaly	6	24	ambiguous genitalia	2	8
irregular teeth	4	16	clitoral hypertrophy	1	4
epicanthic folds	3	12	imperforate anus	1	4
broad nasal bridge	3	12	Other:		
strabismus	3	8	tracheoesophageal fistula	3	12
low hairline	2	8	esophageal atresia	2	8
facial hemangiomata	1	4			
unusual facies (details	3	12	* Not Mutually Exclusive.		
not stated)					

Breast Feeding Summary

No data available.

References

1. German J, Kowan A, Ehlers KH. Trimethadione and human teratogenesis. Teratology 1970;3:349–62.
2. Zackae EH, Mellman WJ, Neiderer B, Hanson JW. The fetal trimethadione syndrome. J Pediatr 1975; 87:280–4.
3. Nichols MM. Fetal anomalies following maternal trimethadione ingestion. J Pediatr 1973;82:885–6.
4. Feldman GL, Weaver DD, Lourien EW. The fetal trimethadione syndrome. Report of an additional family and further delineation of this syndrome. Am J Dis Child 1977;131:1389–92.
5. Rosen RC, Lightner ES. Phenotypic malformations in association with maternal trimethadione therapy. J. Pediatr 1978;92:240–4.
6. Zellweger H. Anticonvulsants during pregnancy: a danger to the developing fetus? Clin Pediatr 1974;13:338–45.
7. Rischbieth RH. Troxidone (trimethadione) embryopathy: Case report with review of the literature. Clin Exp Neurol 1979;16:251–6.
8. Fabro S, Brown NA. Teratogenic potential of anticonvulsants. N Engl J Med 1979;300:1280–1.
9. National Institute of Health. Anticonvulsants found to have teratogenic potential. JAMA 1981;245:36.
10. Dansky L, Andermann E, Andermann F. Major congenital malformations in the offspring of epileptic patients. Genetic and environmental risk factors. In *Epilepsy, Pregnancy and the Child*. Proceedings of a Workshop held in Berlin, September 1980. New York: Raven Press, 1981.
11. Nakane Y, Okuma T, Takahashi R, et al. Multi-institutional study on the teratogenicity and fetal toxicity of antiepileptic drugs: A report of a collaborative study group in Japan. Epilepsia 1980;21:663–80.

Name: **TRIMETHAPHAN**

Class: **Antihypertensive**   Risk Factor: **C**

Fetal Risk Summary

No reports linking the use of trimethaphan with congenital defects have been located. Trimethaphan, a short acting ganglionic blocker which requires continuous infusion for therapeutic effect, has been studied in pregnant patients (1, 2). It is not recommended for use in pregnancy because of adverse hemodynamic effects (3). The drug is not effective in the control of hypertension in toxemic patients (1–3).

Breast Feeding Summary

No data available.

References

1. Assali NS, Douglas RA Jr, Suyemoto R. Observations on the hemodynamic properties of a thiophanium derivative, Ro 2-2222 (Arfonad), in human subjects. Circulation 1953;8:62–9.

2. Assali NS, Suyemoto R. The place of the hydrazinophthalazine and thiophanium compounds in the management of hypertensive complications of pregnancy. Am J Obstet Gynecol 1952;64:1021–36.
3. Assali NS. Hemodynamic effects of hypotensive drugs used in pregnancy. Obstet Gynecol Surv 1954;9:776–94.

Name: **TRIMETHOBENZAMIDE**

Class: **Antiemetic**   Risk Factor: **C**

Fetal Risk Summary

Trimethobenzamide has been used in pregnancy to treat nausea and vomiting (1, 2). No adverse effects in the fetus were observed. In a third study, 193 patients were treated with trimethobenzamide in the 1st trimester (3). The incidence of severe congenital defects at 1 month, 1 year and 5 years were 2.6%, 2.6% and 5.8%, respectively. The 5.8% incidence was increased over non-treated controls (3.2%) ($p < 0.05$) but other factors, including the use of other antiemetics in some patients, may have contributed to the results. The authors concluded that the risk of congenital malformations with trimethobenzamide was low.

Breast Feeding Summary

No data available.

References

1. Breslow S, Belafsky HA, Shangold JE, Hirsch LM, Stahl MB. Antiemetic effect of trimethobenzamide in pregnant patients. Clin Med 1961;8:2153–5.
2. Winters HS. Antiemetics in nausea and vomiting of pregnancy. Obstet Gynecol 1961;18:753–6.
3. Milkovich L, van den Berg BJ. An evaluation of the teratogenicity of certain antinauseant drugs. Am J Obstet Gynecol 1976;125:244–8.

Name: **TRIMETHOPRIM**

Class: **Anti-infective**   Risk Factor: **C**

Fetal Risk Summary

Trimethoprim is available as a single agent and in combination with various sulfonamides (see also Sulfonamides). The drug crosses the placenta, producing similar levels in fetal and maternal serum and in amniotic fluid (1–3). Because trimethoprim is a folate antagonist, caution has been advocated for its use in pregnancy (4). However, case reports and placebo-controlled trials have failed to demonstrate an increase in fetal abnormalities (5–9).

Sulfa-trimethoprim combinations have been shown to cause a drop in the sperm count after 1 month of continuous treatment in males (10). Decreases varied between 7 and 88%. The authors theorized that trimethoprim deprived the spermatogenetic cells of active folate by inhibiting dihydrofolate reductase.

Breast Feeding Summary

Trimethoprim is excreted into breast milk in low concentrations. Following 160 mg twice daily for 5 days, milk concentrations varied between 1.2 and 2.4 μg/ml (average 1.8) with peak levels occurring at 2 to 3 hours (11). No adverse effects were reported in the infants. Nearly identical results were found in a study with 50 patients (12). Mean milk levels were 2.0 μg/ml representing a milk:plasma ratio of 1.25. The authors concluded that these levels represented a negligible risk to the suckling infant.

References

1. Ylikorkala O, Sjostedt E, Jarvinen PA, Tikkanen R, Raines T. Trimethoprim-sulfonamide combination administered orally and intravaginally in the 1st trimester of pregnancy: its absorption into serum and transfer to amniotic fluid. Acta Obstet Gynecol Scand 1973;52:229–34.
2. Reid DWJ, Caille G, Kaufmann NR. Maternal and transplacental kinetics of trimethoprim and sulfamethoxazole, separately and in combination. Can Med Assoc J 1975;112:67s–72s.
3. Reeves DS, Wilkinson PJ. The pharmacokinetics of trimethoprim and trimethoprim/sulfonamide combinations, including penetration into body tissues. Infection 1979;7(Suppl 4):S330–41.
4. McEwen LM. Trimethoprim/sulphamethoxazole mixture in pregnancy. Br Med J 1971;4:490–1.
5. Williams JD, Condie AP, Brumfitt W, Reeves DS. The treatment of bacteriuria in pregnant women with sulphamethoxazole and trimethoprim. Postgrad Med J 1969;45(Suppl):71–6.
6. Ochoa AG. Trimethoprim and sulfamethoxazole in pregnancy. JAMA 1971;217:1244.
7. Brumfitt W, Pursell R. Double-blind trial to compare ampicillin, cephalexin, co-trimoxazole, and trimethoprim in treatment of urinary infection. Br Med J 1972;2:673–6.
8. Brumfitt W, Pursell R. Trimethoprim/sulfamethoxazole in the treatment of bacteriuria in women. J Infect Dis 1973;128(Suppl):S657–63.
9. Brumfitt W, Pursell R. Trimethoprim/sulfamethoxazole in the treatment of urinary infection. Med J Aust 1973;1(Suppl):44–8.
10. Murdia A, Mathur V, Kothari LK, Singh KP. Sulpha-trimethoprim combinations and male fertility. Lancet 1978;2:375–6.
11. Arnauld R, Soutoul JH, Gallier J, Borderon JC, Borderon E. A study of the passage of trimethoprim into the maternal milk. Quest med 1972;25:959–64.
12. Miller RD, Salter AJ. The passage of trimethoprim/sulphamethoxazole into breast milk and its significance. In Progress in Chemotherapy Proceedings of the Eighth International Congress of Chemotherapy, Athens, 1973:687–91.

Name: **TRIPROLIDINE**

Class: **Antihistamine**   Risk Factor: **B**

Fetal Risk Summary

No reports linking the use of triprolidine with congenital defects have been located. The Collaborative Perinatal Project monitored 50,282 mother-child pairs, 16 of which had 1st trimester exposure to triprolidine (1). From this small sample, no evidence was found to suggest a relationship to large categories of major or minor malformations or to individual malformations.

In a 1971 study, infants and mothers who had ingested antihistamines during the 1st trimester actually had fewer abnormalities when compared to controls (2). Triprolidine was the third most commonly used antihistamine. The manufacturer claims that in over 20 years of marketing the drug they have not received any reports of triprolidine teratogenicity (3). Their animal studies have also been negative.

Breast Feeding Summary

No data available.

References

1. Heinonen OP, Slone D, Shapiro S. *Birth Defects and Drugs in Pregnancy.* Littleton: Publishing Sciences Group, 1977:323.
2. Nelson MM, Forfar JO. Associations between drugs administered during pregnancy and congenital abnormalities of the fetus. Br Med J 1971;1:523–7.
3. Personal communication. Frosolono MF, Burroughs Wellcome, 1980.

Name: **TROLEANDOMYCIN**

Class: **Antibiotic**   Risk Factor: **C**

Fetal Risk Summary

Troleandomycin is the triacetyl ester of oleandomycin (see Oleandomycin).

Breast Feeding Summary

(See Oleandomycin).

Name: **UREA**

Class: **Diuretic**   Risk Factor: **C**

Fetal Risk Summary

Urea is an osmotic diuretic that is used primarily to treat cerebral edema. Topical formulations for skin disorders are also available. No reports of its use in pregnancy following intravenous, oral or topical administration have been located. Urea, given by intra-amniotic injection, has been used for the induction of abortion (1).

Breast Feeding Summary

No data available.

Reference

1. Ware A, ed. *Martindale: The Extra Pharmacopoeia*, ed. 27. London: The Pharmaceutical Press, 1977:572.

Name: **UROKINASE**

Class: **Thrombolytic**   Risk Factor: **C**

Fetal Risk Summary

No reports on the use of urokinase in human pregnancy have been located. The drug is not teratogenic in rats or mice (1). The manufacturers consider urokinase contraindicated in pregnancy and the first 10 days postpartum (2, 3).

Breast Feeding Summary

No data available.

References

1. Shepard TH. *Catalog of Teratogenic Agents* ed. 3. Baltimore: Johns Hopkins University Press, 1980:342.
2. Product information. Abbokinase. Abbott Laboratories, 1981.
3. Product information. Breokinase. Breon Laboratories, 1981.

V

Name: **VALPROIC ACID**

Class: **Anticonvulsant**

Risk Factor: **D**

Fetal Risk Summary

Valproic acid is a relatively new anticonvulsant used in the treatment of seizure disorders. There are 3 cases of congenital abnormalities in which valproic acid was used (1–3). In 2 of these reports other anticonvulsants were taken (1,2). Malformations reported are similar to the fetal hydantoin syndrome. Reports of normal births with *in utero* exposure to valproic acid have also been located (4–8). Valproic acid has been shown to cross the placenta and achieve fetal serum concentrations 1.4 times the maternal serum levels (6,9). Mclain has reported a dose-related hepatoxic effect with serum levels exceeding 60 μg/ml (10). Because valproic acid is a potent teratogen in experimental studies and due to reports of possible association between valproic and congenital defects, its use during pregnancy is not recommended. If valproic acid is used, serum concentrations should be maintained below 60 μg/ml.

Author (ref)	No. Pts.	Indica- tion	Gestational Age	Dose	Other Drugs	Fetal Effects	Comment
Gomez (1)	1	Petit mal epilepsy	Through- out	0.5–1.5 g/day	Clonazepam Phenobarbital	Lumbosacral meningocele Sensory motor deficit Microcephaly	
Thomas (2)	1	Grand mal epilepsy	Through- out	1.2 g/day	Primidone Carbamazepine	Prolonged PTT and PT Hypoplastic nails Depressed nasal bridge Cleft lip and high arched palate Wide fontanel Abnormal palmar crease Tetralogy of Fallot	Effects also consistent with primi- done embry- opathy (11)
Dalens (3)	1	Grand mal epilepsy	Through- out	1 g/day	None	Prenatal growth deficiency Microcephaly Bulging frontal eminences Hypoplastic nose and orbital edges Ptosis Low set ears Small mandible Abnormal palmar creases Congenital dislocation of hip Cutaneous symphysis of toes	—

Breast Feeding Summary

Valproic acid is excreted into breast milk in small amounts (6,11). No reports linking the use of valproic acid with adverse effects in the nursing infant have been located.

Author (ref)	No. Pts.	Dose	Serum	Milk	M:P Ratio	Effect on Infant
			Concentrations (μg/ml)			
Reith (9)	Not stated	Not stated	95	1	0.07	—
Dickinson (6)	1	250 mg (single dose)	34.3 (3 hr) 9.9 (16 hr)	0.47 0.17	0.01 0.02	—

References

1. Gomez MR. Possible teratogenicity of valproic acid. J Pediatr 1981;98:508–9.
2. Thomas D, Buchanan N. Teratogenic effects of anticonvulsants. J Pediatr 1981;99:163.
3. Dalens B, Raynaud EJ, Gaulme J. Teratogenicity of valproic acid. J Pediatr 1980;97:332–3.
4. Brown NA, Kaoi J, Babra S. Teratogenic potential of valproic acid. Lancet 1980;1:880–1.
5. Alexander FW. Sodium valproate and pregnancy. Arch Dis Child 1979;54:240–2.
6. Dickenson RG, Harland RC, Lynn RK, Smith NB. Transmission of valproic acid (Depakene) across the placenta: half-life of the drug in mother and baby. J Pediatr 1979;94:832–5.
7. Hiilesmaa VK, Bardy AH, Granstrom ML, Teramo KAW. Valproic acid during pregnancy. Lancet 1980;1:883.
8. Nakane Y, Okuma T, Takahashi R, et al. Multi-institutional study on teratogenicity and fetal toxicity of antiepileptic drugs: a report of a collaborative study group in Japan. Epilepsia 1980;21:663–80.
9. Reith H, Schafer H. Antiepileptic drugs during pregnancy and the lactation period. Pharmacokinetic data. Dtsch Med Wochenschr 1979;104:818–23.
10. Mclain LW Jr. Teratogenic effects of valproic acid. JAMA 1979;242:1672.
11. Radd NL, Freedom RM. A possible primidone embryopathy. J Pediatr 1979;94:835.

Name: **VANCOMYCIN**

Class: **Antibiotic**   Risk Factor: **C**

Fetal Risk Summary

No data available.

Breast Feeding Summary

No data available.

Name: **VASOPRESSIN**

Class: **Pituitary Hormone**   Risk Factor: **B**

Fetal Risk Summary

No reports linking the use of vasopressin with congenital defects have been located. Vasopressin and the structurally related synthetic polypeptides, desmopressin and lypressin, have been used during pregnancy to treat diabetes insipidus, a rare disorder (1–3). No adverse effects on the newborns were reported.

A three-fold increase of circulating levels of endogenous vasopressin has been reported for women in the last trimester and in labor as compared to non-pregnant women (4). Although infrequent, the induction of uterine activity in the 3rd trimester has been reported after intramuscular and intranasal vasopressin (5). The intravenous use of desmopressin, which is normally given intranasally, has also been reported to cause uterine contractions (3).

Breast Feeding Summary

Patients receiving vasopressin, desmopressin or lypressin for diabetes insipidus have been reported to breast feed without apparent problems in the infant (1). Experimental work in lactating women suggests that suckling almost doubles the maternal blood concentration of vasopressin (4).

References

1. Hime MC, Richardson JA. Diabetes insipidus and pregnancy. Obstet Gynecol Surv 1978;33:375–9.
2. Phelan JP, Guay AT, Newman C. Diabetes insipidus in pregnancy: a case review. Am J Obstet Gynecol 1978;130:365–6.
3. van der Wildt B, Drayer JIM, Eske TKAB. Diabetes insipidus in pregnancy as a first sign of a craniopharyngioma. Eur J Obstet Gynecol Reprod Biol 1980;10:269–74.
4. Robinson KW, Hawker RW, Robertson PA. Antidiuretic hormone (ADH) in the human female. J Clin Endocrinol Metab 1957;17:320–2.
5. Oravec D, Lichardus B. Management of diabetes insipidus in pregnancy. Br Med J 1972;4:114–5.

Name: **VERAPAMIL**

Class: **Antiarrhythmic**   Risk Factor: **C**

Fetal Risk Summary

Verapamil is a slow channel calcium inhibitor used as an antiarrhythmic agent. No reports linking its use with congenital defects have been located. Placental passage of verapamil was demonstrated in 2 of 6 patients given 80 mg orally at term (1). Cord levels were 15.4 and 24.5 ng/ml (17 and 26% of maternal serum) in two newborns delivered at 49 and 109 minutes, respectively.

Verapamil could not be detected in the cord blood of 4 infants delivered 173 to 564 minutes after the dose. Intravenous verapamil was administered to patients in labor at a rate of 2 μg/kg/minute for 60 to 110 minutes (2). The serum concentrations of the infants averaged 8.5 ng/ml (44% of maternal serum).

A 33-week fetus with a tachycardia of 240 to 280 beats/minute was treated *in utero* for 6 weeks with β-acetyldigoxin and verapamil (80 mg three times daily) (1). The fetal heart rate returned to normal 5 days after initiation of therapy, but the authors could not determine if verapamil had produced the beneficial effect. At birth, no signs of cardiac hypertrophy or disturbances in repolarization were observed.

The manufacturer has reports of patients treated with verapamil during the 1st trimester without producing fetal problems (3). Animal studies have also not revealed a fetal risk (3,4). However, hypotension (systolic and diastolic) has been observed in 5 to 10% of patients after intravenous therapy (4,5). Although reports are lacking, reduced uterine blood flow with fetal hypoxia (bradycardia) is a potential risk.

Breast Feeding Summary

No data available.

References

1. Wolff F, Breuker KH, Schlensker KH, Bolte A. Prenatal diagnosis and therapy of fetal heart rate anomalies: with a contribution on the placental transfer of verapamil. J Perinat Med 1980;8:203–8.
2. Strigl R, Gastroph G, Hege HG, et al. Nachweis von verapamil in mutterlichen und fetalen blut des menschen. Geburtshilfe Frauenheilkd 1980;40:496–9.
3. Personal communication. Anderson, MS GD Searle and Company, 1981.
4. Product information. Calan. GD Searle and Company, 1981.
5. Product information. Isoptin. Knoll Pharmaceutical Company, 1981.

Name: **VIDARABINE**

Class: **Antiviral**   Risk Factor: **C**

Fetal Risk Summary

Vidarabine has not been studied in human pregnancy. The drug is teratogenic in some species of animals after topical and intramuscular administration (1,2). Daily instillations of a 10% solution into the vaginas of pregnant rats in late gestation had no effect on the offspring.

Breast Feeding Summary

No data available.

References

1. Pavan-Langston D, Buchanan RA, Alford CA Jr, eds. *Adenine arabinoside: an antiviral agent.* New York: Raven Press, 1975:153.

2. Schardein JL, Hertz DL, Petretre JA, Fitzgerald JE, Kurtz SM. The effect of vidarabine on the development of the offspring of rats, rabbits and monkeys. Teratology 1977;15:213–42.

Name: **VINBLASTINE**

Class: **Antineoplastic**   Risk Factor: **D**

Fetal Risk Summary

Vinblastine is an antimitotic antineoplastic agent. The drug has been used in pregnancy, including the 1st trimester, without producing malformations (1–6). Two cases of malformed infants have been reported following 1st trimester exposure to vinblastine (7,8). Garrett reported a case of a 27-year-old woman with Hodgkin's disease who was given vinblastine, mechlorethamine and procarbazine during the 1st trimester (7). At 24 weeks of gestation, she spontaneously aborted a male child with oligodactyly of both feet with webbing of the 3rd and 4th toes. These defects were attributed to mechlorethamine therapy. A mother with Hodgkin's disease treated with vinblastine, vincristine and procarbazine in the 1st trimester (3 weeks after the last menstrual period) delivered a 1900-g male infant at about 37 weeks of gestation who developed fatal respiratory distress syndrome (8). At autopsy, a small secundum atrial septal defect was found. Vinblastine in combination with other antineoplastic agents may produce ovarian dysfunction (9–11). Alkylating agents are the most frequent cause of this problem (11). Ovarian function may return to normal with successful pregnancies possible, depending on the patient's age at time of therapy and the total dose of chemotherapy received (10). Data from one review indicated that 40% of infants exposed to anticancer drugs were of low birth weight (12). This finding was not related to the timing of exposure. Long term studies of growth and mental development in offspring exposed to vinblastine during the 2nd trimester, the period of neuroblast multiplication, have not been conducted (13).

Breast Feeding Summary

No data available.

References

1. Armstrong JG, Dyke RW, Fouts PJ, Jansen CJ. Delivery of a normal infant during the course of oral vinblastine sulfate therapy for Hodgkin's disease. Ann Intern Med 1964;61:106–7.
2. Rosenzweig AI, Crews QE Jr, Hopwood HG. Vinblastine sulfate in Hodgkin's disease in pregnancy. Ann Intern Med 1964;61:108–12.
3. Lacher MJ. Use of vinblastine sulfate to treat Hodgkin's disease during pregnancy. Ann Intern Med 1964;61:113–5.
4. Lacher MJ, Geller W. Cyclophosphamide and vinblastine sulfate in Hodgkin's disease during pregnancy. JAMA 1966;195:192–4.
5. Nordlund JJ, DeVita VT Jr, Carbone PP. Severe vinblastine-induced leukopenia during late pregnancy with delivery of a normal infant. Ann Intern Med 1968;69:581–2.
6. Goguei A. Hodgkin's disease and pregnancy. Nouv Presse Med 1970;78:1507–10.
7. Garrett MJ. Teratogenic effects of combination chemotherapy. Ann Intern Med 1974;80:667.

8. Thomas RPM, Peckham MJ. The investigation and management of Hodgkin's disease in the pregnant patient. Cancer 1976;38:1443–51.
9. Morgenfeld MC, Goldberg V, Parisier H, Bugnard SC, Bur GE. Ovarian lesions due to cytostatic agents during the treatment of Hodgkin's disease. Surg Gynecol Obstet 1972;134:826–8.
10. Ross GT. Congenital anomalies among children born of mothers receiving chemotherapy for gestational trophoblastic neoplasms. Cancer 1976;37:1043–7.
11. Schilsky RL, Lewis BJ, Sherins RJ, Young RC. Gonadal dysfunction in patients receiving chemotherapy for cancer. Ann Intern Med 1980;93:109–14.
12. Nicholson HO. Cytotoxic drugs in pregnancy: review of reported cases. J Obstet Gynaecol Br Commonw 1968;75:307–12.
13. Dobbing J. Pregnancy and leukaemia. Lancet 1977;1:1155.

Name: **VINCRISTINE**

Class: **Antineoplastic**

Risk Factor: **D**

Fetal Risk Summary

Vincristine is an antimitotic antineoplastic agent. Fifteen references have described the use of the drug in 20 pregnancies, 6 during the 1st trimester (1–15). A mother with Hodgkin's disease treated with vincristine, vinblastine and procarbazine in the 1st trimester (3 weeks after the last menstrual period) delivered a 1900-g male infant at about 37 weeks of gestation who developed fatal respiratory distress syndrome (9). At autopsy, a small secundum atrial septal defect was found. In a Hodgkin's case treated with vincristine, mechlorethamine and procarbazine during the 1st trimester, the electively aborted fetus had malformed kidneys (markedly reduced size and malpositioned) (15). The only other apparent adverse effect observed following vincristine use in pregnancy was in a 1000-g male infant born with pancytopenia who was exposed to 6 different antineoplastic agents in the 3rd trimester (1). Data from one review indicated that 40% of the infants exposed to anticancer drugs were of low birth weight (16). This finding was not related to the timing of exposure. Long term studies of growth and mental development in offspring exposed to these drugs during the 2nd trimester, the period of neuroblast multiplication, have not been conducted (17). Vincristine, in combination with other antineoplastic agents, may produce gonadal dysfunction in males and females (18–25). Alkylating agents are the most frequent cause of this problem (22). Ovarian and testicular function may return to normal with successful pregnancies possible, depending on the patient's age at time of treatment and the total dose of chemotherapy received (18).

Breast Feeding Summary

No data available.

References

1. Pizzuto J, Aviles A, Noriega L, Niz J, Morales M, Romero F. Treatment of acute leukemia during pregnancy: presentation of nine cases. Cancer Treat Rep 1980;64:679–83.

2. Colbert N, Najman A, Gorin NC, et al. Acute leukaemia during pregnancy: favourable course of pregnancy in two patients treated with cytosine arabinoside and anthracyclines. Nouv Presse Med 1980;9:175–8.

3. Daly H, McCann SR, Hanratty TD, Temperley IJ. Successful pregnancy during combination chemotherapy for Hodgkin's disease. Acta Haematol (Basel) 1980;64:154–6.

4. Tobias JS, Bloom HJG. Doxorubicin in pregnancy. Lancet 1980;1:776.

5. Garcia V, San Miguel J, Borrasea AL. Doxorubicin in the first trimester of pregnancy. Ann Intern Med 1981;94:547.

6. Dara P, Slater LM, Armentrout SA. Successful pregnancy during chemotherapy for acute leukemia. Cancer 1981;47:845–6.

7. Burnier AM. Discussion. In Plows CW. Acute myelomonocytic leukemia in pregnancy: report of a case. Am J Obstet Gynecol 1982;143:41–3.

8. Lilleyman JS, Hill AS, Anderton KJ. Consequences of acute myelogenous leukemia in early pregnancy. Cancer 1977;40:1300–3.

9. Thomas PRM, Peckham MJ. The investigation and management of Hodgkin's disease in the pregnant patient. Cancer 1976;38:1443–51.

10. Pawliger DF, McLean FW, Noyes WD. Normal fetus after cytosine arabinoside therapy. Ann Intern Med 1971;74:1012.

11. Lowenthal RM, Funnell CF, Hope DM, Stewart IG, Humphrey DC. Normal infant after combination chemotherapy including teniposide for Burkitt's lymphoma in pregnancy. Med Pediatr Oncol 1982;10:165–9.

12. Sears HF, Reid J. Granulocytic sarcoma: local presentation of a systemic disease. Cancer 1976;37:1808–13.

13. Durie BGM, Giles HR. Successful treatment of acute leukemia during pregnancy: combination therapy in the third trimester. Arch Intern Med 1977;137:90–1.

14. Newcomb M, Balducci L, Thigpen JT, Morrison FS. Acute leukemia in pregnancy: successful delivery after cytarabine and doxorubicin. JAMA 1978;239:2691–2.

15. Mennuti MT, Shepard TH, Mellman WJ. Fetal renal malformation following treatment of Hodgkin's disease during pregnancy. Obstet Gynecol 1975;46:194–6.

16. Nicholson HO. Cytotoxic drugs in pregnancy: review of reported cases. J Obstet Gynaecol Br Commonw 1968;75:307–12.

17. Dobbing J. Pregnancy and leukaemia. Lancet 1977;1:1155.

18. Schilsky RL, Sherins RJ, Hubbard SM, Wesley MN, Young RC, DeVita VT Jr. Long-term follow-up of ovarian function in women treated with MOPP chemotherapy for Hodgkin's disease. Am J Med 1981;71:552–6.

19. Schwartz PE, Vidone RA. Pregnancy following combination chemotherapy for a mixed germ cell tumor of the ovary. Gynecol Oncol 1981;12:373–8.

20. Estiu M. Successful pregnancy in leukaemia. Lancet 1977;1:433.

21. Johnson SA, Goldman JM, Hawkins DF. Pregnancy after chemotherapy for Hodgkin's disease. Lancet 1979;2:93.

22. Schilsky RL, Lewis BJ, Sherins RJ, Young RC. Gonadal dysfunction in patients receiving chemotherapy for cancer. Ann Intern Med 1980;93:109–14.

23. Sherins RJ, DeVita VT Jr. Effect of drug treatment for lymphoma on male reproductive capacity. Ann Intern Med 1973;79:216–20.

24. Sherins RJ, Olweny CLM, Ziegler JL. Gynecomastia and gonadal dysfunction in adolescent boys treated with combination chemotherapy for Hodgkin's disease. N Engl J Med 1978;299:12–6.

25. Lendon PRM, Peckham MJ. The investigation and management of Hodgkin's disease in the pregnant patient. Cancer 1976;38:1443–51.

Name: **WARFARIN**

Class: **Anticoagulant**   Risk Factor: **D**

Fetal Risk Summary

See Coumarin Derivatives.

Breast Feeding Summary

See Coumarin Derivatives.

Z

Name: **ZOMEPIRAC**

Class: **Nonsteroidal Anti-inflammatory**   Risk Factor: **B***

Fetal Risk Summary

No reports linking the use of zomepirac with congenital defects have been located. Theoretically, zomepirac, a prostaglandin synthetase inhibitor, could cause constriction of the ductus arteriosus *in utero* (1). Persistent pulmonary hypertension of the newborn should also be considered (2). Drugs in this class have been shown to inhibit labor and prolong pregnancy (2). The manufacturer recommends that the drug not be used during pregnancy (3).

[*Risk Factor D if used in 3rd trimester or near delivery.]

Breast Feeding Summary

No data available. The manufacturer recommends that the drug not be used when breast feeding (4).

References

1. Levin DL. Effects of inhibition of prostaglandin synthesis on fetal development, oxygenation, and the fetal circulation. Semin Perinatol 1980;4:35–44.
2. Fuchs F. Prevention of prematurity. Am J Obstet Gynecol 1976;126:809–20.
3. Product information. Zomax. McNeil Laboratories, 1982.

APPENDIX

A. ANTIHISTAMINES
Brompheniramine (C)
Buclizine (C)
Chlorpheniramine (B)
Cimetidine (B)
Cyclizine (B)
Cyproheptadine (B)
Dexbrompheniramine (C)
Dexchlorpheniramine (B_M)
Dimenhydrinate (B)
Diphenhydramine (C)
Doxylamine (B)
Hydroxyzine (C)
Meclizine (B)
Phenyltoloxamine (C)
Promethazine (C)
Pyrilamine (C)
Trimeprazine (C)
Triprolidine (B)

B. ANTI-INFECTIVES
1. Amebicides
Carbarsone (D)
Diiodohydroxyquin (C)
2. Anthelmintics
Gentian Violet (C)
Piperazine (B)
Pyrantel Pamoate (C)
Pyrvinium Pamoate (C)
3. Aminoglycosides
Amikacin (C_M)
Gentamicin (C)
Kanamycin (D)
Neomycin (C)
Streptomycin (D)
Tobramycin (C)
4. Antifungals
Amphotericin B (B)
Clotrimazole (B)

Flucytosine (C)
Griseofulvin (C)
Miconazole (B)
Nystatin (B)
5. Cephalosporins
Cefaclor (B)
Cefadroxil (B)
Cefamandole (B)
Cefatrizine (B)
Cefazolin (B)
Cefotaxime (B)
Cefoxitin (B)
Cefuroxime (B)
Cephalexin (B)
Cephaloglycin (B)
Cephaloridine (B)
Cephalothin (B)
Cephapirin (B)
Cephradine (B)
6. Penicillins
Amoxicillin (B)
Ampicillin (B)
Bacampicillin (B)
Carbenicillin (B)
Cloxacillin (B)
Cyclacillin (B)
Dicloxacillin (B)
Hetacillin (B)
Methicillin (B)
Nafcillin (B)
Oxacillin (B)
Penicillin G (B)
Penicillin G, Benzathine (B)
Penicillin G, Procaine (B)
Penicillin V (B)
Ticarcillin (B)
7. Tetracyclines
Chlortetracycline (D)
Clomacycline (D)

Demeclocycline (D)
Doxycycline (D)
Methacycline (D)
Minocycline (D)
Oxytetracycline (D)
Tetracycline (D)

8. Other Anti-infectives
Bacitracin (C)
Chloramphenicol (C)
Clindamycin (B)
Colistimethate (B)
Erythromycin (B)
Furazolidone (C)
Lincomycin (B)
Novobiocin (C)
Oleandomycin (C)
Polymyxin B (B)
Spectinomycin (B)
Trimethoprim (C)
Troleandomycin (C)
Vancomycin (C)

9. Antituberculosis
para-Aminosalicyclic Acid (C)
Ethambutol (B)
Isoniazid (C)
Rifampin (C)

10. Antivirals
Amantadine (C)
Idoxuridine (C)
Vidarabine (C)

11. Plasmodicides
Chloroquine (D)
Primaquine (C)
Pyrimethamine (C)
Quinacrine (C)
Quinine (C)

12. Sulfonamides
Mafenide (B/D)
Phthalylsulfacetamide (B/D)
Phthalylsulfathiazole (B/D)
Succinylsulfathiazole (B/D)
Sulfacetamide (B/D)
Sulfachlorpyridazine (B/D)
Sulfacytine (B/D)
Sulfadiazine (B/D)
Sulfadimethoxine (B/D)
Sulfadoxine (B/D)
Sulfaethidole (B/D)
Sulfaguanidine (B/D)
Sulfamerazine (B/D)
Sulfamethazine (B/D)
Sulfamethizole (B/D)

Sulfamethoxazole (B/D)
Sulfamethoxydiazine (B/D)
Sulfamethoxypyridazine (B/D)
Sulfametopyrazine (B/D)
Sulfanilamide (B/D)
Sulfanilcarbamide (B/D)
Sulfaphenazole (B/D)
Sulfapyridine (B/D)
Sulfasalazine (B/D)
Sulfasymazine (B/D)
Sulfathiazole (B/D)
Sulfisoxazole (B/D)
Sulfonamides (B/D)

13. Trichomonacides
Metronidazole (C)

14. Urinary Germicides
Cinoxacin (B)
Mandelic Acid (C)
Methenamine (B)
Methylene Blue (C/D)
Nalidixic Acid (B)
Nitrofurantoin (B)

15. Scabicide/Pediculicide
Benzene Hexachloride, Gamma (B)

C. ANTINEOPLASTICS
Aminopterin (X)
Azathioprine (D)
Bleomycin (D)
Busulfan (D)
Chlorambucil (D)
Cisplatin (D)
Cyclophosphamide (D)
Cytarabine (D)
Dacarbazine (D)
Dactinomycin (D)
Daunorubicin (D)
Doxorubicin (D)
Fluorouracil (D)
Laetrile (C)
Mechlorethamine (D)
Melphalan (D)
Mercaptopurine (D)
Methotrexate (D)
Mithramycin (D)
Procarbazine (D)
Teniposide (D)
Thioguanine (D)
Thiotepa (D)
Vinblastine (D)
Vincristine (D)

D. AUTONOMICS

1. Parasympathomimetics (Cholinergics)
Acetylcholine (C)
Ambenonium (C)
Bethanechol (C)
Carbachol (C)
Demecarium (C)
Echothiophate (C)
Edrophonium (C)
Isoflurophate (C)
Neostigmine (C)
Physostigmine (C)
Pilocarpine (C)
Pyridostigmine (C)

2. Parasympatholytics (Anticholinergic)
Anisotropine (C)
Atropine (C)
Belladonna (C)
Benztropine (C)
Biperiden (C_M)
Clidinium (C)
Cycrimine (C)
Dicyclomine (B)
Diphemanil (C)
Ethopropazine (C)
Glycopyrrolate (C)
Hexocyclium (C)
Homatropine (C)
L-hyoscyamine (C)
Isopropamide (C)
Mepenzolate (C)
Methantheline (C)
Methixene (C)
Methscopolamine (C)
Orphenadrine (C)
Oxyphencyclimine (C)
Oxyphenonium (C)
Piperidolate (C)
Procyclidine (C)
Propantheline (C)
Scopolamine (C)
Thiphenamil (C)
Tridihexethyl (C)
Trihexyphenidyl (C)

3. Sympathomimetics Adrenergic)
Albuterol (B)
Angiotensin (C)
Dobutamine (C)
Dopamine (C)
Ephedrine (C)
Epinephrine (C)
Fenoterol (B)
Isoetharine (C)
Isoproterenol (C)
Isoxsuprine (C)
Levarterenol (D)
Mephentermine (C)
Metaproterenol (B)
Metaraminol (D)
Methoxamine (D)
Phenylephrine (D)
Phenylpropanolamine (C)
Pseudoephedrine (C)
Ritodrine (B)
Terbutaline (B)

4. Sympatholytics
Propranolol (C)
Nadolol (C_M)

5. Skeletal Muscle Relaxants
Chlorzoxazone (C)
Decamethonium (C)

E. COAGULANTS/ANTICOAGULANTS

1. Anticoagulants
Anisindione (D)
Coumarin Derivatives (D)
Dicumarol (D)
Diphenadione (D)
Ethyl Biscoumacetate (D)
Heparin (C)
Nicoumalone (D)
Phenindione (D)
Phenprocoumon (D)
Warfarin (D)

2. Antiheparin
Protamine (C)

3. Hemostatics
Aminocaproic Acid (C)
Aprotinin (D)

4. Thrombolytics
Streptokinase (C)
Urokinase (C)

F. CARDIOVASCULAR DRUGS

1. Cardiac Drugs
Acetyldigitoxin (B)
Bretylium (C)
Deslanoside (B)
Digitalis (B)
Digitoxin (B)

Digoxin (B)
Disopyramide (C)
Gitalin (B)
Lanatoside C (B)
Nadolol (C$_M$)
Ouabain (B)
Propranolol (C)
Quinidine (C)
Verapamil (C)

2. Antihypertensives
Captopril (C)
Clonidine (C)
Diazoxide (D)
Hexamethonium (C)
Hydralazine (B)
Methyldopa (C)
Minoxidil (C)
Nadolol (C$_M$)
Nitroprusside (D)
Pargyline (C)
Prazosin (C)
Propranolol (C)
Reserpine (D)
Trimethaphan (C)

3. Vasodilators
Amyl Nitrite (C)
Cyclandelate (C)
Dioxyline (C)
Dipyridamole (C)
Erythrityl Tetranitrate (C)
Isosorbide Dinitrate (C)
Isoxsuprine (C)
Nicotinyl Alcohol (C)
Nitroglycerin (C)
Nylidrin (C)
Pentaerythritol Tetranitrate (C)
Tolazoline (C)

G. CENTRAL NERVOUS SYSTEM DRUGS

1. Analgesics and Antipyretics
Acetaminophen (B)
Aspirin (C/D)
Aspirin, Buffered (C/D)
Choline Salicylate (C/D)
Ethoheptazine (C)
Magnesium Salicylate (C/D)
Phenacetin (B)
Propoxyphene (C/D)
Salsalate (C/D)
Sodium Salicylate (C/D)

Sodium Thiosalicylate (C/D)
2. Narcotic Analgesics
Alphaprodine (B/D)
Anileridine (B/D)
Butorphanol (B/D)
Codeine (C/D)
Dihydrocodeine Bitartrate (B/D)
Fentanyl (B/D)
Heroin (B/D)
Hydrocodone (B/D)
Hydromorphone (B/D)
Levorphanol (B/D)
Meperidine (B/D)
Methadone (B/D)
Morphine (B/D)
Nalbuphine (B/D)
Opium (B/D)
Oxycodone (B/D)
Oxymorphone (B/D)
Pentazocine (B/D)
Phenazocine (B/D)

3. Narcotic Antagonists
Cyclazocine (D)
Levallorphan (D)
Nalorphine (D)
Naloxone (C)

4. Nonsteroidal Anti-inflammatory drugs
Fenoprofen (B/D)
Ibuprofen (B/D)
Indomethacin (B/D)
Meclofenamate (B/D)
Naproxen (B$_M$/D)
Oxyphenbutazone (D)
Phenylbutazone (D)
Sulindac (B/D)
Tolmetin (B/D)
Zomepirac (B/D)

5. Anticonvulsants
Aminoglutethimide (D)
Bromides (D)
Carbamazepine (D)
Clonazepam (D)
Ethosuximide (C)
Ethotoin (D)
Magnesium Sulfate (B)
Mephenytoin (C)
Mephobarbital (C)
Metharbital (B)
Methsuximide (C)
Paramethadione (X)

Phenobarbital (B)
Phensuximide (C)
Phenytoin (D)
Primidone (D)
Trimethadione (X)
Valproic Acid (D)

6. Antidepressants

Amitriptyline (D)
Amoxapine (C_M)
Butriptyline (D)
Clomipramine (D)
Desipramine (C)
Dibenzepin (D)
Dothiepin (D)
Doxepin (C)
Imipramine (D)
Iprindole (D)
Iproniazid (C)
Isocarboxazid (C)
Maprotiline (B_M)
Mebanazine (C)
Nialamide (C)
Nortriptyline (D)
Opipramol (D)
Phenelzine (C)
Protriptyline (C)
Tranylcypromine (C)

7. Tranquilizers

Acetophenazine (C)
Butaperazine (C)
Carphenazine (C)
Chlorpromazine (C)
Chlorprothixene (C)
Droperidol (C)
Flupenthixol (C)
Fluphenazine (C)
Haloperidol (C)
Hydroxyzine (C)
Lithium (D)
Loxapine (C)
Mesoridazine (C)
Molindone (C)
Perphenazine (C)
Piperacetazine (C)
Prochlorperazine (C)
Promazine (C)
Thiopropazate (C)
Thioridazine (C)
Thiothixene (C)
Trifluoperazine (C)
Triflupromazine (C)

8. Stimulants

Caffeine (B)
Dextroamphetamine (D)
Diethylpropion (B)
Fenfluramine (C)
Mazindol (C)
Methylphenidate (C)
Phendimetrazine (C)
Phentermine (C)

9. Sedatives and Hypnotics

Amobarbital (D)
Aprobarbital (C)
Butalbital (C/D)
Chloral Hydrate (C)
Chlordiazepoxide (D)
Diazepam (D)
Ethanol (D/X)
Ethchlorvynol (D)
Flunitrazepam (C)
Lorazepam (C)
Mephobarbital (C)
Meprobamate (D)
Methaqualone (D)
Metharbital (D)
Oxazepam (C)
Pentobarbital (C)
Phenobarbital (B)
Secobarbital (C)

H. DIAGNOSTIC AGENTS

Evans Blue (C)
Indigo Carmine (B)
Methylene Blue (C/D)

I. ELECTROLYTES

Potassium Chloride (A)
Potassium Citrate (A)
Potassium Gluconate (A)

J. DIURETICS

Acetazolamide (C)
Amiloride (B_M)
Bendroflumethiazide (D)
Benzthiazide (D)
Chlorothiazide (D)
Chlorthalidone (D)
Cyclopenthiazide (D)
Cyclothiazide (D)
Ethacrynic Acid (D)
Furosemide (C)

Glycerin (C)
Hydrochlorothiazide (D)
Hydroflumethiazide (D)
Isosorbide (C)
Mannitol (C)
Methyclothiazide (D)
Metolazone (D)
Polythiazide (D)
Quinethazone (D)
Spironolactone (D)
Triameterene (D)
Trichlormethiazide (D)
Urea (C)

K. ACIDIFYING AGENTS
Ammonium Chloride (B)

L. ANTIDIARRHEALS
Diphenoxylate (C)
Loperamide (C)
Paregoric (B/D)

M. GASTROINTESTINAL AGENTS
1. Antiemetics
Buclizine (C)
Cyclizine (B)
Dimenhydrinate (B)
Meclizine (B)
Prochlorperazine (C)
Trimethobenzamide (C)
2. Laxatives/Purgatives
Casanthranol (C)
Cascara Sagrada (C)
Danthron (C)
Dioctyl calcium sulfosuccinate (C)
Dioctyl potassium sulfosuccinate (C)
Dioctyl sodium sulfosuccinate (C)
Lactulose (C)
Mineral oil (C)
3. Antiflatulents
Simethicone (C)

N. HEAVY METAL ANTAGONISTS
Penicillamine (D)

O. HORMONES
1. Adrenals
Betamethasone (C)
Cortisone (D)
Dexamethasone (C)

Prednisolone (B)
Prednisone (B)
2. Estrogens
Chlorotrianisene (D)
Contraceptives (See Oral Contraceptives)
Dienestrol (D)
Diethystilbestrol (X)
Estradiol (D)
Estrogens, Conjugated (D)
Estrone (D)
Ethinyl Estradiol (D)
Hormonal Pregnancy Test Tablets (D)
Mestranol (D)
Oral Contraceptives (D)
3. Progestogens
Contraceptives (See Oral Contraceptives)
Ethisterone (D)
Ethynodiol (D)
Hydroxyprogesterone (D)
Lynestrenol (D)
Medroxyprogesterone (D)
Norethindrone (D)
Norethynodrel (D)
Norgestrel (D)
Oral Contraceptives (D)
4. Antidiabetic Agents
Acetohexamide (D)
Chlorpropamide (D)
Insulin (B)
Tolazamide (D)
Tolbutamide (D)
5. Pituitary
Corticotropin/Cosyntropin (C)
Desmopressin (B)
Lypressin (B)
Somatostatin (B)
Vasopressin (B)
6. Thyroid
Calcitonin (B)

P. SPASMOLYTICS
Aminophylline (C)
Dyphylline (C)
Oxtriphylline (C)
Theophylline (C)

Q. ANTITUSSIVES AND EXPECTORANTS
1. Antitussives

Codeine (C/D)
2. Expectorants
Guaifenesin (C)

R. MISCELLANEOUS
Camphor (C)
Clofibrate (C)

Clomiphene (C/X)
Colchicine (C)
Cyclamate (C)
Disulfiram (X)
Phenazopyridine (C)
Phencyclidine (X)
Probenecid (B)

INDEX

Beromycin, see Penicillin V
Besacolin, see Bethanechol
Besan, see Pseudoephedrine
Beta-2, see Isoetharine
Betamethasone, 33
Betapen-VK, see Penicillin V
Betasolon, see Betamethasone
Bethanechol, 35
Betnelan, see Betamethasone
Bexophene, see Propoxyphene
Bicillin, see Penicillin G benzathine
Bicillin LA, see Penicillin G benzathine
Bidramine, see Diphenhydramine
Biotet, see Oxytetracycline
Biperiden, 35
Biquin, see Quinidine
Bi-Quinate, see Quinine
Bishydroxycoumarin, see Dicumarol
BL-S640, see Cefatrizine
Blenoxane, see Bleomycin
Bleomycin, 35
Bleph, see Sulfonamides
Bobbamycin, see Oxytetracycline
Bonamine, see Meclizine
Bonine, see Meclizine
Bontril, see Phendimetrazine
Bowtussin, see Guaifenesin
Bramcillin, see Penicillin V
Breokinase, see Urokinase
Breonesin, see Guaifenesin
Brethine, see Terbutaline
Bretylium, 36
Bretylol, see Bretylium
Bricanyl, see Terbutaline
Bristacycline, see Tetracycline
Bristamycin, see Erythromycin
Bristopen, see Oxacillin
Bristuric, see Bendroflumethiazide
Brochicide, see Guaifenesin
Bromamine, see Brompheniramine
Bromatane, see Brompheniramine
Bromides, 36
Bromo Seltzer, see Acetaminophen
Bromopheniramine, 37
Brondaxin, see Oxtriphylline
Bronitin Mist, see Epinephrine
Bronkaid, see Epinephrine
Bronkodyle, see Theophylline
Bronkometer, see Isoetharine
Bronkosol, see Isoetharine
Broserpine, see Reserpine
Brufen, see Ibuprofen
Bucladin-S, see Buclizine
Buclifen, see Buclizine
Buclizine, 38
Buff-A, see Aspirin, buffered
Buffaprin, see Aspirin, buffered
Bufferin, see Aspirin, buffered
Buffex, see Aspirin, buffered
Buffinol, see Aspirin, buffered
Buf-Tabs, see Aspirin, buffered
Bu-Lax, see Dioctyl sodium sulfosuccinate

Buphenine, see Nylidrin
Busulfan, 38
Busulphan, see Busulfan
Butacal, see Phenylbutazone
Butacote, see Phenylbutazone
Butadione, see Phenylbutazone
Butagesic, see Phenylbutazone
Butalan, see Phenylbutazone
Butalbital, 39
Butalgin, see Phenylbutazone
Butaperazine, 40
Butaphen, see Phenylbutazone
Butapirazol, see Phenylbutazone
Butapirone, see Oxyphenbutazone
Butarex, see Phenylbutazone
Butazolidin, see Phenylbutazone
Butazolidin Alka, see Phenylbutazone
Butazone, see Phenylbutazone
Butina, see Phenylbutazone
Butoroid, see Phenylbutazone
Butorphanol, 40
Butoz, see Phenylbutazone
Butozone, see Phenylbutazone
Butrex, see Phenylbutazone
Butriptyline, 41
Buzon, see Phenylbutazone

Caffeine, 42
Calan, see Verapamil
Calcimar, see Calcitonin
Calciopen, see Penicillin V
Calciparin, see Heparin
Calciparine, see Heparin
Calcipen, see Penicillin V
Calcitare, see Calcitonin
Calcitonin, 44
Calcium bromide, see Bromides
Calcium cyclamate, see Cyclamate
Calmazine, see Trifluoperazine
Calmoden, see Chlordiazepoxide
Calmonal, see Meclizine
Calmurid, see Urea
Calmuril, see Urea
Calsynar, see Calcitonin
Cama Inlay-Tabs, see Aspirin, buffered
Camcolit, see Lithium
Campho-phenique, see Camphor
Camphor, 44
Camphorated oil, see Camphor
Canestan, see Clotrimazole
Cantil, see Mepenzolate
Capcycline, see Tetracycline
Capoten, see Captopril
Caps-Pen-V, see Penicillin V
Captopril, 45
Carbacel, see Carbachol
Carbachol, 45
Carbacholine, see Carbachol
Carbamazepine, 46
Carbamide, see Urea
Carbapen, see Carbenicillin
Carbarsone, 47